Medical Coding

Medical Coding

UNDERSTANDING ICD-10-CM AND ICD-10-PCS

Leah A. Grebner, MS, RHIA, CCS, FAHIMA

Midstate College

Angela Suarez, BA, CPC, RMA

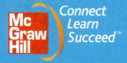

Mc Graw Hill

Connect
Learn
Succeed™

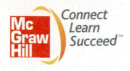

ISBN 978-0-07-340221-5
MHID 0-07-340221-4

Vice president/Director of marketing: *Alice Harra*
Editorial director: *Michael S. Ledbetter*
Senior sponsoring editor: *Natalie J. Ruffatto*
Director, digital products: *Crystal Szewczyk*
Managing development editor: *Michelle L. Flomenhoft*
Development editor: *Raisa Priebe Kreek*
Executive marketing manager: *Roxan Kinsey*
Marketing specialist: *Ada Bjorklund-Moore*
Digital development editor: *Katherine Ward*
Director, Editing/Design/Production: *Jess Ann Kosic*
Project manager: *Jean R. Starr*
Senior buyer: *Michael R. McCormick*

Senior designer: *Srdjan Savanovic*
Senior photo research coordinator: *Lori Hancock*
Photo researcher: *Lori Hancock*
Manager, digital production: *Janean A. Utley*
Media project manager: *Cathy L. Tepper*
Cover design: *George Kokkonas*
Interior design: *Ellen Pettengell*
Typeface: *11/13.5 Palatino*
Compositor: *Laserwords Private Limited*
Printer: *Quad/Graphics*

Credits: The credits section for this book begins on page 604 and is considered an extension of the copyright page.

Library of Congress Cataloging-in-Publication Data

Grebner, Leah A.
   Medical coding : understanding ICD-10-CM and ICD-10-PCS / Leah A. Grebner, Angela R. Suarez.
      p. ; cm.
   Understanding ICD-10-CM and ICD-10-PCS
   Includes bibliographical references and index.
   ISBN-13: 978-0-07-340221-5 (alk. paper)
   ISBN-10: 0-07-340221-4 (alk. paper)
   I. Suarez, Angela R. II. Title. III. Title: Understanding ICD-10-CM and ICD-10-PCS.
[DNLM:1. International statistical classification of diseases and related health problems. 10th revision. Clinical modification.
2. International statistical classification of diseases and related health problems. 10th revision. Procedure coding system.
3. Clinical Coding—methods. 4. Disease—classification. 5. International Classification of Diseases. WX 173]
616.001′2—dc23

2011040060

BRIEF CONTENTS

CONTENTS

LEAH A. GREBNER, MS, RHIA, CCS, FAHIMA, has been employed in the HIM field since 1989 in a wide variety of settings, which include acute care, home health, skilled nursing, physician office, consulting, and education. She serves as director of the Health Information Technology, Medical Coding Specialist, and Medical Transcription programs at Midstate College in Peoria, Illinois. Leah holds a master's degree in health services administration from the University of St. Francis in Joliet, Illinois, and she is currently working on her dissertation for a PhD in health services with a specialization in community health promotion and education.

Leah has presented for regional, state, and national audiences on a variety of topics related to coding, compliance, electronic health records, personal health records, and applied research in HIM. She has also served as a volunteer in various positions since 2001. She was a member of the board of directors for the Illinois Health Information Management Association (ILHIMA) and Central Illinois Health Information Management Association (CIHIMA). In addition, Leah has played an active role in several committees and workgroups for the American Health Information Management Association (AHIMA). She served as co-chair of the ICD-10 Academic Transition Workgroup, which involved contributing to a series of articles in the *Journal of AHIMA* and presentations at the AHIMA Assembly on Education to guide educators and practitioners in preparation for and transition to ICD-10-CM and ICD-10-PCS. Most recently, Leah is currently serving on the AHIMA ICD-10 in the Classroom Workgroup, which has a charge of investigating, evaluating and researching the topic of ICD-10 Transition in the Classroom, in order to develop best practices of a successful implementation.

Outside of her professional activities, Leah enjoys spending time with her husband and two sons, who are all very supportive of her professional and educational endeavors. She is active in choir and other fellowship groups at her church and is a member of a local Middle Eastern dance troupe.

ANGELA R. SUAREZ, BA, CPC, RMA, has worked in healthcare for over 20 years. She earned her bachelor's degree in pre-medical science and clinical psychology from Spalding University and is currently working towards a Master's of Business Administration degree. During her academic studies in the medical sciences, she also gained practical hands-on clinical and administrative experience while working in hospitals, physician offices, and home health agencies. She then continued her education beyond graduation to include several science and healthcare–related courses, which involved writing proposals for healthcare policy and grants in addition to holding the titles and responsibilities of a medical office administrator and educator. Angela has spent the past six years teaching a wide variety of courses in medical coding, billing, health insurance, and medical office administration. Drawing on her strong clinical background, Angela has also taught courses in the sciences, including Anatomy & Physiology, Pathophysiology, and Pharmacology. Angela was evaluated to be the top 1 percent of educators at her educational institution and has an excellent ability to dissect and disseminate knowledge in a way that is easy to understand. Angela enjoys sharing her knowledge and experience with anyone who is interested in learning from her, as well as sharing her knowledge and experience with students seeking entry to healthcare professions.

Angela is a member of the American Academy of Professional Coders (AAPC) and the American Health Information Management Association (AHIMA). She currently lives in Louisville, Kentucky, with her husband and is blessed to have a 21-year-old son who is a musician. Angela enjoys spending her spare time with her family, cooking ethnic foods, traveling the world, and listening to music.

PREFACE

From the careful management of patient information and protection of patient privacy to the payment of insurance claims, the administration of healthcare is an undercurrent in all of our lives. The medical coder plays a vital role in this process, helping translate complex clinical information into data for medical offices and payers. Coders enable reimbursement for services and, by generating trackable data about healthcare encounters, contribute to improving patient care. As a result, medical coding is a healthcare field that continues to be in high demand, projected to grow by 20% between 2008 and 2018.

Becoming a successful medical coder involves developing a variety of skills, from a familiarity with medical language to the ability to navigate several coding systems with ease. Coders must embrace lifelong learning and stay up-to-date in the coding field, but those foundational skills remain. The ICD-10 transition means that coders must develop the skills to navigate new coding systems and, in the case of ICD-10-PCS, to embrace an entirely new way of coding.

But there's no need to fear the transition to ICD-10. Whether you are just starting your professional coding career or have been coding for years, *Medical Coding: Understanding ICD-10-CM and ICD-10-PCS* provides the framework you need to approach ICD-10 with confidence. Beginning with coding basics, then walking through both ICD-10-CM and ICD-10-PCS, *Medical Coding* guides you through the transition by helping you develop the coding skills you need to succeed in 2013 and beyond.

Medical Coding: Understanding ICD-10-CM and ICD-10-PCS creates a roadmap through the entire ICD-9-CM, ICD-10-CM, and ICD-10-PCS coding systems. The book not only presents students with the basics of how to select codes and follow coding guidelines, but also provides a more in-depth look at conditions and procedures that are classified throughout the coding systems. By becoming more familiar with all of the conditions and procedures that are classified within each section, the coding student not only enhances their knowledge of medical terminology and pathophysiology, but also develops a greater level of understanding of how each section is classified. Leah uses this approach when teaching her coding classes. Students often react with statements that include, "I've never heard of that condition before. I think I will look that one up to learn more about it when I get home," and "Wow! I never would have thought that there would be a code for something like that."

Here's What Instructors and Students Can Expect from *Medical Coding: Understanding ICD-10-CM and ICD-10-PCS*

- A balanced approach to medical coding from authors with both AAPC and AHIMA certifications
- Comprehensive coverage of ICD-10-CM and ICD-10-PCS in one book
- Overview of both physician/outpatient coding and hospital/inpatient coding, with multiple chapters on procedure coding systems and the specifics of ICD-10-PCS
- Clear, readable language that demystifies the coding process
- Exercises to practice coding and opportunities to go beyond the code by thinking critically about code selection and the implications of choosing those codes
- Spotlights on anatomy, physiology, pathophysiology, and medical terminology in light of new clinical needs in ICD-10-CM

Here's What Instructors Have Said about *Medical Coding*

"Eases the student into the new coding [systems] and gives a thorough explanation of the reasoning for the change."

BARBARA WORLEY, RMA, DPM, KING'S COLLEGE

"A comprehensive transitional tool for students needing ICD-9 now and ICD-10 in the near future."

JERRI ROWE, MA, CPC, MEDVANCE INSTITUTE

"The approach to how the book is laid out is well thought out and is flexible in the way that it is arranged."

KATHERINE BAUS, RHIA, CCS-P, AHIMA-APPROVED CERTIFIED **ICD-10-PCS** TRAINER, SOUTHWEST FLORIDA COLLEGE

Organization of *Medical Coding*

Medical Coding: Understanding ICD-10-CM and ICD-10-PCS consists of four parts:

Part	Coverage
I: Introduction to Medical Coding	Part I provides an overview of medical coding, including the origins of ICD-9-CM and ICD-10-CM. It explains the basics of medical billing and reimbursement, discusses types of medical records, and walks through how to abstract information from medical records in order to code accurately.
II: ICD-10-CM	Part II is a comprehensive walkthrough of ICD-10-CM. Chapters on body systems, neoplasms, signs and symptoms, health status, and injuries explain how to code in ICD-10-CM, pointing out differences from ICD-9-CM for coders.
III: Introduction to Medical Procedure Coding	Part III introduces procedure coding and explains the various code sets used in healthcare settings to report procedures. It includes a chapter on ICD-9-CM, Volume 3, to orient new coders before transitioning to ICD-10-PCS.
IV: ICD-10-PCS	Part IV provides an in-depth guide to the completely new format and function of coding in ICD-10-PCS.

Chapter-by-Chapter Content Highlights

- **Chapter 1** discusses the history of medical coding by outlining the development of the ICD classification system.
- **Chapter 2** differentiates among various diagnostic coding systems and formats.
- **Chapter 3** explains the basics of data and billing, including how data sets relate back to medical documentation and affect coding.
- **Chapter 4** discusses the types of medical documentation that coders may encounter in various healthcare settings, including electronic health records.
- **Chapter 5** lays the foundation for coding by explaining how to translate documentation into codes. It discusses the key terms and notes that coders should look for.
- **Chapter 6** explains the coding process for signs, symptoms, and abnormal findings.
- **Chapter 7** details how to assign codes for factors influencing health status and contact with health services, such as pregnancy.
- **Chapter 8** explains how to code for infectious and parasitic diseases.
- **Chapter 9** provides a comprehensive framework for coding neoplasms.
- **Chapter 10** discusses the coding process for endocrine, nutritional, and metabolic diseases, including an in-depth explanation of how diabetes coding has changed in ICD-10-CM.
- **Chapter 11** explains how to code diseases of blood, blood-forming organs, and the immune mechanism (including the spleen).

- **Chapter 12** discusses the details of coding mental and behavioral disorders, emphasizing the importance of carefully reviewing clinical documentation and querying when coding has social implications.
- **Chapter 13** explains how to code for diseases of the nervous system and sense organs, including major sections on the eye and ear.
- **Chapter 14** discusses the coding process for diseases of the circulatory system, with detailed sections on hypertension and heart disease.
- **Chapter 15** explains the ins and outs of coding for respiratory diseases, including respiratory failure. It clarifies the relationships between respiratory conditions and other disorders, which must be considered when assigning codes.
- **Chapter 16** walks through the coding process for disorders of the digestive system, including hernias.
- **Chapter 17** provides an in-depth look at how to code for diseases of the genitourinary system, including reproductive conditions and types of kidney failure.
- **Chapter 18** begins a series of chapters on pregnancy and newborns by explaining the coding process for pregnancy, childbirth, and the puerperium.
- **Chapter 19** explains how to code conditions that arise in the newborn (perinatal) period, even if these conditions do not surface until adulthood.
- **Chapter 20** discusses the coding process for congenital malformations, deformations, and chromosomal abnormalities.
- **Chapter 21** explains the coding of skin conditions, ranging from eczema and acne to burns and procedural complications.
- **Chapter 22** shows the wide variety of conditions related to the musculoskeletal system and connective tissue in explaining the coding process for these conditions, noting instances where ICD-10-CM requires greater specificity because of its emphasis on laterality and acuity.
- **Chapter 23** explains how to code injuries, poisonings, and other consequences of external causes.
- **Chapter 24** complements the coverage of Chapter 23 in discussing how to code the causes of injury, poisoning, and morbidity, given that two codes are needed for these medical events.
- **Chapter 25** introduces the various procedure coding systems and conventions in use, covering ICD-9-CM Volume 3, CPT, HCPCS, and more.
- **Chapter 26** walks through the process of selecting procedure codes from ICD-9-CM, Volume 3.
- **Chapter 27** introduces ICD-10-PCS and explains the new structure, format, and table conventions of the coding system, stressing the need to build each code individually, rather than memorize or refer to specific codes for particular procedures.
- **Chapter 28** explains the coding process for procedures classified within Sections 0–4 of ICD-10-PCS, including a discussion of each character's values.
- **Chapter 29** continues the ICD-10-PCS walkthrough with a discussion of coding from Sections 5–9 of ICD-10-PCS.
- **Chapter 30** explains how to select codes from Sections B–H of ICD-10-PCS.

To the Instructor

McGraw-Hill knows how much effort it takes to prepare for a new course. Through focus groups, symposia, reviews, and conversations with instructors like you, we have gathered information about what materials you need in order to facilitate successful courses. We are committed to providing you with high-quality, accurate instructor support. If you would like to participate in future product reviews or events, be sure to let your McGraw-Hill sales representative know!

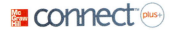

Instructor Resources

You can rely on the following materials to help you and your students work through the exercises in the book:

- Instructor edition of the Online Learning Center (OLC) at **www.mhhe.com/ grebner**. Your McGraw-Hill sales representative can provide you with access and show you how to "go green" with our online instructor support. The OLC contains a number of resources to assist you in teaching your course:

Resource	Description
Instructor's manual (organized by learning outcomes)	- Lesson plans and sample syllabi - Answer keys for end-of-section and end-of-chapter questions - Additional critical thinking questions for extra practice - Key medical and anatomic terms for further A&P study
PowerPoints (organized by learning outcomes)	- Key terms - Key concepts - Teaching notes

Electronic testbank	- EZ Test online (computerized)
	- Word version
	- Questions are tagged with
	  • Learning outcome
	  • Level of difficulty
	  • Level of Bloom's Taxonomy
	  • Feedback
	  • Industry standards

Tools to plan course	- Correlations of the learning outcomes to accrediting bodies, such as CAHIIM, ABHES, and CAAHEP - Sample syllabi and lesson plans - Asset map—clickable PDF with links to all key supplements, broken down by learning outcomes

- *Connect Plus:* McGraw-Hill's *Connect Plus* is a revolutionary online assignment and assessment solution, providing instructors and students with tools and resources to maximize their success. Through *Connect Plus,* instructors enjoy simplified course setup and assignment creation. Robust, media-rich tools and activities, all tied to the textbook learning outcomes, ensure you'll create classes geared toward achievement. You'll have more time with your students and spend less time agonizing over course planning.

Connect Plus for *Medical Coding* contains the following activities:

- End-of-section and end-of-chapter material
- Interactive, engaging activities that reinforce key terms, A&P knowledge, and coding skills
- Case studies with clinical documentation for more coding practice and analytical skill building

CodeitRightOnline™: Your Online Coding Tool

So that your students can gain experience with the use of an online coding tool, they will have access to a 14-day period to CodeitRightOnline, produced by Contexo Media, a division of Access Intelligence. CodeitRightOnline is available online at **www.codeitrightonline.com**.

Features

These are the general features that are offered with a subscription:

- CodeitRightOnline Search—Provides the ability to find a CPT, HCPCS Level II, and ICD-9-CM code either using the index or tabular search sections, by code terminology, description, keyword, or code number to locate the correct code. Plus, the Single Search Feature allows you to locate all codes related to a particular term.
- Fully customizable—Provides note capability, LCD customization, personalized searches and fee schedules, and specialty-specific code sets.
- Coding Crosswalks—Essential coding links from CPT codes to ICD-9-CM to HCPCS Level II codes and Anesthesia codes.
- Articles compiled from CMS, OIG, carriers, intermediaries, payers, and other government websites, along with newsletter articles from AMA, AHA, Decision Health, Coding Institute, and others.
- LCD/NCD codes for a local state carrier, Medicare's payment policy indicators, and, of course, CPT®, HCPCS Level II, and ICD-9-CM codes with full descriptions and our Plain English Definitions.
- ICD-10-CM/PCS Code Sets—Help you prepare for 2013 mandatory implementation with ICD-10-CM/PCS full code sets and descriptions
- NCCI Edits Validator™—Validates codes to help you remain in compliance with the correct coding guidelines established by the Centers for Medicare & Medicaid Services (CMS).
- Automatic Updates—Ensure that CodeitRightOnline contains the most up-to-date, real-time information.
- Build-A-Code™—Allows students to build codes from the ground up, helping them understand how ICD-10 codes are constructed.
- Click-A-Dex™—Helps index searches for easy future reference.
- Comprehensive Medicare Resource—Contains local coverage determination (LCD) and national coverage determination (NCD) information, contact information for comprehensive lists of Medicare providers, and information on how to bill for procedures allowed by Medicare's Physician Quality Reporting Initiative (PQRI) program.

- ABC Codes and Descriptions—Provide access to the alternative medicine codes you need to describe services, remedies, and/or supplies required during patient visits.
- Educational Games and Learning Tools—Games and interactive tools that help reinforce the student's knowledge of anatomy.

Using the Online Coding Tool

Go to **www.codeitrightonline.com** to complete the steps needed to begin. The following screen will appear:

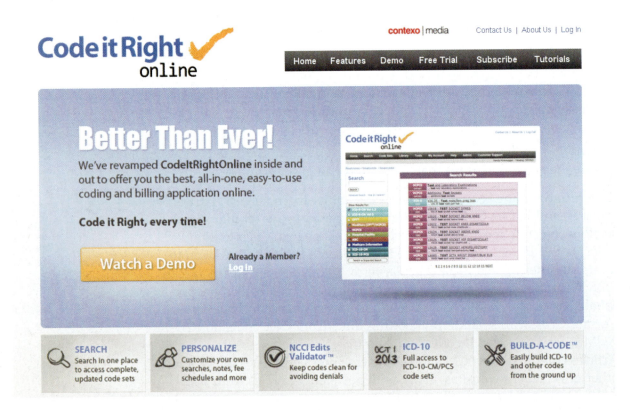

Click on the Free Trial tab at the top right-hand corner of the screen. On the page that appears, enter your name, e-mail address, school, phone, and address. Next, click on "Use account contact information" for your account administrator information, a one-time process that optimizes CodeitRightOnline for your location. Choose a username and password you will remember. Next, read the Terms and Conditions, including the AMA Agreement. After accepting these Terms and Conditions, click "Continue." You will then receive an e-mail containing an activation link. Clicking on the link will activate your account. From that page, follow the "Click here" link to sign in with the account information you selected. This will take you to the CodeitRightOnline home page—you're in!

These actions set up your trial subscription. Now, to use the online coding tool to locate codes, click "Search" and select the appropriate code set. Next, choose the start point for your code search. For example, select

ICD-9-CM Vol 1, 2 and Vol 3 in the Show Results For box, enter the term "Fracture," and click "Search." CodeitRightOnline will return a list of the various fracture entries for your selection. To see how it works, choose Fracture of Ribs, Closed, and click the code number to review the tabular list entry.

Do More Now

Do More

McGraw-Hill Higher Education and Blackboard have teamed up. What does this mean for you?

1. **Your life, simplified.** Now you and your students can access McGraw-Hill's *Connect Plus* and Create right from within your Blackboard course—all with one sign-on. Say goodbye to the days of logging in to multiple applications.
2. **Deep integration of content and tools.** Not only do you get single sign-on with *Connect Plus* and Create, but you also get deep integration of McGraw-Hill content and content engines right in Blackboard. Whether you're choosing a book for your course or building *Connect Plus* assignments, all the tools you need are right where you want them—inside Blackboard.
3. **Seamless gradebooks.** Are you tired of keeping multiple gradebooks and manually synchronizing grades into Blackboard? We thought so. When a student completes an integrated *Connect Plus* assignment, the grade for that assignment automatically (and instantly) feeds your Blackboard grade center.
4. **A solution for everyone.** Whether your institution is already using Blackboard or you just want to try Blackboard on your own, we have a solution for you. McGraw-Hill and Blackboard can now offer you easy access to industry-leading technology and content, whether your campus hosts it or we do. Be sure to ask your local McGraw-Hill representative for details.

Need Help with the Book or Online Course? Contact McGraw-Hill Higher Education's Customer Experience Team

Visit our Customer Experience Team Support website at **www.mhhe.com/support**. Browse our FAQs (Frequently Asked Questions) and product documentation, and/or contact a Customer Experience Team representative.

The Customer Experience Team is available Sunday through Friday.

GUIDED TOUR

Many pedagogical tools have been incorporated throughout the book to help students learn.

Chapter Opener

The **chapter opener** sets the stage for what will be learned in the chapter.

Learning Outcomes are written to reflect the revised version of Bloom's Taxonomy and to establish the key points the student should focus on in the chapter. In addition, major chapter heads are structured to reflect the Learning Outcomes and are numbered accordingly.

Key Terms are first introduced in the chapter opener, so the student can see them all in one place.

Learning Aids

Key Terms are bolded and defined in the margin, so that students will become familiar with the language of coding. These are reinforced in the **Glossary** at the end of the book.

remission Absence of malignant cells following treatment.

Tips

Coding Tips highlight helpful information for students.

CODING TIP ▸

If anemia is documented as being an adverse effect of treatment by chemotherapy, radiation therapy, or immunotherapy, the coder should first assign the appropriate code for the adverse effect, then assign the codes for anemia and the neoplastic condition.

Spotlight on A&P features emphasize medical terminology, anatomy, physiology, and pathophysiology to help coders navigate ICD-10's greater code specificity.

Spotlight on A&P

A variety of names are used for neoplastic conditions classified as being of unspecified or uncertain behavior. Become familiar with these terms, so that you can recognize and code these conditions correctly.

9 NEOPLASMS

Think About It 9.4

also available in
connect plus+

Assign ICD-10-CM codes for the following situations, applying any appropriate sequencing guidelines.

1. Intracranial nevus _____
2. Intra-abdominal hemangioma _____
3. Subserosal leiomyoma of the uterus _____
4. Cystic lymphangioma _____
5. Mammary myxoid fibroma of the right breast _____

Beyond the Code: Why is it pertinent to report an additional code to identify the functional activity of endocrine glands with benign neoplasm?

Exercises within the chapter provide students with hands-on coding practice. *Beyond the code* questions encourage students to think critically about code sets and clinical information.

End-of-Chapter Resources

The **Chapter Summary** is in a tabular, step-by-step format with page references to help with review of the materials.

The **Chapter Review** contains the following questions, all tagged by Learning Outcomes: code assignment, multiple-choice, short answer (code manual navigation and code selection), Online Activities, and Real-World Application: Case Studies to strengthen the links between education and professional coding.

CHAPTER 9 REVIEW

Chapter Summary

Learning Outcome	Key Concepts/Examples
9.1 Apply general neoplasm coding guidelines. (pages 125–128)	• Neoplasms are classified primarily by site or topography, within subsections to identify behavior as malignant, in situ, benign, uncertain, or unspecified. • If the reason for the encounter is solely for the administration of chemotherapy, immunotherapy, or radiation therapy, a code from the Z51 category should be assigned as the principal or first-listed diagnosis, with the malignancy assigned as an additional code.
9.2 Discuss aspects of coding malignant neoplasms. (pages 128–131)	• For malignant neoplasms, many of the categories have instructions to assign additional codes to identify any alcohol abuse and dependence, history of tobacco use, tobacco dependence, or tobacco use. • If Kaposi's sarcoma is associated with human immunodeficiency virus (HIV) disease, code B20 should be assigned prior to the code for Kaposi's sarcoma in category C46.
9.3 Identify terms used to document in situ neoplasms. (pages 131–132)	• In situ neoplasms are non-invasive. • The term *dysplasia* is often used when documenting in situ neoplasms.
9.4 Classify conditions related to benign neoplasms. (page 132)	• When reporting benign neoplasm of the pancreas, ovary, testis, thyroid, and other endocrine glands, an additional code should be assigned to identify functional activity.
9.5 Describe neoplasms of uncertain behavior and neoplasms of unspecified behavior. (page 133)	• Uncertain behavior means that histologic confirmation regarding whether the neoplasm is malignant or benign cannot be made. • When reporting post-transplant lymphoproliferative disorder (PTLD), a code from category T86 should be assigned to identify a complication of transplanted organs and tissue, followed by code D47.z1.

Applying Your Skills

For each condition, assign the appropriate code(s) using ICD-9-CM and ICD-10-CM.

Condition	ICD-9-CM	ICD-10-CM
1. *[LO 9.2]* Osteosarcoma of the left fibula	_____	_____
2. *[LO 9.2]* Melanoma of the right forearm	_____	_____
3. *[LO 9.2]* Adenocarcinoma of the distal esophagus	_____	_____
4. *[LO 9.3.]* Ductal carcinoma in situ (DCIS) of the left breast axillary tail in a female patient	_____	_____
5. *[LO 9.1.]* Multiple myeloma in remission	_____	_____

Checking Your Understanding

Select the letter that best answers the question or completes the sentence.

1. *[LO 9.2]* What is the correct coding assignment for a patient with AIDS-related Kaposi's sarcoma of the skin of the right lower leg?
   a. B20, C44.71 b. C46.0
   c. C46.0, B20 d. B20, C46.0

2. *[LO 9.4]* What should be reported with an additional code when coding benign neoplasm of the pancreas, ovary, testis, thyroid, and other endocrine glands?
   a. risk factors b. functional activity
   c. symptoms d. sequelae

3. *[LO 9.1]* Which of the following is not a behavioral classification of neoplasms?
   a. benign b. in situ
   c. malignant d. transitional

Real-World Application

[LO 9.5] Assign ICD-10-CM codes for the following admission for chemotherapy:

Discharge Summary

Diagnoses:

1. Diffuse large B-cell lymphoma following renal transplant.
2. Stage 3 Chronic renal insufficiency.

History of Present Illness: This 46-year-old white male was diagnosed with post-transplant lymphoproliferative disorder following complaints of abdominal pain, weight loss, and anorexia. He did not seek medical attention immediately. Large-cell lymphoma was diagnosed after lymph node biopsy in the groin.

Hospital Course: Patient was admitted for administration of fourth cycle of chemotherapy with rituximab plus cyclophosphamide, daunorubicin, vincristine, and prednisone was started. Treatment was tolerated well with no nausea, vomiting, or fatigue.

Laboratory Findings: WBC 9.8 with normal differential, ANC 7600, hemoglobin 8.6, hematocrit 26.8, MCV 110, and platelet count of 220,000.

Discharge Instructions: Patient was discharged home to follow up in office next week. Continue medications as prescribed.

Online Activity

[LO 9.1] Visit the Surveillance, Epidemiology and End Results (SEER) website of the National Cancer Institute. Discuss how neoplasm coding fits into cancer registry activities. Summarize your findings in a brief report.

ACKNOWLEDGMENTS

Suggestions have been received from faculty and students throughout the country. We rely on this vital feedback with all of our books. Each person who has offered comments and suggestions has our thanks.

The efforts of many people are needed to develop and improve a product. Among these people are the reviewers and consultants who point out areas of concern, cite areas of strength, and make recommendations for change. In this regard, the following instructors provided feedback that was enormously helpful in preparing the first edition of *Medical Coding: Understanding ICD-10-CM and ICD-10-PCS.*

Workshops

In 2010 and 2011, McGraw-Hill conducted 13 health professions workshops, providing an opportunity for more than 700 faculty members to gain continuing education credits, as well as to provide feedback on our products.

Book Reviews

Many instructors participated in manuscript reviews throughout the development of the book.

Gina M. Augustine, MLS, RT,
  RHIT, CPC, CPC-H, CPhT
Fortis College

Katherine E. Baus, RHIA, CCS-P
Southwest Florida College

Sue Butler, CPC, CIMC
Lansing Community College

Tiffany B. Cooper, CPC
Isothermal Community College

Patricia De La Rosa, CPC, CBCS,
  CMAA
Keiser Career College

Angela G. Hennessy, MS
Corning Community College

Judy Hurtt, MEd
East Central Community
  College

J. Kelly, PhD, CPC
Davenport University

JanMarie C. Malik, MBA, RHIA
Shasta Community College

Sandra Metcalf, ME
Grayson County College

Kathleen O'Gorman, BS, CPC
Tunxis Community College

Lois Lorraine Patterson-Fluker,
  NRCCS
Virginia College

Deborah J. Phillips, AS, CPC, CPC-H
Virginia College

Staci R. Porter, AA, MA
San Joaquin Valley College

Marie J. Pyram, CBCS, MBAHSA
Keiser Career College

Jerri Rowe, MA, CPC
MedVance Institute

Mary Jo Slater
Community College of Beaver County

Deanna L. Stephens, RMA, CMOA, NCICS
Virginia College

Pam Ventgen, CMA (AAMA), CCS-P, CPC, CPC-I
University of Alaska Anchorage

Sharvette Walker, CPC, AHIMA-Approved ICD-10-CM/PCS trainer
South Suburban College & Olive Harvey College

Cindy Ward, CPC, CPC-H, CEMC, CPMA, CCC
MedTech College

Barbara S. Worley, BS, RMA (AAMT)
King's College

Technical Editing/Accuracy Panel

A panel of instructors completed a technical edit and review of all content in the book page proofs to verify its accuracy, as well as the supplements.

Kathleen O'Gorman, BS, CPC
Tunxis Community College

Andrea Potteiger, CCS, CCS-P, CPC

Deanna L. Stephens, CMOA, NCICS, RMA, AABA
Virginia College

Barbara Wilson, CPC, CCS-P, RHIT
Southeastern Institute

Amy D. Lawrence, MBA/HR, CPC, CCA, CMAA, CBCS
Ultimate Medical Academy

Acknowledgments from the Authors

We want to thank the editorial team at McGraw-Hill—Michael Ledbetter, Natalie Ruffatto, Raisa Kreek, and Michelle Flomenhoft—for their willingness and ability to develop us as writers.

The EDP staff was also outstanding: senior designer Srdj Savanovic created a terrific design, which was implemented through the production process by Jean Starr, project manager; Kara Kudronowicz, buyer; Lori Hancock, photo research coordinator; and Cathy Tepper, media project manager.

Special thanks to Roxan Kinsey, executive marketing manager, for her tireless efforts in advocating for students and instructors.

Last but not least, thanks to our families for their love and support.

Leah Grebner and Angela Suarez

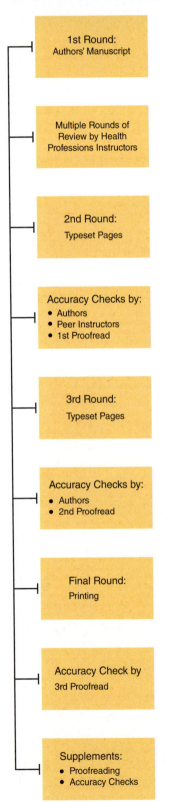

You have a right to expect an accurate textbook, and McGraw-Hill invests considerable time and effort to make sure that we deliver one. Listed below are the many steps we take to make sure this happens.

Our Accuracy Verification Process

First Round—Development Reviews

STEP 1: Numerous **health professions instructors** review the draft manuscript and report on any errors that they may find. The authors make these corrections in their final manuscript.

Second Round—Page Proofs

STEP 2: Once the manuscript has been typeset, the **authors** check their manuscript against the page proofs to ensure that all illustrations, graphs, examples, and exercises have been correctly laid out on the pages and that all codes have been updated correctly.

STEP 3: An outside panel of **peer instructors** completes a review of content in the page proofs to verify its accuracy. The authors add these corrections to their review of the page proofs.

STEP 4: A **proofreader** adds a triple layer of accuracy assurance in pages by looking for errors; then a confirming, corrected round of page proofs is produced.

Third Round—Confirming Page Proofs

STEP 5: The **author team** reviews the confirming round of page proofs to make certain that any previous corrections were properly made and to look for any errors they might have missed on the first round.

STEP 6: The **project manager,** who has overseen the book from the beginning, performs **a final check** to make sure that no new errors have been introduced during the production process.

Final Round—Printer's Proofs

STEP 7: The **project manager** performs a **final check** of the book during the printing process, providing a final accuracy review. In concert with the main text, all supplements undergo a proofreading and technical editing stage to ensure their accuracy.

Results

What results is a textbook that is as accurate and error-free as is humanly possible. Our authors and publishing staff are confident that the many layers of quality assurance have produced books that are leaders in the industry for their integrity and correctness. *Please view the Acknowledgments section for more details on the many people involved in this process.*

INTRODUCTION TO MEDICAL CODING

PART I

Chapter Summary

Learning Outcome	Key Concepts/Examples
1.1 Outline the history of medical coding system development. **(pages 3–4)**	• The roots of medical coding can be traced back to the London Bills of Mortality, which was used to track deaths in the early 1600s. • The need for tracking medical statistics was more widely recognized in the 1800s. • It is recommended that the disease classification system be revised every 10 years, which was done until 1985. • The WHO changed the planned 1985 revision meeting to 1989 due to extensive expansion of the system and a need for restructuring.
1.2 Explain clinical modifications to the International Classification of Diseases. **(page 4)**	• The abbreviation *CM* represents the clinical modification the United States made to the International Classification of Diseases. • Addition of classification of procedures is a part of the clinical modifications the United States made.
1.3 Describe how the International Classification of Diseases is maintained in the United States. **(page 5)**	• The cooperating parties for maintaining official coding guidelines for ICD-9-CM are the American Hospital Association (AHA), American Health Information Management Association (AHIMA), Centers for Medicare and Medicaid Services (CMS), and National Center for Health Statistics (NCHS). • Official ICD-9-CM coding advice is disseminated in the quarterly publication *Coding Clinic* for ICD-9-CM, with a special edition to present guidelines for new codes each year.
1.4 Identify aspects of ICD-11 to consider as ICD-10-CM and ICD-10-PCS are being implemented in the United States. **(pages 6–7)**	• The final draft of ICD-11 should be submitted to the World Health Assembly by 2014. • ICD-11 will have three distinct versions, referred to as uses, defined by the levels of care, which are specified as primary care, clinical, and research.

Checking Your Understanding

Select the letter that best answers the question or completes the sentence.

1. *[LO 1.1]* Why was the 1985 revision meeting postponed?
   a. lack of need to update
   b. scheduling conflicts
   c. need for restructuring due to extensive expansion
   d. extensive changes due to classifying diseases, rather than just mortality

2. *[LO 1.4]* When should the final draft of ICD-11 be submitted to the World Health Assembly?
   a. 2013
   b. 2014
   c. 2020
   d. 2023

3. *[LO 1.1]* What was the intended use for the classification of diagnoses in the early 1600s?
   a. reimbursement
   b. tracking of deaths
   c. collection of statistics for healthcare facilities
   d. medical research

4. *[LO 1.2]* What does the abbreviation *CM* represent in ICD-9-CM and ICD-10-CM?
   a. coding methods
   b. classification of medicine
   c. coordination and maintenance
   d. clinical modification

5. *[LO 1.3]* What organizations are the cooperating parties for maintaining official coding guidelines for ICD-9-CM?
   a. AHA, AHIMA, CMS, NCHS
   b. AHA, AMA, CMS, NCHS
   c. AHA, AMA, CMS, HHS
   d. AHA, AAPC, AHIMA, CMS

6. *[LO 1.4]* How many parameters are included in the content model for ICD-11?
   a. 3
   b. 7
   c. 10
   d. 13

7. *[LO 1.1]* How frequently should the ICD classification system be revised, as recommended by the WHO?

 a. annually, for implementation January 1
 b. annually, for implementation October 1
 c. every other year
 d. every 10 years

8. *[LO 1.1]* The need to track medical statistics became more widely recognized in

 a. 1562.
 b. the early 1600s.
 c. 1785.
 d. the 1800s.

9. *[LO 1.2]* Which of the following is the result of the clinical modification of the International Classification of Diseases?

 a. development of a procedure coding system
 b. increased specificity
 c. ability to expand
 d. statistical data collection

10. *[LO 1.3]* How many editions of *Coding Clinic* for ICD-9-CM are published each year?

 a. one
 b. two
 c. four
 d. five

Fill in the word(s) to complete each sentence.

11. *[LO 1.1]* The roots of medical coding can be traced back to the _____ in the early 1600s.

12. *[LO 1.1]* The International Classification of Diseases was updated every _____ years until 1985.

13. *[LO 1.1]* ICD-10 was endorsed by the 43rd _____ in 1990.

14. *[LO 1.2]* The abbreviation *CM* stands for _____.

15. *[LO 1.2]* The *PCS* in ICD-10-PCS stands for _____.

16. *[LO 1.3]* Proposed and final rulings for changes to ICD in the United States are published in the _____.

17. *[LO 1.3]* Coding changes, additions, and deletions are effective on _____ of each year.

18. *[LO 1.4]* The final draft of ICD-11 should be submitted to the World Health Assembly by _____.

Provide short answers for questions 19 and 20.

19. *[LO 1.2]* What similarities and differences exist between the classification of causes of death and the classification of diseases?

20. *[LO 1.3]* What are the pros and cons of revising the coding system on a regular basis?

Online Activity

[LO 1.3] Visit the websites for the WHO, CMS, and NCHS to learn more about the role of each organization in ICD-9-CM and ICD-10-CM/PCS. What are the similarities between the ways that each organization is involved in these code sets? What are the differences?

Real-World Application

[LO 1.3] Put yourself in the place of a representative of one of the cooperating parties for maintaining the coding system in the United States. What are some of the variables you might consider when making recommendations for changes each year?

2 FORMATS AND CONVENTIONS OF DIAGNOSIS CODING SYSTEMS

Learning Outcomes
After completing this chapter, students should be able to

2.1 Explain the layout of the ICD-9-CM and ICD-10-CM manuals.

2.2 Differentiate between the organization of the ICD-9-CM and ICD-10-CM manuals.

2.3 Define the terms and phrases used in ICD-9-CM and ICD-10-CM that provide instructions for coding and sequencing.

2.4 Explain how punctuation in the code book provides guidance for the coder.

2.5 Interpret abbreviations that are used in the code book.

Key Terms
alphabetic index
and
brackets
category
code also
code first
colon
conventions
excludes
excludes1
excludes2
guidelines
includes
nonessential modifiers
Not Elsewhere Classifiable (NEC)
Not Otherwise Specified (NOS)
parentheses
placeholder
sections
see
see also
tabular list
use additional code
with

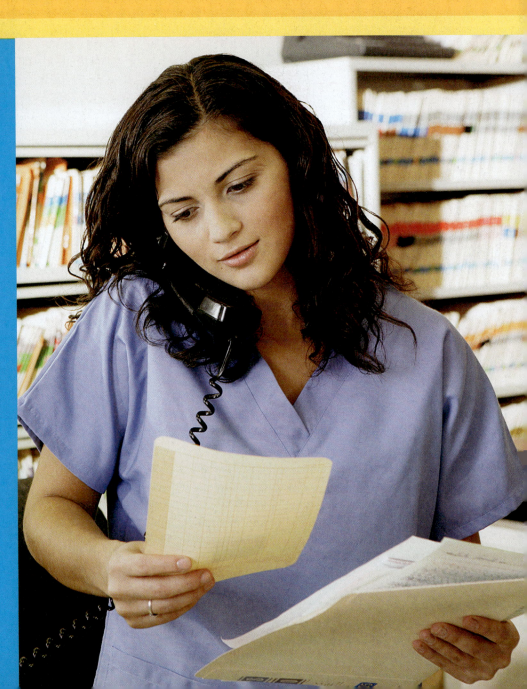

Introduction

Coding requires the use of a code book, or coding manual, an organized list of codes with helpful instructions about each code. This chapter will show you the basic organization of both the ICD-9-CM and the ICD-10-CM manuals and point out what has changed in ICD-10-CM. Because coding also makes use of medical language, which can have different terms, abbreviations, or punctuation than regular written language, this chapter will also introduce you to the instructional terminology, phrases, punctuation, and abbreviations that are used in these manuals.

2.1 Layout of the Code Book

When learning how to code, your first step is to get to know your code book. The code book is full of tools to assist you in complete and accurate reporting. Most coders have never read a code book from cover to cover. However, it is important to become familiar with everything between those two covers, so that you will know what you are looking for and how to find it.

Official **conventions** and **guidelines** are located in the front of most ICD-9-CM, ICD-10-CM, and ICD-10-PCS code books. ICD-9-CM consists of three volumes. Volume 2 is the **Alphabetic Index** to Diseases and Injuries, organized alphabetically by main term. Contained within Volume 2 is also the Table of Drugs and Chemicals (Section II) and the Index to External Causes of Injury E Codes (Section III). Volume 1 is the **Tabular List** of Diseases. It contains a chronological listing of all diagnosis codes (001.0–999.9). Also contained within the Tabular are two supplementary classifications. V Codes describe Factors influencing Health Status and Contact with Health Services (V01.0–V91.99). E Codes describe External Causes of Injury and Poisoning (E000.0–E999.1). Volume 3 contains both an Alphabetic Index and Tabular List of procedure codes. Procedure codes are surgical in nature, requiring anesthesia and performed in an inpatient setting. This volume is only used by hospitals to report surgeries performed in their facilities. Volume 2 and Volume 1 can be used by both outpatient and hospital providers.

In contrast, ICD-10-CM includes only the alphabetic index and tabular list for diagnoses (Volumes 1 and 2 in ICD-9-CM). Volume 3 has been replaced by ICD-10-PCS, which consists of a system for building procedure codes. Coding guideline *I.A.1. The Alphabetic Index and Tabular List* in your code book addresses the presence of these parts of the coding system.

Within Volume 1—Tabular List of Diseases—chapters are subdivided into **sections** grouping different categories of codes. There are 17 chapters, all organized by etiology (cause of disease) or body system. ICD-9-CM

conventions Guidelines for how codes are selected and sequenced.

guidelines Instructions in the code book that provide helpful notes about how to assign codes in certain cases.

alphabetic index Alphabetic list of diagnoses and their associated codes.

tabular list Chronological list of codes.

sections Groupings of several categories of codes created by the subdivisions of chapter classifications.

CODING TIP ▶

ICD-9-CM consists of three volumes, whereas ICD-10-CM consists of only two volumes. This is due to the development of ICD-10-PCS.

Table 2.1 Comparison of Chapter Titles and Code Ranges in ICD-9-CM and ICD-10-CM

ICD-10-CM Chapter Title	ICD-10-CM	ICD-9-CM
Certain Infectious and Parasitic Diseases	A00–B99	001–139
Neoplasms	C00–D49	140–239
Diseases of the Blood and Blood-Forming Organs and Certain Disorders Involving the Immune Mechanism	D50–D89	280–289 (only includes diseases of blood and blood-forming organs)
Endocrine, Nutritional, and Metabolic Diseases	E00–E89	240–279 (also includes immunity disorders)
Mental and Behavioral Disorders	F01–F99	290–319
Diseases of the Nervous System	G00–G99	320–389 (Diseases of the Nervous System and Sense Organs)
Diseases of the Eye and Adnexa	H00–H59	
Diseases of the Ear and Mastoid Process	H60–H95	
Diseases of the Circulatory System	I00–I99	390–459
Diseases of the Respiratory System	J00–J99	460–519
Diseases of the Digestive System	K00–K94	520–579
Diseases of the Skin and Subcutaneous Tissue	L00–L99	680–709
Diseases of the Musculoskeletal System and Connective Tissue	M00–M99	710–739
Diseases of the Genitourinary System	N00–N99	580–629
Pregnancy, Childbirth, and the Puerperium	O00–O9a	630–677 (Complications of Pregnancy, Childbirth, and the Puerperium)
Certain Conditions Originating in the Perinatal Period	P00–P96	760–779
Congenital Malformations, Deformations, and Chromosomal Abnormalities	Q00–Q99	740–759 (Congenital Anomalies)
Symptoms, Signs, and Abnormal Clinical Laboratory Findings, Not Elsewhere Classified	R00–R99	780–799 (Symptoms, Signs, and Ill-Defined Conditions)
Injury Poisoning and Certain Other Consequences of External Causes	S00–T98	800–999 (Injury and Poisoning)
External Causes of Morbidity	V00–Y98	E800–E999 Supplementary Classification of External Causes of Injury and Poisoning
Factors Influencing Health Status and Contact with Health Services	Z00–Z99	V01–V83 Supplementary Classification of Factors Influencing Health Status and Contact with Health Services

codes may contain up to five digits. ICD-10-CM codes may contain as many as seven digits. The expansion of the codes was done to allow for greater specificity in the coding system. The first three digits are referred to as the **category** and are followed by a decimal point. In ICD-9-CM there may be a 4th or 5th digit required to fully explain the diagnostic condition. In ICD-10-CM there may be a 4th, 5th, 6th or 7th digit required for subcategory level coding. Some codes with six or seven characters may require the use of a **placeholder** character, *X*, if there is not a 5th or 6th character. Official instructions related to sections, categories, and characters in ICD-10-CM codes are found in the following coding guidelines:

- *I.A.2. Format and structure*
- *I.A.3. Use of codes for reporting purposes*
- *I.A.4. Placeholder character*
- *I.A.5. 7th Characters*

category The first three characters of both ICD-9-CM and ICD-10-CM diagnosis codes.

placeholder The character *X* is inserted to hold the places of the 5th or 6th character in codes with six or seven characters if there is not a 5th or 6th character.

Think About It 2.1

also available in **connect** (plus+)

Some codes with six or seven characters require the use of a placeholder character of *X* if there is not a 5th or 6th character. Why shouldn't the code just skip the placeholder(s) and have fewer characters?

2.2 Comparison of ICD-9-CM and ICD-10-CM

As coders are making the transition from ICD-9-CM to ICD-10-CM, it is helpful to compare the layout of the code books to note the similarities and differences. When comparing the titles of the chapters in the two coding systems, you may notice that the names of many chapters are identical or similar in wording. As shown in Table 2.1, the overall layout of the coding systems for diagnosis coding is very similar between ICD-9-CM and ICD-10-CM, as is the method of looking up codes. The codes themselves, however, look very different.

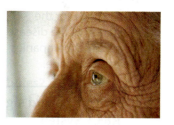

One change from ICD-9-CM to ICD-10-CM is the inclusion of separate chapters for diseases of the eye, ear, and nervous system.

CODING TIP ▶

Even though the codes themselves are different, the overall layout and method of looking up codes are very similar between ICD-9-CM and ICD-10-CM.

Think About It 2.2

also available in **connect** (plus+)

What differences do you notice in the comparison of the chapters between ICD-9-CM and ICD-10-CM? Which factors may have contributed to these differences?

7. *[LO 2.5]* What does the abbreviation NEC represent?
   a. other specified
   b. unspecified
   c. no extra code
   d. need extra code

8. *[LO 2.3]* Which term or phrase instructs the coder to assign another code prior to the code being referenced?
   a. code also
   b. code first
   c. use additional code
   d. with

9. *[LO 2.4]* What is a nonessential modifier?
   a. a term that may coexist with the main term but may change the code assignment for the condition
   b. a term that may coexist with the main term but does not change the code assignment for the condition
   c. a term that changes the code assignment for the condition if it coexists with the main term
   d. a term that must coexist with the main term in order to assign the code for the condition

10. *[LO 2.1]* What is a placeholder?
    a. The character *X* is inserted to hold the place of the 5th and/or 6th character in codes with six or seven characters if there is not a 5th and/or 6th character.
    b. Since all ICD-10-CM codes are to be seven characters in length, if the code does not specify out to seven characters, the character *X* is inserted to hold the place of missing characters.
    c. If the coder is awaiting clarification on documentation from a physician, the character *X* is inserted in the areas awaiting additional specification in the documentation.
    d. A code composed of the character *X* in all positions is used to report a code in the case that there is an instructional notation to "code first," but no appropriate condition is documented.

Online Activity

[LO 2.1] ICD-10-CM official conventions and guidelines are available to anybody for free through the Centers for Disease Control and Prevention (CDC), along with additional ICD-10-CM resources. Visit the CDC website and search for the ICD-10-CM information. Describe what you find in your search.

Real-World Application

[LO 2.1] You have been hired as a coding supervisor at an acute care hospital. One of the first things you discover in your new position is that the facility does not have a coding policies and procedures manual. Write a section for a policies and procedures manual that addresses the use of official conventions and guidelines for ICD-10-CM coding.

3 DATA AND BILLING BASICS

Learning Outcomes *After completing this chapter, students should be able to*

3.1 Outline the evolution of medical billing and reimbursement systems.

3.2 Describe the inpatient prospective payment system.

3.3 Explain the outpatient prospective payment system.

3.4 Identify prospective payment systems for other healthcare settings.

3.5 Relate data sets to medical documentation.

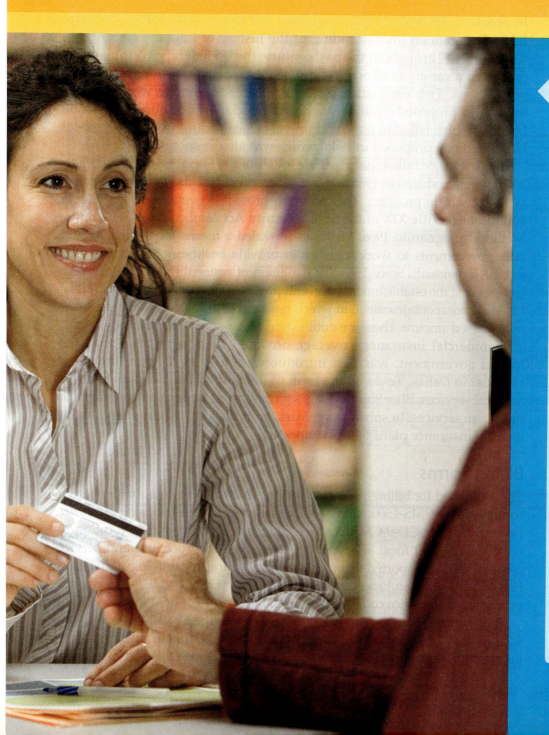

Key Terms

ambulatory payment classifications (APCs)

commercial insurance

Data Elements for Emergency Department Systems (DEEDS)

home health resource groups (HHRGs)

inpatient prospective payment system (IPPS)

Medicaid

Medicare

Medicare severity diagnosis-related groups (MS-DRGs)

National Electronic Disease Surveillance System (NEDSS)

National Hospital Ambulatory Medical Care Survey (NHAMCS)

Outcome and Assessment Information Set (OASIS)

Prospective payment system (PPS)

Resource-Based Relative Value Scale (RBRVS)

Social Security Act

Title XVIII

Title XIX

Uniform Ambulatory Care Data Set (UACDS)

Uniform Hospital Discharge Data Set (UHDDS)

1. Personal identification
2. Date of birth
3. Sex
4. Race and ethnicity
5. Residence
6. Hospital identification
7. Admission date
8. Type of admission
9. Discharge date
10. Physician identification—attending physician
11. Physician identification—operating physician
12. Principal diagnosis
13. Other diagnoses
14. Qualifier for other diagnoses
15. External cause-of-injury code
16. Birth weight of neonate
17. Procedures and dates
18. Disposition of the patient
19. Patient's expected source of payment
20. Total charges

Each MS-DRG is associated with a standardized basic payment amount, which is based on the average resources used to treat Medicare patients for diagnoses and procedures within that MS-DRG, using the ICD-9-CM diagnosis and procedure codes. This standardized payment has two parts, a labor-related share and a non-labor share. The labor-related share is adjusted according to the wage index for the location of the facility to account for variation in hospital labor costs. Once the base payment rate is calculated, it is multiplied by the MS-DRG relative weight, which accounts for differences in the case mix of patients treated across facilities. There are several add-on payments associated with IPPS, including add-ons for

- facilities that serve a disproportionate share of low-income patients,
- facilities incurring indirect costs of medical education,
- cases utilizing approved technologies under the technology add-on payment criteria, and
- outlier payments for cases that are unusually costly.

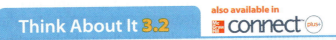

Think About It 3.2 also available in McGraw Hill **connect** plus+

What do you think are the pros and cons of reimbursement through IPPS?

3.3 Outpatient Prospective Payment System (OPPS)

The outpatient prospective payment system (OPPS) does not have any basis on ICD-10-CM or ICD-10-PCS codes; instead, CPT and HCPCS codes are used. This does not mean that coders do not assign diagnosis codes from ICD-10-CM. The diagnosis codes must be linked to the CPT and HCPCS codes to justify medical necessity, but the payment is completely driven by the CPT and HCPCS codes.

All hospital outpatient services are classified into **ambulatory payment classifications (APCs).** Each CPT and HCPCS code for procedures or services provided in the outpatient setting is assigned an associated APC. Procedures and services assigned to each APC are similar in medical purpose and resource utilization. Each APC is assigned a payment rate, and hospitals may be paid for more than one APC per encounter, based on the procedures and services provided. Diagnoses are reported using ICD-9-CM (and eventually ICD-10-CM after October 1, 2013) codes.

> ### Think About It 3.3
>
> also available in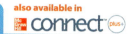
>
> Why do you think OPPS is set up so that more than one APC payment may be made per encounter, rather than basing the payment system on calculation of one procedure or service?

3.4 Prospective Payment Systems for Other Healthcare Settings

Along with the IPPS and OPPS, coders should also be aware of the other prospective payment systems (PPSs) that exist. Never limit yourself in your career by only learning about one specific area of the healthcare field. You never know when an opportunity may appear in a different type of healthcare setting. Figure 3.3 shows a timeline of the development of these prospective payment systems, and Table 3.1 describes the factors associated with each PPS.

Physician Office

In 1992, Medicare implemented a **Resource-Based Relative Value Scale (RBRVS)** physician fee schedule. This payment system determines a relative value for physician services, which is based on resources generally used for each level of service. Three values of work expense, practice expense, and professional liability insurance expense are associated with CPT codes for physician service levels. These three values for the specific CPT code are calculated with a geographic adjustment in order to determine the payment.

Home Health

On October 1, 2000, the home health prospective payment system (HH PPS) was implemented. HH PPS consists of base payment, which is adjusted for health condition and care needs, and geographic differences in wages. HH PPS payments are provided for each 60-day episode of care. The **Outcome and Assessment Information Set (OASIS)** instrument is used to document assessment of the patient's condition. Data collected in the OASIS are used to determine the case-mix adjustment to the standard payment rate. There are 80 case-mix groups, which are called **home health resource groups (HHRGs),** available for patient classification based on clinical presentation, functional factors, and service utilization.

4 ELEMENTS OF MEDICAL DOCUMENTATION

Learning Outcomes *After completing this chapter, students should be able to*

4.1 Discuss how methods of documentation and obtaining data may vary according to setting or type of record in general and for the facesheet.

4.2 Recognize elements of documentation that are normally included in commonly dictated reports.

4.3 Explore elements of surgical procedure documentation.

4.4 Identify components of physician orders and progress notes.

4.5 Apply knowledge of coding guidelines to documentation by nonphysician providers.

Key Terms

assessment

consultation report

demographic

discharge summary (final summary)

electronic health record (EHR)

facesheet

history and physical (H&P)

medication administration records

nursing notes

objective

operative report

pathology report

physician orders

plan

progress notes

SOAP note

subjective

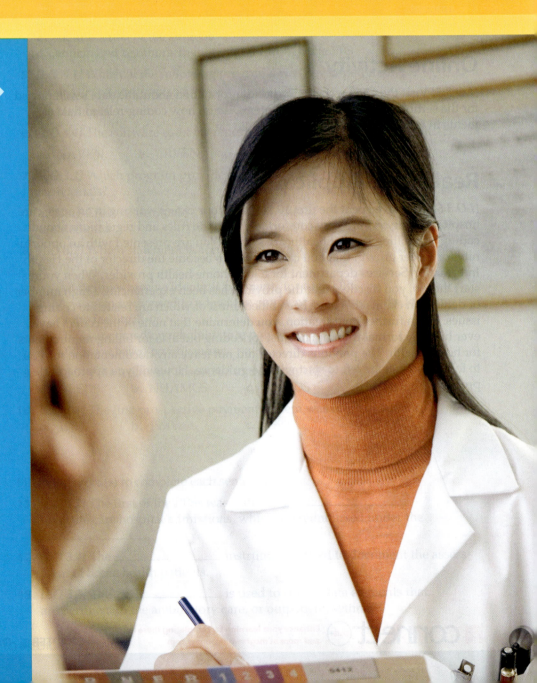

Introduction

Coders use patient encounter information to assign codes. But where does this information come from? This chapter provides an introduction to the types of documentation found on healthcare records, any of which you may see at some point in your coding career, no matter the setting where you code. Note that the examples of documentation in this chapter are representative of the basic format that may be encountered, but different facilities create the documents slightly differently.

If this is your first exposure to medical documentation, you may find it beneficial to seek opportunities to gain additional familiarity with forms you may encounter as a coder. Although samples of forms can be found on the Internet, it is more beneficial to gain exposure to forms that are used by facilities in your own community, where you may be seeking employment in the future. Some facilities allow students to do job shadowing, which provides an excellent opportunity to not only see what the forms look like but also see them in action as records are used at various points in the healthcare process.

> **Spotlight on A&P**
>
> Due to the detailed nature of ICD-10-CM and ICD-10-PCS coding, coders must adequately comprehend medical terminology, anatomy, and physiology to interpret operative reports and translate them into ICD-10-CM and ICD-10-PCS codes.

4.1 Introduction to Health Record Documentation

A variety of forms and formats are used in medical documentation. Some are unique to specific settings, whereas others are more universal. The conversion from traditional paper records to **electronic health records (EHRs)** is another variable that impacts the appearance and format of documentation. In this chapter, you will see examples of various forms that will be found on records in paper format. Keep in mind that electronic health records collect the same documentation, just in a different medium. Screens in electronic health records are often designed to resemble paper documents. Although there is variation in the appearance of the screens and icons in electronic health records, there are many similarities between them.

Some electronic health record systems are also associated with computer-assisted coding (CAC) systems. Many coding students perceive computer-assisted coding as something that will completely replace coding jobs, but it is important to recognize that there is no replacement for human decision making in the unlimited number of unique situations that occur in healthcare. Computer-assisted coding is helpful to identify

electronic health records (EHRs) Automated health record documentation that includes digital images, point-of-care documentation by providers, clinical decision support, and the ability to be accessed by multiple users at the same time.

> **CODING TIP ▶**
>
> Forms and elements of documentation may vary across different types of healthcare settings.

documentation and it provides some guidance, but coders may be able to identify additional elements to be coded or recognize when the computer-assisted coding system has inappropriately coded an item.

A **facesheet** is a document that is generally filed first or at the top of many types of healthcare encounters. Facesheets are found on inpatient, outpatient, and long-term care records. Most inpatient facesheets include a patient's identification information, account number, medical record number, **demographic** information, insurance information, attending physician, and admitting physician, as well as other pertinent data as determined by the facility. Physician office patient information forms collect patient demographic information, employer information, insurance information, emergency contact information, and other pertinent data as identified by the provider. Aside from patient identification, coders may also find documentation of diagnoses and physician information on the facesheet. The facesheet's equivalent in the physician office is known as a patient information form or patient registration form.

Facilities that are using true electronic health records may not have an actual facesheet for a record. Instead, the data elements are entered into the computer and are stored in a database. A facesheet or report with information normally found on a facesheet may be printed or displayed through a database query. Figure 4.1 provides an example of a facesheet.

facesheet Document that contains patient information, found on inpatient, outpatient, and long-term care records.

demographic Characteristics of individuals such as age, gender, and address, which are used for statistical purposes.

Think About It 4.1

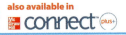
also available in **connect** plus+

Reflect on a time that you or one of your family members received medical care. When were the data elements for the facesheet collected, and how was the documentation obtained?

4.2 Dictated Reports

A variety of dictated reports appear in health records, in addition to the brief handwritten (or physician-entered in the EHR) progress notes. These include the history and physical, discharge summary, consultation report, operative report, pathology report, and radiology report. A physician dictates these reports; then a transcriptionist listens to the dictation and types what is dictated.

A **history and physical (H&P)** report is generally dictated by the physician and transcribed for the health record. This document normally includes the chief complaint or reason for admission, past medical history, social history, surgical history, family history, review of systems, physical examination, assessment of the patient's problems, and plans for treatment. Documentation in the history and physical provides the coder with information about why the patient presented for care. This information helps identify the principal diagnosis.

history and physical (H&P) Document that normally includes the chief complaint or reason for admission, past medical history, social history, surgical history, family history, review of systems, physical examination, assessment of the patient's problems, and plans for treatment.

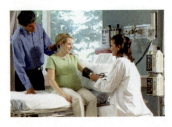

During healthcare encounters, the physician records the patient's history and conducts various examinations. These records are referred to as the history and physical, or H&P. The H&P is the basis of what coders use to assign codes.

FAMILY CARE CLINIC

285 Stephenson Boulevard
Stephenson, OH 60089–4000
614-555-0000

PATIENT INFORMATION FORM

Patient				
Last Name	First Name	MI	Sex __ M __ F	Date of Birth / /
Address	City		State	Zip
Home Ph # ( )	Cell Ph # ( )	Marital Status		Student Status
SS# Email		Allergies		
Employment Status	Employer Name	Work Ph # ( )		Primary Insurance ID #
Employer Address	City		State	Zip
Referred By		Ph # of Referral ( )		

Responsible Party (Complete this section if the person responsible for the bill is not the patient)

Last Name	First Name	MI	Sex __ M __ F	Date of Birth / /
Address	City	State	Zip	SS#
Relation to Patient __ Spouse __ Parent __ Other	Employer Name		Work Phone # ( )	
Spouse, or Parent (if minor):			Home Phone # ( )	

Insurance (If you have multiple coverage, supply information from both carriers)

Primary Carrier Name	Secondary Carrier Name
Name of the Insured (Name on ID Card)	Name of the Insured (Name on ID Card)
Patient's relationship to the insured __ Self __ Spouse __ Child	Patient's relationship to the insured __ Self __ Spouse __ Child
Insured ID #	Insured ID #
Group # or Company Name	Group # or Company Name
Insurance Address	Insurance Address
Phone #	Copay $ Deductible $	Phone #	Copay $ Deductible $

Other Information

Is patient's condition related to: __ Employment __ Auto Accident (if yes, state in which accident occurred: __) __Other Accident	Reason for visit:
Date of Accident: / / Date of First Symptom of Illness: / /	

Financial Agreement and Authorization for Treatment

I authorize treatment and agree to pay all fees and charges for the person named above. I agree to pay all charges shown by statements, promptly upon their presentation, unless credit arrangements are agreed upon in writing.	I authorize payment directly to FAMILY CARE CLINIC of insurance benefits otherwise payable to me. I hereby authorize the release of any medical information necessary in order to process a claim for payment in my behalf.
Signed: _____	Date: _____

figure 4.1 Patient Information Form
The patient information collected in a physician office is very similar to that contained on an inpatient facesheet.

Figure 4.2 (p. 40) provides an example of an H&P document.

An electronic format that provides similar information to an H&P, using Medisoft EHR is illustrated in Figure 4.3 (p. 41).

A **discharge summary** (sometimes called a **final summary**) is found on inpatient records for patients who have been discharged. It provides a summary of a hospitalization, starting with the chief complaint or reason for admission and providing information about diagnostic testing, surgical procedures, and other treatments provided during the hospitalization. Information is also documented about the discharge disposition of the patient and follow-up care. The coder can use this information to analyze the circumstances of the admission to determine the principal diagnosis.

discharge summary (final summary) Summary of a hospitalization, generally completed by the attending physician, starting with the chief complaint or reason for admission and providing information about diagnostic testing, surgical procedures, and other treatments provided during the hospitalization; found on inpatient records for patients who have been discharged.

CHAPTER 4 REVIEW

Chapter Summary

Learning Outcome	Key Concepts/Examples
4.1 Discuss how methods of documentation and obtaining data may vary according to setting or type of record in general and for the facesheet. **(pages 37–38)**	• Forms and documentation vary with different types of healthcare settings. • Facesheets normally include the patient's identification information, account number, medical record number, demographic information, and insurance information, as well as documentation of diagnoses and procedures.
4.2 Recognize elements of documentation that are normally included in commonly dictated reports. **(pages 38–41)**	• The history and physical report normally includes the chief complaint or reason for admission, past medical history, social history, surgical history, family history, review of systems, physical examination, assessment of the patient's problems, and plans for treatment. • A discharge summary provides a summary of a hospitalization, starting with the chief complaint or reason for admission and providing information about diagnostic testing, surgical procedures, other treatments provided during the hospitalization, discharge disposition of the patient, and follow-up care. • A consultation report is formatted similarly to a history and physical and is completed by a specialist who has been asked to provide an opinion or coverage for an aspect of care related to the consulting physician's area of specialization.
4.3 Explore elements of surgical procedure documentation. **(pages 42–43)**	• Operative reports may appear on inpatient or outpatient records and normally include the preoperative diagnosis, postoperative diagnosis, surgeon(s) who performed the procedure, type of anesthesia, name of the procedure, specimens sent to pathology, detailed narrative description of the procedure, condition of the patient at the conclusion of the procedure, and disposition of the patient at the conclusion of the procedure. • A pathology report generally includes information about the type and size of the specimen submitted, a summary of gross and microscopic findings, detailed findings, and a pathological diagnosis.

Learning Outcome	Key Concepts/Examples
4.4 Identify components of physician orders and progress notes. **(pages 44–45)**	• Progress notes and orders are written by both physician and nonphysician providers. • SOAP is an acronym for subjective, objective, assessment, and plan.
4.5 Apply knowledge of coding guidelines to documentation by nonphysician providers. **(pages 46–47)**	• Although most coding activities are focused on physician documentation, some elements of nonphysician documentation also need to be reviewed in the coding process. • Body mass index (BMI) and pressure ulcer stage code assignment may be based on documentation by nonphysician providers, since this information is typically documented by other clinicians involved in the care of the patient.

Checking Your Understanding

Select the letter that best answers the question or completes the sentence.

1. *[LO 4.1]* Which of the following does not impact the content or format of health record documentation?

   a. paper records   **b.** electronic health records
   c. type of healthcare setting   **d.** demographic information

2. *[LO 4.3]* What document is the best place to find information about the morphology of a specimen that was removed during a surgical procedure?

   a. operative report   **b.** consultation report
   c. pathology report   **d.** discharge summary

3. *[LO 4.2]* What document is the best place to find information about the reason a patient presented for treatment and the pertinent medical history?

   a. discharge summary   **b.** history and physical
   c. consultation report   **d.** operative report

4. *[LO 4.4]* What does the acronym SOAP stand for?

   a. statement, objective, assessment, plan
   b. subjective, observation, assessment, plan
   c. subjective, objective, assessment, plan
   d. subjective, objective, assessment, procedure

5. *[LO 4.5]* Which of the following can be coded from documentation by a non-physician provider?

   a. stage of a pressure ulcer
   b. insulin dependence for diabetes

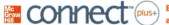

    c. presence of a pressure ulcer

    d. diagnosis of obesity

6. *[LO 4.2]* If an attending physician contacts a gastroenterologist for further assessment of a gastrointestinal problem, what kind of documentation provides the details of the assessment?

    a. consultation report   **b.** progress note

    c. discharge summary   **d.** physician order

7. *[LO 4.1]* Which of the following items is not normally found on a facesheet?

    a. patient name

    b. demographic data

    c. name of anesthesiologist for a surgical procedure

    d. account number

8. *[LO 4.4]* Which part of a SOAP note includes documentation of a diagnosis?

    a. subjective   **b.** objective

    c. assessment   **d.** plan

9. *[LO 4.3]* ICD-10-PCS requires significant documentation of the details for surgical procedures that are performed. Where are these details located?

    a. discharge summary   **b.** progress note

    c. operative report   **d.** pathology report

10. *[LO 4.5]* Which of the following nonphysician healthcare professionals may document information in the record that can be used for coding body mass index or the stage of a pressure ulcer?

    a. RN   **b.** surgical technician   **c.** social worker   **d.** CNA

Fill in the blank with the word(s) to complete the statement.

11. *[LO 4.3]* A(n) _____ provides information about the preoperative diagnosis, postoperative diagnosis, surgeon(s) who performed the procedure, type of anesthesia, name of the procedure, specimens sent to pathology, and detailed narrative description of the procedure.

12. *[LO 4.2]* A(n) _____ is on the record if the attending physician requests a specialist to see the patient.

13. *[LO 4.4]* A(n) _____ is used to document prescribed medications, therapies, consultation requests, and other treatments.

14. *[LO 4.4]* A(n) _____ documents pertinent information during a hospital or long-term care stay.

15. *[LO 4.5]* _____ provide a list of medications that have been ordered for the patient.

16. *[LO 4.3]* A(n) _____ generally includes information about the type and size of a specimen submitted and a summary of gross and microscopic findings.

17. *[LO 4.2.]* A(n) _____ normally includes the chief complaint or reason for admission, past medical history, social history, surgical history, family history, review of systems, physical examination, assessment of the patient's problems, and plans for treatment.

18. *[LO 4.2]* A(n) _____ provides a summary of a hospitalization.

19. *[LO 4.5]* Codes for _____ and _____ may be determined based on documents from nonphysician providers, such as dieticians or nurses.

20. *[LO 4.5]* _____ include nursing assessments and treatments.

Online Activity

[LO 4.5] Search online for examples of health record documentation and the forms used for health record documentation in healthcare settings besides the physician office or hospital. Discuss what forms you located, what kind of provider documents information on the form, and what kind of information on the form may be useful to you as a coder.

Real-World Application

[LO 4.1] You are in the position of a coding manager at a facility that is converting to electronic health records, and you are assigned the task of submitting a document to the IT department to provide a list of documents your staff needs to perform their jobs, along with a justification of why they need to access each document. Create an example of what this list might look like, including the justification for each document.

McGraw Hill **connect** ™ plus+ **Enhance your learning by completing these exercises and more at mcgrawhillconnect.com**

CHAPTER 4   MEDICAL DOCUMENTATION   51

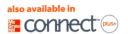
In each of the following scenarios, underline the diagnoses and circle the procedures that should be coded.

1. A patient has an EGD in an ambulatory surgery setting with documentation from the physician citing indigestion, epigastric pain, and possible peptic ulcer disease.

2. A patient is discharged after a five-day hospitalization. The patient was admitted with complaints of left arm pain and chest tightness and was determined to have an acute myocardial infarction. While in the hospital, the patient had a cardiac catheterization and PTCA. Additional documentation reflected hypertension and NIDDM.

3. A patient with IDDM was discharged from ICU following admission for complaints of dizziness and confusion. Testing during hospitalization resulted in documentation of ketoacidosis.

4. A patient with CAD and hypertension was admitted for CABG.

5. A patient presents to the emergency department with arm pain following a fall from a tree. It is determined that the patient has a closed fracture of the radial shaft, and a closed reduction is performed.

5.2 What Should Be Coded?

For any case that is being coded, it is necessary to accurately identify the diagnosis to be coded. Sometimes, physicians overdocument diagnoses or provide information about past conditions or diagnoses that are not pertinent to the episode of care being coded.

When reviewing medical documentation, it is important to note that not every diagnosis or symptom documented is necessarily appropriate to code. If a definitive diagnosis has been established, it is not appropriate to assign codes for signs and symptoms of that diagnosis. If there are other conditions considered to be an integral part of a disease process that is being coded, those other conditions are not to be coded. However, be aware of additional signs, symptoms, and other conditions not associated with diseases being coded, as they should be coded if present and pertinent to care provided at an encounter. Sometimes guidance is provided about other conditions that should be coded through "code first" and "use additional code" directions. For additional details, refer to coding guidelines *I.B.4. Signs and symptoms, I.B.5. Conditions that are an integral part of a disease process*, and *I.B.6. Conditions that are not an integral part of a disease process.*

Figure 5.1 demonstrates the use of "code first" and "use additional code." As shown, when using codes in subclassification R65.1-, the coder should sequence first a code for the underlying condition, such as heatstroke or injury and trauma. If code R65.11 is assigned, then an additional code should be assigned, following R65.11, to identify specific acute organ dysfunction, such as acute kidney failure or acute respiratory failure.

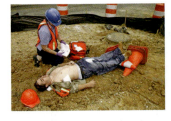

Not every diagnosis or symptom documented is always appropriate to code. For example, when SIRS is documented, code first for the underlying condition, such as heatstroke or trauma.

R65 Symptoms and signs specifically associated with systemic inflammation and infection

R65.1 Systemic inflammatory response syndrome (SIRS) of non-infectious origin

Code first underlying condition, such as:

heatstroke (T67.0)

injury and trauma (S00–T88)

Excludes1: sepsis- code to infection

severe sepsis (R65.2)

R65.10 Systemic inflammatory response syndrome (SIRS) of non-infectious origin without acute organ dysfunction

Systemic inflammatory response syndrome (SIRS) NOS

R65.11 Systemic inflammatory response syndrome (SIRS) of non-infectious origin with acute organ dysfunction

Use additional code to identify specific acute organ dysfunction, such as:

acute kidney failure (N17.-)

acute respiratory failure (J96.0-)

figure 5.1 Example of "Code First" and "Use Additional Code" Notes in ICD-10-CM

Coding rules also differ among inpatient and outpatient settings. There are times when a definite diagnosis may not yet be identified by the physician. When assigning codes in an outpatient setting, if a diagnosis is listed as being "possible," "probable," "questionable," "rule out," or any other method of suggesting that the physician has not made a definite decision regarding the diagnosis, it is not appropriate to assign a code for the condition listed; rather, the coder should assign any signs or symptoms of the condition that are documented as reasons that the physician is considering the diagnosis. For example, if a physician orders a CBC to be done in an outpatient lab and documents the reason for the test as "fatigue, rule out anemia," the code should be assigned for fatigue.

However, the opposite of this rule applies in the inpatient setting. In inpatient situations, the coder should assign the code for the possible, probable, questionable, or otherwise suggested condition, rather than coding the associated signs and symptoms. If documentation of a final diagnosis for an inpatient admission is stated as "probable peptic ulcer disease," it is appropriate to assign the code for peptic ulcer disease.

> **CODING TIP ▸**
>
> If a definitive diagnosis has been established, it is not appropriate to assign codes for signs and symptoms of that diagnosis.

> **CODING TIP ▸**
>
> Coding can differ in the inpatient and outpatient settings. Diagnoses listed as being "possible," "probable," "questionable," or "rule out" should be coded in the inpatient setting, but they should not be coded in outpatient settings.

Think About It 5.2

also available in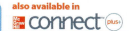

Why is it inappropriate to assign codes for signs and symptoms if a definitive diagnosis is coded?

5.3 Helpful Resources for Coders

Many situations can create confusion for new coders, especially those who lack detailed knowledge of pathophysiology. For example, if the physician documents that a patient presents with shortness of breath and determines that the patient has congestive heart failure and pulmonary edema, an inexperienced coder may recognize that shortness of breath is a symptom but may not realize that pulmonary edema is also a symptom of congestive heart failure because of how the physician has documented it. "Excludes" notes are often helpful in these kinds of situations, but the best practice is to look up any term that is unfamiliar. Reference materials are invaluable resources for coders; their worth may be justified by recognizing that using them can prevent errors in reimbursement through the promotion of accurate coding.

> **CODING TIP** ▸
>
> Reference materials are invaluable resources for coders. When considering whether to purchase a reference item, keep in mind that using it can help you prevent errors in reimbursement or delay in payment by coding correctly the first time.

Learning is a lifelong process for coders. If you are in a very short coding diploma certificate program, the course you are taking right now may be near the end of your program. However, you still have much more to learn in your career. As you go through your coding course, keep in mind that you are being provided with the tools you will need to guide you through coding decisions that may be more complex in nature. No coding course or textbook can provide every coding scenario you will encounter, and no coder knows how to code everything perfectly without seeking guidance at some point. The key to success as a coder is developing a strong knowledge base and knowing where to turn for the answers you need beyond that.

There are numerous options for continuing education for coders. Continuing education seminars and conferences are available through professional organizations, such as the American Health Information Management Association (AHIMA) and the American Academy of Professional Coders (AAPC). Although these are national organizations, they also have state and regional associations or chapters, which serve the needs of members at a more local level for those who may not be able to attend larger national conferences.

Another option for continuing education is in the form of audio seminars. These allow multiple coders in a single setting to attend the educational opportunity without the expense of travel or lost productivity associated with taking an education day to attend a conference or seminar. Recorded audio seminars can also be purchased for later reference or attendance by coders who were not available at the time they were originally presented.

Professional journals are continually publishing educational articles about hot topics that are coding-related. These may be useful if you work at an institution that does not provide the benefit of sending coders to continuing

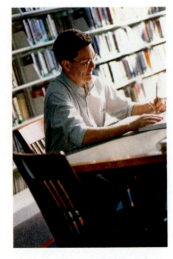

For a coder, education is a lifelong process. Stay up-to-date about the coding field by reading articles, becoming professionally certified, and interacting with other coders. Part of the process involves maintaining required continuing education units (CEUs) for coding credentials.

education seminars or conferences. For credentialed coders, there are even some journal articles accompanied by continuing education quizzes, which may be used to accumulate **continuing education units (CEUs).** CEUs are required for coders who have successfully passed a coding credential examination. Obtaining a professional coding credential is a method of demonstrating that you have achieved competence in the coding career field.

AHIMA and AAPC are two organizations that provide examinations to obtain credentials. When you reach the point in your coding career that you feel you are ready to take one of these examinations, you may wonder which one will be more beneficial to you. This is where developing a professional network in your area becomes valuable. Do some research on both large and small employers of healthcare professionals in your area to determine which credentials are more widely recognized, as this varies by geographic region. AHIMA coding credentials include the following:

- Certified Coding Associate (CCA)
- Certified Coding Specialist (CCS)
- Certified Coding Specialist–Physician-based (CCS-P)

The credentials obtainable through AAPC are the following:

- Certified Professional Coder (CPC®)
- Certified Professional Coder–Outpatient Hospital (CPC-H®)
- Certified Professional Coder-Payer (CPC-P®)
- Certified Interventional Radiology Cardiovascular Coder (CIRCC®)
- Various specialty credentials

Both sets of credentials are equally well respected in the coding profession.

continuing education units (CEUs) Credits that are required to maintain credentials for coders who have successfully passed a coding credential examination.

CODING TIP ▸

Obtaining a professional coding credential shows that you have achieved coding competence.

Think About It 5.3

also available in **McGraw Hill connect** plus+

Which books or other resource materials have you encountered in previous courses that may be good to use for reference materials as a coder?

5.4 Communication

Excellent written and verbal communication skills are critical for coders, because they must communicate in a professional manner with others, not just within their department but also with individuals in other departments, third-party payers, and physician providers. Communication with any of these people can take many forms: an informal written note, a formal letter, e-mail, face-to-face verbal communication, telephone communication, or voice mail. As our society becomes increasingly accepting of more informal communication through text messaging, it is imperative to keep a heightened awareness of maintaining professionalism in communication in the workplace. This includes, but is not limited to, the use of correct spelling, grammar, and punctuation.

Think About It 5.5

also available in

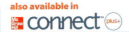 connect plus+

Why should you always cross-reference the tabular list when looking up codes?

5.6 Diagnosis Coding in the Inpatient Setting

Inpatient coding is performed in an acute care hospital setting. The information presented in this section will outline the basic guidance that you will need to identify diagnoses to be coded and to report the appropriate sequence in the inpatient setting. Official coding guidelines for the situations discussed in this section are found in *Section II, Selection of Principal Diagnosis* of the coding guidelines.

A **principal diagnosis** is defined in the Uniform Hospital Discharge Data Set (UHDDS) as "that condition established after study to be chiefly responsible for occasioning the admission of the patient to the hospital for care." If a definitive diagnosis has been established, it is not appropriate to assign a code for a symptom, signs, or an ill-defined condition as a principal diagnosis.

If two conditions are interrelated and both potentially meet the definition of principal diagnosis, then it is appropriate to sequence either condition If two or more conditions are interrelated and both potentially meet the definition of principal diagnosis, then it is appropriate to sequence either condition first. The only exception would be if the coding guidelines suggest alternate sequencing or the admission circumstances dictate otherwise. If multiple diagnoses equally meet the criteria for principal diagnosis, and no additional instructions impact sequencing, any of the diagnoses may be sequenced as principal. When two or more contrasting or comparative diagnoses, often referred to as **differential diagnoses,** are documented as "either/or" or "diagnosis A versus diagnosis B," the diagnoses are coded as if they were confirmed, and they are sequenced according to the circumstances of admission. If no further determination can be made regarding which diagnosis should be principal, then either diagnosis may be sequenced first. For example, if documentation stated "peptic ulcer disease versus acute cholecystitis," both conditions would be coded, and the circumstances of admission would be evaluated to determine if there is a reason that one should be sequenced prior to the other.

Occasionally, a patient presents for an outpatient encounter that results in inpatient admission. If the inpatient admission is due to a complication of care from the outpatient setting, the code for the complicating condition should be listed as the principal diagnosis. If the patient is admitted for further care for or evaluation of the condition being treated or evaluated in the outpatient setting, that condition should be reported as the principal diagnosis.

principal diagnosis
Condition established after study to be chiefly responsible for occasioning the admission of the patient to the hospital for care.

differential diagnoses
Two or more contrasting or comparative diagnoses.

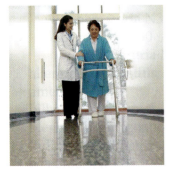

Coding in the inpatient setting has its own set of rules and guidelines. For example, guidelines about coding for signs and symptoms are opposite those in the outpatient setting.

Secondary diagnoses are those that impact patient care because they extend the length of stay or require clinical evaluation, therapeutic treatment, diagnostic procedures, or increased care and/or monitoring. This is defined in item 11b of the UHDDS. Reporting of historical conditions as secondary codes is appropriate if there is an impact on current care or treatment. An example of a secondary diagnosis is a patient admitted for a total knee replacement for osteoarthritis of the knee and the physician documents that the patient has diabetes mellitus. The presence of diabetes mellitus should be coded as a secondary diagnosis, because it has an impact on care during the total knee replacement due to the potential for issues with healing. *Section III. Reporting Additional Diagnoses* in the coding guidelines addresses the details.

Abnormal findings from diagnostic testing are normally not coded simply from the fact that they are documented. However, if the attending physician relates the abnormal findings to a diagnosis, additional testing or treatment, it may be appropriate to query the provider to determine if they should be reported. For example, if a patient has a screening mammogram and a mass is noted, which results in ordering a breast sonogram for further evaluation, depending on the documentation, it may be appropriate to query the physician to determine if the abnormal finding should be reported. Refer to coding guideline *III.B. Abnormal findings* for additional instructions.

In the inpatient setting, uncertain diagnoses, which are often reflected by documentation as "possible" or "probable," should be reported as though they were truly established. Note that this guideline is pertinent only to inpatient short-term admissions, acute care admissions, long-term care admissions, and psychiatric hospital admissions. The coder should exercise caution with documentation to notice the difference between "rule out" and "ruled out," because a condition that has been "ruled out" should not be coded, but a condition documented as "rule out" should be coded. This instruction is detailed in coding guideline *III.C. Uncertain Diagnosis.*

secondary diagnoses
Diagnoses that impact patient care because they extend the length of stay or require clinical evaluation, therapeutic treatment, diagnostic procedures, or increased care and/or monitoring.

7. *[LO 5.7]* Which of the following statements is correct regarding coding for ambulatory surgery?

   a. If the postoperative diagnosis is different from the preoperative diagnosis, only the postoperative diagnosis should be reported, since it was confirmed by the procedure.

   b. If the postoperative diagnosis is different from the preoperative diagnosis, they should both be reported, with the postoperative diagnosis sequenced first.

   c. If the postoperative diagnosis is different from the preoperative diagnosis, they should both be reported, with the preoperative diagnosis sequenced first.

   d. If the postoperative diagnosis is different from the preoperative diagnosis, only the preoperative diagnosis should be reported, since the postoperative diagnosis cannot be confirmed.

8. *[LO 5.5]* When is it appropriate to assign a three-digit code?

   a. in the outpatient setting only

   b. if there is not sufficient documentation to report greater specificity

   c. if the code is not further subdivided to report greater specificity

   d. never

9. *[LO 5.6]* The condition established after study to be chiefly responsible for occasioning the admission of the patient to the hospital for care is the

   a. admission diagnosis.   b. principal diagnosis.

   c. first-listed diagnosis.   d. final diagnosis.

10. *[LO 5.4]* Which of the following is an appropriately written physician query?

    a. On June 15, serum calcium was reported as 4.2 and an order was written for administration of calcium gluconate. Is there a specific diagnosis that you wish to report for either or both of these items that were documented in the record?

    b. Documentation in the record suggests that this patient probably has acute respiratory failure. Do you wish to document that diagnosis?

    c. You documented that this patient has pneumonia. The sputum culture on October 2 indicated the presence of *Staphylococcus aureus*. Does this patient have *Staph aureus* pneumonia?

    d. Does this patient have congestive heart failure?

Online Activity

[LO 5.3] Explore the AHIMA and AAPC websites regarding membership and credentials. Outline the benefits of membership and credentials.

Real-World Application

[LO 5.6] Assume you have been hired as coding supervisor for an acute care facility. During your first day on the job, you discover that there is no policies and procedures manual. Write a brief policy and procedure that addresses general coding guidelines and how they will be incorporated into coding processes.

ICD-10-CM

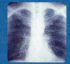
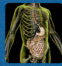

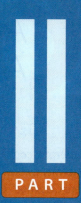

PART II

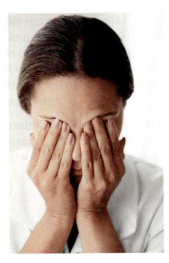

Some signs and symptoms, such as fatigue and pain, are more general. If a sign or symptom is associated with an underlying condition, code and sequence the causal condition first.

- Syncope and collapse
- Convulsions
- Shock
- Hemorrhage
- Enlarged lymph nodes
- Edema
- Hyperhidrosis
- Lack of expected normal physiological development
- Symptoms and signs concerning food and fluid intake
- Cachexia
- Systemic inflammatory response syndrome (SIRS)
- Hypothermia
- Fussy infant
- Dry mouth
- Clubbing of fingers
- Early satiety
- Decreased libido
- Chills

If a fever is associated with an underlying condition, such as leukemia, neutropenia, or sickle cell disease, the causal condition should be sequenced first. Fatigue associated with a neoplasm should be reported with the neoplasm code sequenced first, followed by code R53.0, neoplastic-related fatigue. Generalized hyperhidrosis should be sequenced following N95.1 if it is associated with menopause. The symptom code for functional quadriplegia, R53.2, should be assigned only if specifically documented and it is not associated with neurologic deficit or injury. The official guideline for functional quadriplegia coding is *I.C.18.f. Functional quadriplegia.*

> **CODING TIP ▸**
>
> The symptom code for functional quadriplegia, R53.2, should be assigned only if specifically documented and it is not associated with neurologic deficit or injury.

systemic inflammatory response syndrome (SIRS) Systemic response to infection, burns, trauma, or other severe insult. Symptoms may include fever, tachycardia, tachypnea, and leukocytosis (elevated white blood cell count).

severe sepsis Sepsis associated with acute organ dysfunction.

The reporting of underweight as a symptom should have an additional code from Z68.- assigned if body mass index is documented. When reporting cachexia, the underlying condition should be reported first, if documented. Code R68.13, apparent life-threatening event in infant (ALTE), requires additional codes to report associated signs and symptoms.

Coders should be aware of the coding guidelines for **systemic inflammatory response syndrome (SIRS)** and **severe sepsis** and should understand the disease processes involved. There are also a significant number of instructions in the code book to support the guidelines and assist the coder in code selection and sequencing.

SIRS may be non-infectious in origin. In this case, the first code assigned should be the underlying condition, followed by either R65.10 or R65.11. If R65.11 is assigned, an additional code should also be reported to identify any documented acute organ dysfunction. Official guidance for coding SIRS of non-infectious origin is provided in guideline *I.C.18.g. SIRS due to Non-infectious Process.*

Severe sepsis can be documented in a variety of ways, including, but not limited to, infection with associated acute organ dysfunction, sepsis with acute organ dysfunction, sepsis with multiple organ dysfunction, and SIRS due to infectious process with acute organ dysfunction. Sequencing is important in coding severe sepsis. The first code assigned should identify the underlying infection. The second code is either R65.20, severe sepsis without septic shock, or R65.21, severe sepsis with septic shock. Additional code assignment should identify specific organ dysfunction.

Think About It 6.4

also available in McGraw Hill **connect** (plus+)

Assign ICD-10-CM codes for the following situations, applying any appropriate sequencing guidelines.

1. Weakness in an elderly patient _____

2. Underweight 24-year-old patient with BMI of 17 _____

3. Functional quadriplegia with no noted neurologic deficit or history of injury _____

4. SIRS caused by acute gallstone pancreatitis, resulting in acute renal medullary necrosis _____

5. Cachexia due to abnormal loss of weight _____

What is the proper sequencing for the following example?

_____ R65.21, Severe sepsis with septic shock

_____ J96.0, Acute respiratory failure

_____ A41.51, Sepsis due to *Escherichia coli*

6.5 Abnormal Findings

When there is no definitive diagnosis, it is necessary and appropriate for coders to report abnormal findings on examinations of blood, urine, and other body fluids, substances, or tissues. Additionally, abnormal findings on diagnostic imaging, function studies, and tumor markers not leading to a definitive diagnosis should also be reported. Finally, coders should be aware of the guidelines for classification of death without an established diagnosis, signs, or symptoms. In ICD-10-CM, the codes used to report these situations are classified in categories R70–R99.

Spotlight on A&P

Coders must have an understanding of the diagnostic tests performed in ancillary departments in order to code for their findings.

Applying Your Skills

For each condition, assign the appropriate code(s) from ICD-9-CM and ICD-10-CM.

Condition	ICD-9-CM Code	ICD-10-CM Code
1. [LO 6.3] Dizziness	_____	_____
2. [LO 6.5] Abnormal TB test	_____	_____
3. [LO 6.5] Abnormal EEG	_____	_____
4. [LO 6.4] Atypical febrile seizures	_____	_____
5. [LO 6.2] Right lower quadrant abdominal pain	_____	_____
6. [LO 6.3] Coma with eyes open to pain at arrival to ER	_____	_____
7. [LO 6.4] Generalized pain	_____	_____
8. [LO 6.2] Localized mass/lump on left forearm	_____	_____
9. [LO 6.2] Epigastric tenderness	_____	_____
10. [LO 6.2] Ataxic gait	_____	_____
11. [LO 6.2] Pleurodynia	_____	_____
12. [LO 6.4] Localized edema	_____	_____
13. [LO 6.2] Splitting of urinary stream	_____	_____
14. [LO 6.2] Heartburn	_____	_____
15. [LO 6.5] PAP smear of vagina with high-grade squamous intraepithelial lesion (HGSIL)	_____	_____
16. [LO 6.2] Periumbilical rebound tenderness	_____	_____
17. [LO 6.5] Finding of cocaine in blood	_____	_____
18. [LO 6.4] Child with short stature/lack of growth	_____	_____
19. [LO 6.5] Microcalcification on diagnostic mammogram	_____	_____

Checking Your Understanding

1. [LO 6.5] Which of the following scenarios is appropriate for the assignment of code R99?

    a. A patient presents to ER with chest pain, is determined to be having an acute myocardial infarction, and expires in the ER prior to admission to the hospital.

    b. A patient presents to ER with chest pain and expires in the ER prior to admission to the hospital.

    c. A patient is brought to ER and pronounced dead upon arrival.

    d. A patient presents to ER with chest pain, is determined to be having an acute myocardial infarction, and expires immediately after transfer to ICU and admission to the hospital.

2. [LO 6.1] Which of the following is considered a symptom?

    a. fever

    b. elevated blood pressure

    c. decreased white blood count

    d. dizziness

3. *[LO 6.3]* Where can documentation be obtained for reporting codes associated with the Glasgow coma scale?

   a. EMT, ER nurse, or physician documentation on   presentation
   b. physician documentation of the final diagnosis
   c. physician documentation, which must be used in order for codes to be assigned
   d. history obtained from the patient or an individual accompanying the patient

4. *[LO 6.4]* What else should be reported with generalized hyperhidrosis?

   a. neoplasm   b. menopause
   c. neurologic deficit   d. injury

5. *[LO 6.2]* What is the appropriate code assignment for a patient with dysphagia resulting from a cerebral infarction?

   a. R13.10   b. I69.391
   c. R13.10, I69.391   d. I69.391, R13.10

6. *[LO 6.5]* What else should be coded when reporting findings of alcohol in blood?

   a. level of alcohol in the blood **b.** blood type
   c. BMI   d. BMI and level of alcohol in the blood

7. *[LO 6.1]* Which of the following is considered to be a sign of a disease process?

   a. heartburn   b. pain
   c. proteinuria   d. dry mouth

8. *[LO 6.3]* What is the correct code assignment and sequencing for a patient with a coma and a skull fracture?

   a. The coma is the only condition that should be coded, as there are codes available to indicate cause.
   b. The skull fracture is the only condition that should be coded, as the code includes specifications for complications of coma.
   c. The skull fracture should be sequenced first, followed by the code to report the coma.
   d. The coma should be sequenced first, followed by the code to indicate the skull fracture as the underlying cause.

9. *[LO 6.1]* Which of the following statements is correct regarding a symptom code with a definitive diagnosis code?

   a. A symptom code may be reported, followed by a definitive diagnosis as a secondary code, if that symptom is not routinely associated with that diagnosis.
   b. A symptom code may be reported as a secondary code with a definitive diagnosis code if that symptom is not routinely associated with that diagnosis.
   c. It is never appropriate to assign a symptom code if there is a definitive diagnosis.
   d. Definitive diagnosis codes are reported first, followed by codes for any associated symptoms of the condition.

10. *[LO 6.4]* Which of the following is not appropriate to report with a code from category R50?

    a. fever following surgery   b. fever with chills
    c. febrile convulsions   d. drug-induced fever

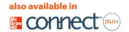
7.3 Genetic Disease Factors, Drug Resistance, Estrogen Receptor, Foreign Body, and Health Hazards for Communicable Diseases

A variety of conditions need to be reported in which patients are genetic carriers of disease, have a genetic susceptibility to a disease, have infections that are drug resistant, or have been exposed to (or are suspected to have been exposed to) a communicable disease. These need to be reported as reasons for seeking healthcare services, receiving precautionary treatment, reporting as a health risk, and for public health reporting. Codes associated with this learning objective are classified in categories Z14–Z28.

Z14–Z15 Genetic Carrier and Genetic Susceptibility to Disease

Codes in this range correspond with the ICD-9-CM codes V83–V84, Genetics. Codes in the Z14–Z17 categories are considered to be status codes, which report that the patient either is a carrier of a specific disease or has residual conditions from previously having had a disease or condition, but are different from history codes because history codes are appropriate only if the patient no longer has a condition or any residual effects of the condition. The Z14 category codes are used to report that the patient is a carrier of a gene for a disease, such as cystic fibrosis, but does not actually have the disease for that gene and is not at risk of developing the disease.

The Z15 category is similar to Z14. However, these codes are used to report that the patient is a carrier of a gene for a disease and is considered to be at risk of developing the disease, such as if a genetic marker were determined to be present. Z15 codes are for use as secondary codes only. If the encounter being coded is for the purpose of genetic counseling, Z31.5 should be listed first.

The concept of "status" is introduced in category Z17, which reports estrogen receptor status. The term "status" is used to report that the patient either is a carrier of a disease or has the sequelae or residual of a past disease or condition. The condition may be the presence of a prosthetic or mechanical device, or the patient might have previously had a significant surgical procedure. Conditions reported with status codes may impact future treatment, which makes status different from history, which indicates that the condition no longer exists. Extensive information about reporting status, including listing of categories and codes for status, can be found in coding guideline *I.C.21.c.3) Status*.

Code Z16, infection with drug-resistant microorganisms, corresponds with the ICD-9-CM code category V09, infection with drug-resistant microorganisms. Note that there is currently only one code to report resistance in ICD-10-CM, whereas category V09 in ICD-9-CM provided multiple codes to specify the drug to which the organism was resistant and resistance to multiple drugs. Codes in the Z17, estrogen receptor status category correspond with the ICD-9-CM code V86, Estrogen Receptor Status.

Z20–Z28 Persons with Potential Health Hazards Related to Communicable Diseases

Codes in this range correspond with ICD-9-CM codes V07–V09, Personal with Need for Isolation, Other Potential Health Hazards and Prophylactic Measures, and V01–V06, Personal with Potential Health Hazards Related to Communicable Diseases. The Z20 category codes are assigned for patients who have been exposed to, or are suspected to have been exposed to, a communicable disease but do not have any symptoms of the disease. These codes may be listed either first or as secondary codes, depending on the circumstances of the episode of care. Coding guideline *I.C.21.c.1) Categories of Z Codes, Contact/Exposure* is the source of instruction for the assignment of codes in category Z20.

Z21 is appropriate to assign if the patient is HIV positive but has never manifested any signs or symptoms of AIDS. Codes in the Z22 category are reported if the patient is a carrier of the causal organism for a disease, has not manifested any symptoms, but is capable of transmitting the disease to others.

Codes in category Z23 are assigned to report patient encounters for the purpose of receiving a prophylactic vaccination. Codes in this category may

Chapter Summary

Learning Outcome	Key Concepts/Examples
7.1 Explain general coding guidelines related to factors influencing health status and contact with health services. **(pages 92–94)**	• Z codes may be listed first or as secondary codes, depending on the circumstances of the encounter. • Z codes are not procedure codes; rather, they provide a reason for the encounter with healthcare services.
7.2 Discuss coding guidelines for persons encountering health services for examinations. **(pages 94–96)**	• Codes in the Z00–Z13 subsection allow for the description of encounters for routine examinations, such as a general checkup, and examinations for administrative purposes, such as pre-employment physicals, and are not to be used if the examination is for the diagnosis of a suspected condition or for treatment purposes. • Observation Z codes are for use in very limited circumstances: when a patient is being observed for a suspected condition that is ruled out and there are no signs, symptoms, or injury related to the suspected condition present.
7.3 Identify reportable situations that involve genetic disease factors, drug resistance, estrogen receptor, foreign body, and health hazards for communicable diseases. **(pages 96–98)**	• Status codes indicate that a patient either is a carrier of a disease or has the sequelae or residual of a past disease or condition. • Codes in category Z23 are assigned to report patient encounters for the purpose of receiving a prophylactic examination.
7.4 Apply code-sequencing guidelines for encounters related to reproduction and other specific healthcare needs. **(pages 98–100)**	• Code Z33.1 is assigned only as a secondary code to reflect that the patient is pregnant but the pregnancy is not related in any way to the reason for the encounter. If the pregnancy is related to the reason for the encounter, it is more appropriate to assign a code from the obstetric chapter. • There are two times when codes in the category for aftercare are to be assigned during the acute treatment phase of a disease process—when a patient is seen for the purpose of receiving radiation therapy to treat a neoplasm and when a patient is seen for the purpose of receiving chemotherapy or immunotherapy.
7.5 Interpret the guidelines for coding history and other factors influencing health status and contact with health services. **(pages 101–103)**	• Personal history codes are used to report that a patient has a pertinent history of a medical condition that is no longer active and the patient is no longer receiving treatment for the condition, but there may be potential for recurrence or the history of the condition impacts current treatment of another condition. • When assigning codes for history, the coder should pay close attention to whether the condition being reported is for personal history or family history.

Applying Your Skills

Assign codes from ICD-9-CM and ICD-10-CM.

	ICD-9-CM	ICD-10-CM
1. *[LO 7.5]* Presence of previously implanted cardiac pacemaker		
2. *[LO 7.5]* Personal history of cancer of the rectosigmoid junction		
3. *[LO 7.4]* Encounter for antineoplastic chemotherapy		
4. *[LO 7.4]* Supervision of normal first pregnancy in the second trimester		
5. *[LO 7.2]* Screening for malignant neoplasm of breast via mammography		
6. *[LO 7.4]* Liveborn infant twin (mate stillborn) delivered by cesarean section in hospital (code for newborn chart)		
7. *[LO 7.3]* Prophylactic combined vaccination against diphtheria, tetanus, and pertussis		
8. *[LO 7.5]* Patient living in extreme poverty		
9. *[LO 7.5]* Family history of lung cancer		
10. *[LO 7.5]* Blood type AB+		
11. *[LO 7.5]* High-risk bisexual behavior		
12. *[LO 7.4]* Twins, one liveborn and one stillborn (outcome of delivery for mother's chart)		
13. *[LO 7.4]* Encounter for sterilization of female via tubal ligation.		
14. *[LO 7.2]* Routine general adult medical examination without abnormal findings		
15. *[LO 7.5]* Adult BMI 33.5		
16. *[LO 7.2]* Encounter for osteoporosis screening		
17. *[LO 7.4]* Encounter for colostomy closure		
18. *[LO 7.5]* Allergy to penicillin		
19. *[LO 7.5]* Noncompliance with medical treatment in the form of medication underdosing due to financial hardship		
20. *[LO 7.5]* Presence of bilateral prosthetic knee replacement devices		

Checking Your Understanding

Select the letter that best answers the question or completes the sentence.

1. *[LO 7.4]* Which code or category is assigned only as a secondary code to reflect that the patient is pregnant but the pregnancy is not related in any way to the reason for the encounter?

   a. Z33.1   **b.** Z34.-   **c.** Z37.-   **d.** Z38.-

2. *[LO 7.1]* Which of the following statements is true?

   a. Z codes should not be assigned if there is a procedure performed during the encounter.
   b. Z codes may be assigned first or as secondary codes, depending on the circumstances of the encounter.
   c. Z codes may only be listed first.
   d. Z codes are only for use as secondary codes.

3. *[LO 7.5]* What are codes in category Z79 used to report?

   a. treatment of withdrawal symptoms
   b. detoxification
   c. use of a prescribed medication for treatment or prophylaxis for a brief period of time
   d. use of a prescribed medication for treatment or prophylaxis for a long period of time

4. *[LO 7.2]* What should not be reported with the Z codes for routine and administrative examinations?

   a. diagnosis for a suspected condition
   b. diagnosis discovered during a routine exam
   c. chronic conditions that exist but are not the focus of the encounter
   d. history codes, which are not the focus of the encounter

5. *[LO 7.3]* Which codes are used to report that the patient is a carrier of a gene for a disease and is considered to be at risk of developing the disease?

   a. Z14   **b.** Z15   **c.** Z80   **d.** Z85

6. *[LO 7.1]* Which of the following may be used only as the principal or first-listed diagnosis?

   a. Z15.03   **b.** Z37.0   **c.** Z92.82   **d.** Z99.12

7. *[LO 7.5]* Which of the following should be reported as an additional code with categories Z77–Z99?

   a. screening   **b.** observation
   c. follow-up examination   **d.** counseling

8. *[LO 7.4]* Which record(s) should have codes in category Z52, donors of organs and tissues, assigned?

   a. only the donor record
   b. only the recipient record
   c. both the donor and recipient records
   d. the recipient record or donor record, depending on who is paying for the donation

9. *[LO 7.2]* When is it appropriate to assign observation Z codes?

   a. when signs or symptoms are present
   b. when an injury-related diagnosis is present
   c. when the patient is being observed for a suspected condition that is ruled out
   d. when a diagnosis has been determined

10. *[LO 7.3]* When is it appropriate to assign code Z21?
    a. The patient has AIDS.
    b. The patient is HIV positive but has never manifested any signs or symptoms of AIDS.
    c. The patient has been exposed to HIV.
    d. The patient presents for a screening HIV test.

Online Activity

[LO 7.1] Search online to find information about reimbursement and coding issues related to factors that influence health status and contact with health services. Write a brief summary of your findings.

Real-World Application

[LO 7.1] Assume that you are writing a policies and procedures manual for an acute care hospital. Write the section that informs employees about factors influencing health status and contact with health services.

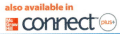
Assign ICD-10-CM codes for the following situations, applying any appropriate sequencing guidelines.

1. Lyme disease, causing meningoencephalitis _____

2. Primary oral syphilis _____

3. Chlamydial conjunctivitis _____

4. Q fever _____

5. Trichomonal urethritis _____

Beyond the Code: Why are chlamydial infections that are sexually transmitted not reported with codes in the A70–A74 subsection?

8.3 Viral Diseases Except for HIV

Coding of viral infections is relatively simple, as they are organized by type of virus. Some codes in this section have instructional notes for the assignment of additional codes. Viral diseases are reported with codes in categories A80–B34, with the exception of B20, human immunodeficiency virus (HIV) disease. Because of the complex nature of HIV coding, HIV is addressed in a section of its own.

A80–A89 Viral and Prion Infections of the Central Nervous System

prion A protein-based infectious agent, which is not viral, bacterial, or fungal, which infects the nervous system.

A **prion** is a protein-based infectious agent, which is not viral, bacterial, or fungal. Prion infections generally infect the nervous system. Codes in this subsection of ICD-10-CM do not correspond with any one specific subsection of ICD-9-CM, as the categories included in this subsection of ICD-10-CM are scattered throughout Chapter 1 of ICD-9-CM. Conditions coded in this subsection include acute poliomyelitis, atypical **virus** infections of the central nervous system, rabies, mosquito-borne viral encephalitis, tick-borne encephalitis, and viral meningitis. Note the instructions associated with category A81 for the coder to assign an additional code to report any dementia accompanying the condition.

virus Pathogen composed of nucleic acid within a protein shell; it can grow and reproduce only after infecting a host cell.

A90–A99 Arthropod-Borne Viral Fevers and Viral Hemorrhagic Fevers

arthropod-borne Of the Arthropoda phylum, referring to a source of one type of infectious manifestation. An infection transmitted by insects, spiders, crustaceans, scorpions and centipedes.

Arthropod-borne infections are those transmitted by insects, spiders, crustaceans, scorpions and centipedes. Codes in this subsection of ICD-10-CM correspond with those in categories 060–066 of ICD-9-CM. Conditions classified in this subsection include dengue fever, dengue hemorrhagic fever, mosquito-borne viral fevers, West Nile fever, yellow fever, and other viral hemorrhagic fevers. West Nile virus infection with neurologic manifestations or other complications requires at least two codes, so that the manifestations or other complications are identified through the secondary codes.

B00–B09 Viral Infections Characterized by Skin and Mucous Membrane Lesions

Codes in this subsection of ICD-10-CM correspond with those in categories 050–059 of ICD-9-CM. Conditions classified to this subsection include herpesviral infections (see Figure 8.1), varicella, zoster, smallpox, monkeypox, measles (see Figure 8.2), rubella, viral warts, and other viral infections characterized by skin and mucous membrane lesions.

B10 Other Human Herpesviruses

Codes in this subsection of ICD-10-CM correspond with those in category 058 of ICD-9-CM. Conditions classified to this subsection are human herpesviruses.

Note that there are no categories B11–B14.

B15–B19 Viral Hepatitis

Codes in this subsection of ICD-10-CM correspond with those in category 070 of ICD-9-CM. Conditions classified to this subsection are acute and chronic viral hepatitis. The most notable difference between ICD-9-CM and ICD-10-CM is that ICD-9-CM had fifth-digit subclassifications for acute, chronic, and hepatitis delta, whereas ICD-10-CM has that specificity built into the codes.

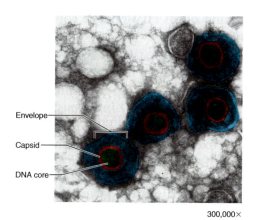

300,000×

figure 8.1 Electron Microscopy of Herpesvirus

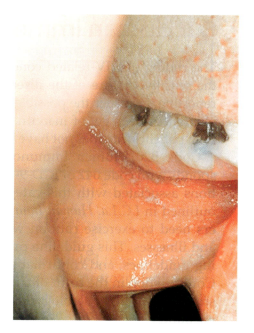

figure 8.2 Koplik Spots on the Buccal Mucosa Early in Measles

remission Absence of malignant cells following treatment.

leukemia Malignancy of blood cells, which originates in the bone marrow.

rather than history. In the case of leukemia, it is important for the coder to identify documentation that specifies whether the patient is in **remission** or if it is truly considered to be a historical condition. The **leukemia** and multiple myeloma categories have codes to report remission; plus codes Z85.6, Personal history of leukemia and Z85.79, Personal history of other malignant neoplasms or lymphoid, hematopoietic and related tissues are available to report history. Anytime the coder is unable to determine the difference with documentation, a physician query may be necessary.

---

also available in

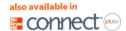

Think About It 9.1

Assign ICD-10-CM codes for the following situations, applying any appropriate sequencing guidelines.

1. Female patient with cancer in the axillary tail of the left breast admitted for administration of chemotherapy _____

2. Anemia associated with left upper lobe lung cancer _____

3. Personal history of malignant neoplasm of ovary _____

4. Patient with osteosarcoma admitted for treatment of pathological fracture of right fibula _____

5. Patient with multiple myeloma and associated pathological vertebral fracture admitted for treatment of multiple myeloma _____

Beyond the Code: Why should a primary malignancy code be used until treatment is completed when a primary malignancy has been excised but further treatment, such as additional surgery for the malignancy, radiation therapy, or chemotherapy, is directed to that site?

9.2 Malignant Neoplasms

The coding of malignant, or cancerous, neoplasms is the focus of this section. These neoplasms are classified in categories C00–C96. When coding malignant neoplasms, follow sequencing guidelines, especially when it comes to additional code assignments. Anatomic terminology is used to identify malignant neoplasms of lymphoid, hematopoietic, and related tissues; coders should review and note any terms they are unfamiliar with.

Codes in this subsection of are coded to ICD-10-CM categories C00–C96 and correspond with those in ICD-9-CM categories 140–208. Conditions coded in this subsection include malignant neoplasms of the following sites:

Spotlight on A&P

When coding malignant neoplasms, knowledge of pathophysiology and terminology helps the coder determine morphology, based on the documentation. Knowledge of anatomy is necessary to identify the exact location of the neoplasm, especially for organs that have codes to report in great detail regarding the part of the organ affected.

- Lip
- Oral cavity

- Male genital organs
- Urinary tract

- Pharynx
- Digestive organs
- Respiratory organs
- Intrathoracic organs
- Bone
- Articular cartilage
- Skin
- Mesothelial tissue
- Soft tissue
- Breast
- Female genital organs
- Eye
- Brain
- Other parts of central nervous system
- Thyroid gland
- Other endocrine glands
- Neuroendocrine tumors
- Ill-defined sites
- Other secondary sites
- Unspecified sites
- Lymphoid tissue
- Hemopoietic tissue

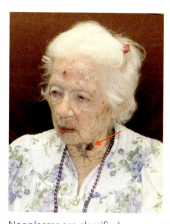

Neoplasms are classified according to site and behavior. For example, the lesion illustrated in this photo would be reported with code C44.4, malignant neoplasm of skin of scalp and neck.

Individual codes in this subsection specify the exact sites of the neoplasm, including laterality. For malignant neoplasms, many of the categories have instructions to assign additional codes to identify any alcohol abuse and dependence, history of tobacco use, tobacco dependence, or tobacco use. Other instructional notes also require the identification of codes for exposure to environmental tobacco smoke, exposure to tobacco smoke in the perinatal period, and occupational exposure to environmental tobacco smoke.

Codes in category C22 for malignant neoplasm of liver and intrahepatic bile ducts have an instructional note to assign additional codes to identify alcohol abuse and dependence, hepatitis B, and hepatitis C. Reporting of malignant neoplasms of bone and articular cartilage of limbs in category C40 requires additional code assignment to identify documentation of major osseous defects. If Kaposi's sarcoma is associated with human immunodeficiency virus (HIV) disease, code B20 should be assigned prior to the code for **Kaposi's sarcoma** in category C46.

Breast cancer codes in category C50 should be followed by an additional code to identify estrogen receptor status, using code Z17.0 or Z17.1. Functional activity should be reported along with codes from category C62 for malignant neoplasm of the testis, category C73 for malignant neoplasm of the thyroid gland, or category C7B for secondary **neuroendocrine tumors.** Malignant neuroendocrine tumors, reported in category C7A, have two instructional notes for additional codes. These are to identify documentation of associated endocrine syndrome, such as carcinoid syndrome or multiple endocrine neoplasia (MEN) syndromes.

Secondary neoplasms are specified in categories C77–C79. Determination of the principal diagnosis when a secondary site is present is based on the focus of treatment. If the treatment is directed only at the secondary site, the principal diagnosis should be the secondary neoplasm. Coding guideline *I.C.2.b. Treatment of secondary site* addresses coding for secondary neoplasms. Figure 9.1 illustrates an example of metastatic (secondary) neoplasm from a primary breast neoplasm.

Three codes in category C80 report malignant neoplasms without specified sites. Code C80.0 reports **disseminated malignant neoplasm,** which includes **carcinomatosis,** or generalized cancer. This code is to be assigned

Kaposi's sarcoma Malignant neoplasm of the connective tissue, that is often associated with AIDS.

CODING TIP ▶

If Kaposi's sarcoma is associated with human immunodeficiency virus (HIV) disease, code B20 should be assigned, followed by the code for Kaposi's sarcoma in category C46.

neuroendocrine tumors Neoplasms originating from nervous and endocrine cells as an integrated functioning mechanism.

disseminated malignant neoplasm Malignant neoplasm has spread throughout the body.

carcinomatosis Generalized cancer.

Checking Your Understanding

Select the letter that best answers the question or completes the sentence.

1. *[LO 9.2]* What is the correct coding assignment for a patient with AIDS-related Kaposi's sarcoma of the skin of the right lower leg?

   a. B20, C44.71
   b. C46.0
   c. C46.0, B20
   d. B20, C46.0

2. *[LO 9.4]* What should be reported with an additional code when coding benign neoplasm of the pancreas, ovary, testis, thyroid, and other endocrine glands?

   a. risk factors
   b. functional activity
   c. symptoms
   d. sequelae

3. *[LO 9.1]* Which of the following is not a behavioral classification of neoplasms?

   a. benign
   b. in situ
   c. malignant
   d. transitional

4. *[LO 9.3]* *Dysplasia* is a term often used to document what kind of neoplasms?

   a. benign
   b. in situ
   c. of uncertain behavior
   d. unspecified

5. *[LO 9.2]* What is the appropriate code assignment for a patient with advanced metastatic disease and no known primary or secondary sites are specified?

   a. C80.0
   b. C80.1
   c. C76.7
   d. C79.9

6. *[LO 9.1]* What is the principal diagnosis if a patient is admitted for administration of chemotherapy for malignancy of a metastatic site?

   a. encounter for antineoplastic chemotherapy
   b. the primary neoplasm
   c. the secondary neoplasm
   d. A physician query must be performed to determine the principal diagnosis.

7. *[LO 9.3]* Non-invasive neoplasms are classified as

   a. benign.
   b. in situ.
   c. of uncertain behavior.
   d. unspecified.

8. *[LO 9.5]* What condition should be coded prior to assigning a code for post-transplant lymphoproliferative disorder?

   a. complication of transplanted organs and tissue
   b. abnormal CBC findings
   c. specific site of biopsy for diagnosis
   d. status post-transplant

9. *[LO 9.4]* Which of the following should be reported with an additional code when coding benign neuroendocrine tumors?

   a. functional activity
   b. symptoms
   c. multiple endocrine neoplasia
   d. residual effects

10. *[LO 9.1]* If a patient has had a malignancy surgically removed and no further treatment is needed, it is coded as

    a. a primary malignancy.
    b. history.
    c. remission.
    d. a secondary malignancy.

Online Activity

[LO 9.1] Visit the Surveillance, Epidemiology and End Results (SEER) website of the National Cancer Institute. Discuss how neoplasm coding fits into cancer registry activities. Summarize your findings in a brief report.

Real-World Application

[LO 9.5] Assign ICD-10-CM codes for the following admission for chemotherapy:

Discharge Summary

Diagnoses:

1. Diffuse large B-cell lymphoma following renal transplant.
2. Stage 3 Chronic renal insufficiency.

History of Present Illness: This 46-year-old white male was diagnosed with post-transplant lymphoproliferative disorder following complaints of abdominal pain, weight loss, and anorexia. He did not seek medical attention immediately. Large-cell lymphoma was diagnosed after lymph node biopsy in the groin.

Hospital Course: Patient was admitted for administration of fourth cycle of chemotherapy with rituximab plus cyclophosphamide, daunorubicin, vincristine, and prednisone was started. Treatment was tolerated well with no nausea, vomiting, or fatigue.

Laboratory Findings: WBC 9.8 with normal differential, ANC 7600, hemoglobin 8.6, hematocrit 26.8, MCV 110, and platelet count of 220,000.

Discharge Instructions: Patient was discharged home to follow up in office next week. Continue medications as prescribed.

10

ENDOCRINE, NUTRITIONAL, AND METABOLIC DISEASES

Learning Outcomes *After completing this chapter, students should be able to*

10.1 Identify disorders of the thyroid gland.

10.2 Apply coding guidelines for diabetes mellitus.

10.3 Compare disorders of glucose regulation, pancreatic internal secretion, and other endocrine glands.

10.4 Use documentation to report codes for malnutrition, other nutritional deficiencies, obesity, and other hyperalimentation.

10.5 Discuss classification of metabolic disorders and postprocedural complications.

Key Terms

body mass index (BMI)
diabetes mellitus
endocrine
goiter
hyperalimentation
malnutrition
metabolic
nutritional
obesity
thyroid
thyrotoxic crisis or storm
type I diabetes mellitus
type II diabetes mellitus

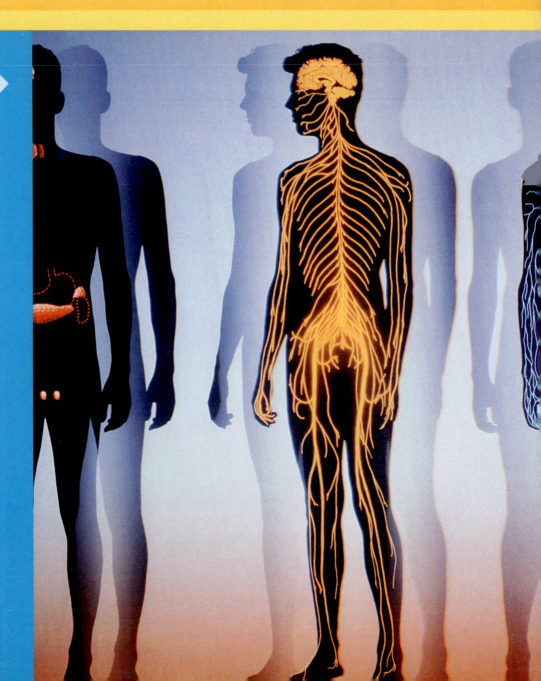

Introduction

In ICD-9-CM and ICD-10-CM, diseases of the **endocrine** system are classified together with **nutritional** and **metabolic** diseases. These include such conditions as:

- thyroid disorders,
- diabetes mellitus,
- disorders of glucose regulation, pancreatic internal secretion, and other endocrine glands,
- malnutrition, overweight, obesity, hyperalimentation, and other nutritional deficiencies, and
- metabolic disorders and postprocedural complications.

ICD-9-CM classifies these conditions in Chapter 3, "Endocrine, Nutritional, and Metabolic Diseases, and Immunity Disorders." This chapter includes codes 240.0–279.9. ICD-10-CM classifies these conditions in Chapter 4, "Endocrine, Nutritional, and Metabolic Diseases," which includes code categories E00–E89.

10.1 Diseases of the Thyroid Gland

Diseases of the **thyroid** gland (illustrated in figure 10.1) are classified in categories E00–E07 of ICD-10-CM. In ICD-9-CM, these conditions were classified as categories 240–246.

E00–E07 Disorders of Thyroid Gland

When assigning codes for hypothyroidism, the coder needs to be aware of the cause, as the condition may be congenital or acquired as a result of medical treatment or other factors. Coding of hyperthyroidism requires attention to the documentation of the presence of **goiter, thyrotoxic crisis, or thyrotoxic storm.**

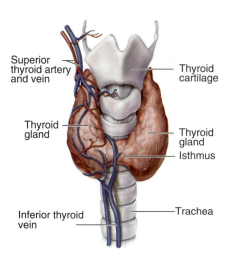

figure 10.1 Anatomy of the Thyroid Gland

endocrine Pertaining to glands and hormones.

nutritional Pertaining to the metabolic processes involved in consumption and physiological utilization of food by which growth, repair, and maintenance of activities in the body as a whole or in any of its parts are accomplished.

metabolic Pertaining to anabolic and catabolic chemical reactions occurring within the body

Spotlight on A&P

Coding diseases in Chapter 4 of ICD-10-CM requires knowledge of the endocrine glands. Many codes in this chapter identify functional changes resulting from glandular disorders. Review the function of each gland and identify hormones secreted by each.

thyroid Endocrine gland located in the center of the neck consisting of two lobes and an isthmus of tissue connecting the lower two-thirds of each lobe; secretes hormones responsible for regulation of heart rate, blood pressure, body temperature, and metabolism of nutrients.

goiter Enlargement of the thyroid gland.

thyrotoxic crisis or storm Hypermetabolic state, which may be life-threatening, caused by excessive secretions from overactivity of the thyroid gland.

If there is documentation of mental retardation along with congenital iodine deficiency syndrome, an additional code from categories F70–F79 should be assigned following the code from category E00. When hypothyroidism is due to a drug or other substance, a code from categories T36–T65 should be assigned and sequenced prior to code E03.2 to identify the causal substance. Acute thyroiditis due to an infectious agent requires an assignment of a secondary code from categories B95–B97 to report the infectious agent. A code from categories T36–T65 should also be assigned and sequenced prior to code E06.4.

Think About It 10.1

also available in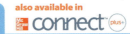

Assign ICD-10-CM codes for the following situations, applying any appropriate sequencing guidelines.

1. Pyogenic thyroiditis due to streptococcus constellatus _____

2. Graves' disease with diffuse goiter _____

3. Hashimoto's thyroiditis _____

4. Multinodular goiter related to iodine deficiency _____

5. Euthyroid sick syndrome _____

Beyond the Code: Which documentation considerations are related to the relationship between thyroid disease and physiological functions in other body systems?

10.2 Diabetes Mellitus and Associated Conditions

diabetes mellitus Chronic metabolic disorder marked by hyperglycemia caused by disorder of insulin secretion.

Coding **diabetes mellitus** and associated conditions is an area where ICD-10-CM differs significantly from ICD-9-CM. Most of the differences have to do with sequencing and combination codes. Codes in this range correspond with the ICD-9-CM codes in categories 249–250.

E08–E13 Diabetes Mellitus

Extensive instructions are provided in coding guideline *I.C.4.a. Diabetes mellitus*. Coders will note that multiple codes are often required when using ICD-9-CM, whereas combination codes are used widely in ICD-10-CM. However, the presence of combination codes does not mean that the use of multiple codes does not occur in ICD-10-CM in this category. In fact, if a patient has multiple diabetic-related conditions, several codes may need to be assigned. Multiple code assignment may be necessary when reporting diabetic-related conditions in order to identify all the complications of the disease.

Determining a patient's type of diabetes mellitus can be challenging. When the type is not documented, the default code is **type II diabetes mellitus**. **Type I diabetes mellitus** is often referred to as juvenile-onset diabetes mellitus due to the fact that most type I diabetics are diagnosed during childhood, but this is not always the case and should not be the sole factor to establish the diagnosis. If the documentation does not specify that a patient has type I diabetes, the default code should come from category E11.-, Type II diabetes mellitus. Type I diabetics require long-term use of insulin and currently there is no cure. The use of insulin is not sufficient to make the assumption of insulin dependence, as type II diabetics may require long-term insulin, or they may use insulin briefly to regain control. If a type II diabetic uses insulin long term, code Z79.4, long term (current) use of insulin should be assigned. The coder should scan documentation looking for the following common abbreviations that will indicate whether or not the patient is insulin dependent. IDDM means Insulin Dependent Diabetes Mellitus. NIDDM means Non-Insulin Dependent Diabetes Mellitus.

Some insulin-dependent diabetics rely on an insulin pump. Pump failure may be accompanied by complications of underdosing or overdosing of insulin. In these cases, a code from subcategory T38.3x6- should be assigned, followed by a code from T38.3x- to rzeport the underdosing or poisoning from overdosing, followed by additional diabetes codes and associated complications.

Diabetes mellitus may be due to an underlying condition, such as drug reaction or other condition. Sequencing instructions for these combinations is provided in the tabular list of the code book for categories E08 and E09. This disease is referred to as Secondary Diabetes Mellitus.

Note that the instructions for sequencing codes with secondary diabetes mellitus differ between ICD-9-CM and ICD-10-CM. The guideline for ICD-9-CM requires the code from category 249 to be sequenced first, with the associated condition listed secondarily, whereas ICD-10-CM requires the underlying condition to be sequenced first, with the code from category E08 listed secondarily. The topic of diabetes mellitus in pregnancy and gestational diabetes will be addressed in Chapter 18 of this book.

E14

Note that there is no category E14.

type II diabetes mellitus
Diabetes mellitus resulting from insulin resistance, with inadequate insulin secretion to sustain normal metabolism, often referred to as non-insulin-dependent diabetes mellitus or adult-onset diabetes mellitus.

type I diabetes mellitus
Diabetes mellitus resulting from failure of the pancreas to produce insulin, often referred to as insulin-dependent diabetes mellitus or juvenile-onset diabetes mellitus.

CODING TIP ▸

The use of insulin is not sufficient to make the assumption of insulin dependence, as type 2 diabetics may require long-term insulin or may use it only briefly to regain control.

CODING TIP ▸

ICD-10-CM requires the underlying condition to be sequenced first. The code from category E08 should be listed secondarily.

When determining a patient's type of diabetes, do not rely solely on the documentation of a patient's use of insulin. Either type of diabetes can require the use of insulin at certain stages, so this is not sufficient information for choosing a code.

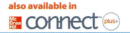
Assign ICD-10-CM codes for the following situations, applying any appropriate sequencing guidelines.

1. Type II diabetes mellitus with left heel and midfoot ulcer with necrosis of muscle _____

2. Type II diabetes with severe nonproliferative diabetic retinopathy with macular edema; patient uses insulin _____

3. Type I diabetes mellitus with gastroparesis _____

4. Diabetes mellitus due to recurring chronic pancreatitis with ketoacidosis and coma, requiring insulin _____

5. Type II diabetes with peripheral angiopathy without gangrene _____

Beyond the Code: Compare the instructions for sequencing codes with secondary diabetes mellitus and explain the differences between ICD-9-CM and ICD-10-CM.

10.3 Disorders of Glucose Regulation, Pancreatic Internal Secretion, and Other Endocrine Glands

Coding for disorders of glucose regulation, pancreatic internal secretion, and other endocrine glands is relatively straightforward. There are no coding guidelines specific to the categories in this section. However, coders should be aware of the ICD-10 manual's instructional notes for guidance. Figures 10.2 and 10.3 diagram the endocrine glands and associated anatomic structures.

E15–E16 Other Disorders of Glucose Regulation and Pancreatic Internal Secretion

Codes in this range correspond with the ICD-9-CM codes in category 251 in ICD-9-CM. The disorders coded in these categories include the following:

- Non-diabetic drug-induced insulin coma
- Hyperinsulinism with hypoglycemic coma
- Hypoglycemic coma
- Functional hyperinsulinism
- Hyperplasia of pancreatic islet beta cells
- Increased secretion of glucagon
- Increased secretion of gastrin
- Zollinger-Ellison syndrome
- Other specified disorders of pancreatic internal secretion

Spotlight on A&P

Many endocrine disorders have significant impact on physiological functions. Increased and decreased function of the endocrine glands cause very different disease processes, so coders must have a thorough comprehension of both the normal physiological functions of the anatomic structures involved and the pathophysiological processes.

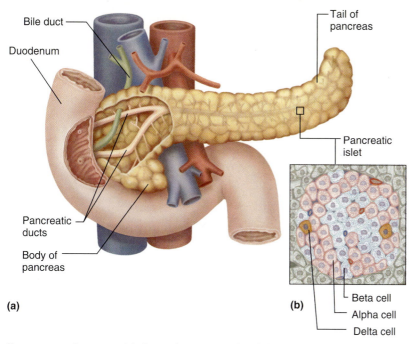

figure 10.2 Pancreas. (a) General anatomy. (b) Alpha, beta, and delta cells.

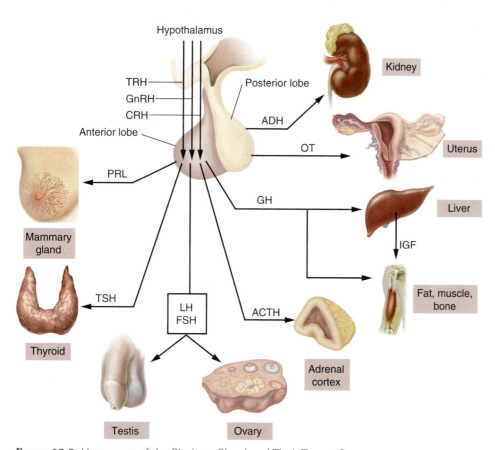

figure 10.3 Hormones of the Pituitary Gland and Their Target Organs

Drug-induced hypoglycemia with coma requires an identification of the causal agent from T36–T50 to be sequenced first, followed by code E16.0.

E17–E19

Note that there are no categories E17–E19.

E20–E35 Disorders of Other Endocrine Glands

The codes in this range correspond with the ICD-9-CM categories 252–259. Disorders coded in these categories include the following:

- Hypoparathyroidism
- Hyperparathyroidism
- Hyperfunction of pituitary gland
- Hypofunction of pituitary gland
- Cushing's syndrome
- Disorders of adrenal gland
- Ovarian dysfunction
- Testicular dysfunction
- Puberty disorders
- Polyglandular dysfunctions
- Thymus disorders
- Other endocrine disorders

When reporting drug-induced hypopituitarism or drug-induced adrenocortical insufficiency, a code form T36–T50 should be sequenced first to identify the drug, followed by E23.1 or E27.3 as a secondary code. If documented as being associated with Conn's syndrome, adrenal adenoma should be identified by assigning D35.0 as a secondary code, following code E26.01. There is an instructional note associated with codes for multiple endocrine neoplasia (MEN) syndrome in subclassification E31.2, which directs the coder to also assign secondary codes if any associated malignancies and other associated conditions are documented.

Code E35 is only for use as a secondary code, following the code for the underlying disease. Category E36 is used for reporting intraoperative complications of the endocrine system. An additional code should be assigned to further specify the complicating disorder.

Think About It 10.3

also available in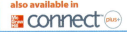

Assign ICD-10-CM codes for the following situations, applying any appropriate sequencing guidelines.

1. Addison's disease   _____

2. Precocious thelarche   _____

3. Zollinger-Ellison syndrome   _____

4. Constitutional gigantism   _____

5. Cushing's disease due to overproduction of pituitary ACTH   _____

Beyond the Code: Identify three endocrine glands and compare the impact of increased and decreased function of each.

10.4 Malnutrition, Other Nutritional Deficiencies, Obesity, and Other Hyperalimentation

This section addresses coding for **malnutrition,** overweight, **obesity, hyperalimentation,** and other nutritional deficiencies. The conditions discussed are reported with codes in categories E40–E68. As in categories E15–E16, coding of these conditions is straightforward, although coders can find guidance in instructional notes.

E40–E46 Malnutrition

Codes in this range correspond with the ICD-9-CM codes in categories 261–263. Disorders coded in these categories include kwashiorkor, malnutrition marasmus, protein-calorie malnutrition, and retarded development due to protein-calorie malnutrition.

E47–E49

Note that there are no categories E47-E49.

E50–E64 Other Nutritional Deficiencies

Codes in this range correspond with the ICD-9-CM codes in categories 264–269. These categories include codes for deficiencies of vitamins, minerals, fatty acids, and other specified nutrients. Category E64 codes are used to report sequelae and late effects of nutritional deficiencies. When reporting sequelae, the code to identify the condition resulting from malnutrition and other nutritional deficiencies should be assigned first, with a code from category E64 assigned as a secondary code.

E65–E68 Overweight, Obesity, and Other Hyperalimentation

Codes in this range correspond with the ICD-9-CM codes in category 278. Conditions reported in this subsection include localized adiposity, overweight and obesity, hyperalimentation, and sequelae of hyperalimentation. Obesity codes are categorized by the type and extent of obesity. A code from subclassification O99.21- should be assigned prior to the code from category E66 if obesity is documented as a complicating factor in pregnancy. If **body mass index (BMI)** is documented, an additional code from category Z68 should be added as a secondary code.

Coding guideline *I.B.14. Documentation for BMI and Pressure Ulcer Stages*, previously introduced in Chapter 4 of this text, provided details regarding assignment of codes based on documentation

malnutrition Condition resulting from inadequate nutrients.

obesity Abnormally high accumulation of body fat and weight that is greater than what is defined as healthy for height and body frame.

hyperalimentation Consumption of an excessive amount of nutrients, which may result from overeating or administration of nutrients by other routes.

Spotlight on A&P

Nutritional deficiencies are often documented by terms other than the specific deficiency, which requires coders to be familiar with the terminology used to describe the conditions.

body mass index (BMI) Calculation based on height and weight to determine body fatness and screen for obesity.

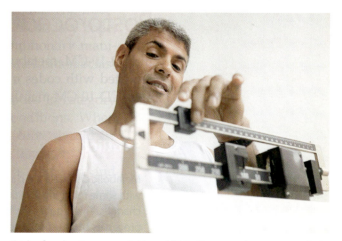

Codes for obesity, overweight, and BMI often must be accompanied by other codes to report associated conditions or characteristics of the patient.

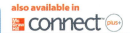
Assign ICD-10-CM codes for the following situations, applying any appropriate sequencing guidelines.

1. Myoclonic epilepsy associated with ragged-red fibers, intractable without status epilepticus _____

2. Metabolic acidosis _____

3. Group C hyperlipidemia _____

4. Lowe's syndrome with associated glaucoma _____

5. Potassium overload _____

Beyond the Code: Why do you think that gout used to be classified in this section in ICD-9-CM but was moved to Chapter 13, "Diseases of the Musculoskeletal System and Connective Tissue," in ICD-10-CM?

Chapter Summary

Learning Outcome	Key Concepts/Examples
10.1 Identify disorders of the thyroid gland. (**pages 139–140**)	• Coding of hyperthyroidism requires attention to documentation of the presence of goiter or thyrotoxic crisis or storm. • Anatomy, physiology, and pathophysiology knowledge needs for coding of thyroid disorders is related to the causal relationships that exist between thyroid diseases and physiological functions in other body systems.
10.2 Apply coding guidelines for diabetes mellitus. (**pages 140–142**)	• Use of insulin is not sufficient to make the assumption of insulin dependence, as type 2 diabetics may require long-term insulin or may use it briefly to regain control. • ICD-10-CM requires the underlying condition to be sequenced first, with the code from category E08 listed secondarily.
10.3 Compare disorders of glucose regulation, pancreatic internal secretion, and other endocrine glands. (**pages 142–144**)	• Increased and decreased functions of the endocrine glands cause very different disease processes, making it necessary for coders to have a thorough comprehension of both the normal physiological function of the anatomic structures involved and the pathophysiological processes.
10.4 Address documentation for coding of malnutrition, other nutritional deficiencies, obesity, and other hyperalimentation. (**pages 145–146**)	• If body mass index (BMI) is documented, an additional code from category Z68 should be added as a secondary code.
10.5 Discuss classification of metabolic disorders and postprocedural complications. (**pages 146–148**)	• Although elevated uric acid in the blood is classified in this section, gout is classified in Chapter 13, "Diseases of the Musculoskeletal System and Connective Tissue," in category M1a.

Applying Your Skills

For each condition, assign the correct code(s) from ICD-9-CM and ICD-10-CM.

Condition	ICD-9-CM Codes	ICD-10-CM Codes
1. *[LO 10.5]* Postsurgical hypothyroidism	_____	_____
2. *[LO 10.2]* Type I diabetes mellitus with diabetic nephrosis	_____	_____
3. *[LO 10.5]* Autosomal recessive ocular albinism	_____	_____
4. *[LO 10.4]* Morbid obesity with alveolar hypoventilation with BMI 52	_____	_____
5. *[LO 10.1]* Toxic multinodular goiter with thyrotoxic crisis	_____	_____
6. *[LO 10.5]* Hypokalemia	_____	_____
7. *[LO 10.2]* Hyperosmotic nonketotic coma in uncontrolled type II diabetes	_____	_____
8. *[LO 10.3]* Hypoglycemia	_____	_____
9. *[LO 10.2]* Diabetic neuropathy in type II diabetic; patient requires insulin	_____	_____
10. *[LO 10.5]* Elevated cholesterol with elevated triglycerides	_____	_____
11. *[LO 10.2]* Ketoacidosis and coma in diabetes mellitus due to pituitary-dependent Cushing's disease	_____	_____
12. *[LO 10.1]* Hashimoto's thyroiditis	_____	_____
13. *[LO 10.5]* Respiratory acidosis	_____	_____
14. *[LO 10.5]* Pulmonary cystic fibrosis due to pseudomonas (two codes, must be in correct sequence)	_____	_____
15. *[LO 10.5]* Hyperuricemia not associated with gouty arthritis	_____	_____
16. *[LO 10.4]* Autosomal recessive ocular albinism	_____	_____
17. *[LO 10.5]* Congenital lactose intolerance	_____	_____
18. *[LO 10.3]* Syndrome of inappropriate ADH secretion (SIADH)	_____	_____
19. *[LO 10.3]* Overproduction of pituitary ACTH	_____	_____
20. *[LO 10.2]* Hyperglycemia	_____	_____

Checking Your Understanding

Select the letter that best answers the question or completes the sentence.

1. *[LO 10.2]* Which of the following is true regarding the determination of the type of diabetes mellitus?

   a. Age at diagnosis is the sole factor for determining type I versus type II.

   b. Long-term use of insulin is the best factor for determining type I versus type II.

   c. Type of diabetes for coding purposes is based on documentation, and the default is type I if the type is not documented.

   d. Type of diabetes for coding purposes is based on documentation, and the default is type II if the type is not documented.

2. *[LO 10.1]* Which of the following does not impact code assignment for hyperthyroidism?

   a. diabetes   b. goiter

   c. thyrotoxic crisis   d. thyrotoxic storm

3. *[LO 10.4]* Which of the following should be sequenced first for a patient with obesity complicating pregnancy?

   a. a code for obesity from category E66
   b. a code for pregnancy from subclassification O99.21
   c. a code to identify body mass index from category Z68
   d. The sequencing is dependent upon the circumstances of the admission.

4. *[LO 10.3]* Which of the following should not be sequenced as a principal diagnosis or first-listed code?

   a. E31.21   **b.** E21.1
   c. E35   **d.** E36.8

5. *[LO 10.5]* How many codes would be assigned to report post-pancreatectomy hyperglycemia, manifested as diabetes mellitus requiring insulin?

   a. one   **b.** two
   c. three   **d.** four

6. *[LO 10.1]* Which code is sequenced first when reporting drug-induced thyroiditis?

   a. E06.4
   b. a code from categories T36.–T65
   c. A physician query must be performed each time this combination is reported.
   d. It depends on the circumstances of admission.

7. *[LO 10.5]* Hemochromatosis is a disorder of _____ metabolism.

   a. calcium   **b.** copper
   c. iron   **d.** magnesium

8. *[LO 10.2]* A patient has diabetes mellitus due to chronic pancreatitis with diabetic chronic kidney disease. Which condition is sequenced first when assigning codes?

   a. a diabetes code from category E08
   b. a chronic kidney disease code from category N18
   c. a pancreatitis code from category K86
   d. The sequencing should be clarified through a physician query.

9. *[LO 10.4]* Beriberi is a deficiency of

   a. vitamin D.
   b. riboflavin.
   c. thiamin.
   d. folate.

10. *[LO 10.3]* Which of the following is coded only for male patients?

    a. E28.1
    b. E29.1
    c. E31.21
    d. all of the above

Online Activity

[LO 10.2] Search online to find information about reimbursement issues related to diabetes mellitus. Identify ways that documentation and/or coding can affect any of these issues.

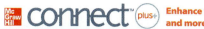

Real-World Application: Case Study

[LO 10.2, LO 10.5] Assign codes for the following physician office progress note.

HISTORY OF PRESENT ILLNESS: This 48-year-old female patient presents for follow-up for acquired hypothyroidism s/p total thyroidectomy. She denies any significant changes in health but has complaint of daytime fatigue. No complaints of intolerance to temperature, muscle weakness, nausea, vomiting, diarrhea, constipation, palpitations, or tremors.

CURRENT MEDICATIONS:
1. Levothyroxine 125 micrograms p.o. once daily.
2. Glucotrol 10 mg b.i.d.
3. Synthroid.

REVIEW OF SYSTEMS: Denies fever, chills, sweats, polydipsia, polyuria, chest pain, shortness of breath, dyspnea, nausea, vomiting, diarrhea, constipation, palpitations, or tremors.

PHYSICAL EXAMINATION:

General: Obese woman, in no acute distress.

Vital Signs: Temperature 98.8, pulse 84, respirations 18, blood pressure 126/68, and weight 182 pounds.

Neck: Well-healed surgical scar on the neck. No palpable thyroid tissue noted on examination. No lymphadenopathy noted.

Thorax: Lungs clear to auscultation.

Cardiovascular: Regular rate and rhythm with no murmurs noted.

Extremities: Deep tendon reflexes 2+/4, no delayed relaxation phase.

Integumentary: Unremarkable.

LABORATORY: Lab values on 06/25/20xx included. Quantitative thyroglobulin less than 0.5, thyroglobulin antibody less than 20, free T4 1.30, TSH 0.120.

ASSESSMENT:
1. Acquired hypothyroidism.
2. Type II diabetes mellitus.
3. Status post total thyroidectomy in 20xx for papillary carcinoma of the thyroid gland.

PLAN:
1. Continue to monitor thyroglobulin levels.
2. Obtain a free T4, TSH, and thyroglobulin levels today.
3. Follow up in approximately 6 months or sooner, if symptoms develop.

11

BLOOD, BLOOD-FORMING ORGANS, AND CERTAIN DISORDERS INVOLVING THE IMMUNE MECHANISM

Learning Outcomes *After completing this chapter, students should be able to*

11.1 Discuss aspects of coding for nutritional and hemolytic anemias.

11.2 Assign codes for aplastic and other anemias and other bone marrow failure syndromes in the appropriate sequence.

11.3 Apply knowledge of the pathophysiology of coagulation defects, purpura, and other hemorrhagic conditions in order to correctly assign codes.

11.4 Explain documentation needs for coding other disorders of blood and blood-forming organs.

11.5 Assign codes for certain disorders involving the immune mechanism.

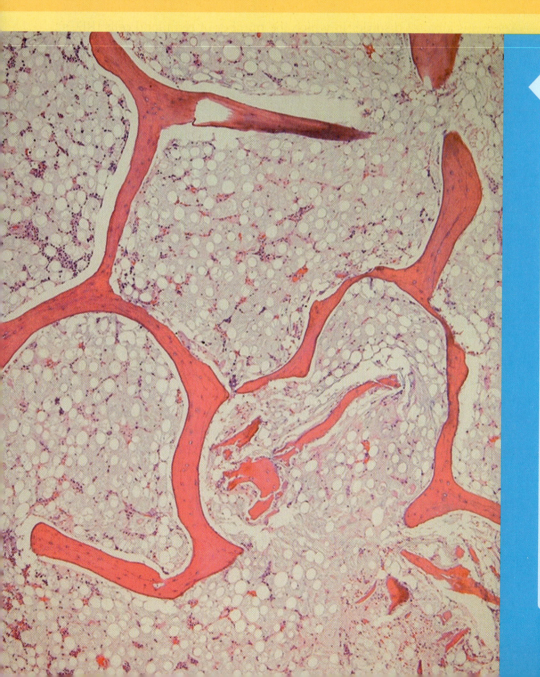

Key Terms

aplastic anemias
coagulation defects
coagulopathy
extrinsic circulating
    anticoagulants
hemolytic anemia
immunodeficiency
intrinsic circulating
    anticoagulants
iron deficiency anemia
nutritional anemias
posthemorrhagic anemias
purpura
sickle cell anemia
sickle cell disease

Introduction

In ICD-9-CM and ICD-10-CM, diseases of the blood and blood-forming organs are classified into one chapter. Blood disorders include anemias, **coagulation defects,** and disorders of the various components of blood. The spleen, a blood-forming organ, is the root of the disorders that constitute the rest of this chapter in the coding manual.

This chapter of the manual, unlike many others, is short and is not divided into subsections. ICD-9-CM classifies these conditions in Chapter 4, "Diseases of the Blood and Blood-Forming Organs," which includes codes 280.0–289.9. ICD-10-CM classifies these conditions, along with others, in Chapter 3, "Diseases of the Blood and Blood-forming Organs and Certain Disorders Involving the Immune Mechanism," which includes code categories D50–D89.

11.1 Nutritional and Hemolytic Anemias

Anemia is a blood disorder in which the number of red blood cells (RBCs), or the amount of hemoglobin each RBC carries, is reduced. There are many kinds of anemias, all of which fall into various types. Two of these types, **nutritional anemias** (deficiency anemias) and **hemolytic anemia,** are disorders whose coding is significantly different in ICD-10-CM. ICD-10-CM allows for the reporting of greater specificity of these anemias than was previously available in ICD-9-CM, especially for types of nutritional anemias. This greater specificity in codes generates a need for increased detail in documentation by providers. For example, rather than just documenting that a patient has vitamin B_{12} deficiency anemia, documentation of the cause of that deficiency is needed in order to code it. Deficiency anemias, blood-loss anemias, **sickle cell disease,** and thalassemia are among the disorders discussed.

D50–D53 Nutritional Anemias

Codes in this range of codes of ICD-10-CM correspond with those in categories 280–281 in ICD-9-CM. These codes classify anemia conditions that are due to a variety of deficiencies, including deficiencies of iron, vitamins, protein, minerals, and other nutrients.

One commonly used category in this section is D50, Iron deficiency anemia. Coders must exercise caution when assigning codes for **iron deficiency anemia** secondary to blood loss, because reimbursement issues may arise if acute and chronic **posthemorrhagic anemias** are confused in the coding process. Similar to the previously mentioned vitamin deficiency example, the assignment of code D62, acute posthemorrhagic anemia, must be clearly documented. If the documentation does not specify acuity, the default code is for chronic, which is classified as D50.0, iron deficiency anemia secondary to blood loss (chronic). Coding of acute versus chronic blood-loss anemia has been an area of focus for compliance audits for several years, since it is an area where errors are common and increased reimbursement may be received inappropriately as a result.

If folate deficiency anemia is drug-induced, code D52.1, drug-induced folate deficiency anemia should be assigned. This code should be followed by a code from T36–T50 to report the causal agent of the anemia.

---

coagulation defects Defects or disorders of blood clotting.

nutritional anemias Also known as deficiency anemias; anemic conditions due to a variety of deficiencies, including iron, vitamins, protein, minerals, and other nutrients.

hemolytic anemia Anemic condition that is the result of red blood cells being destroyed.

sickle cell disease Disease process that causes the red blood cells to be formed in a crescent (sickle) shape, contain abnormal amounts of hemoglobin, and often block blood flow due to the abnormal shape.

iron deficiency anemia Anemia caused by a decreased number of red blood cells and inability of the body to absorb sufficient iron, or insufficient nutritional intake of iron-rich foods.

posthemorrhagic anemias Anemias occurring as the result of hemorrhage.

Spotlight on A&P

Coders are often called upon to interpret documentation and recognize when it is necessary to query a physician about an anemia disorder. This makes it important for coders to have a strong knowledge of pathophysiology and the language of laboratory findings.

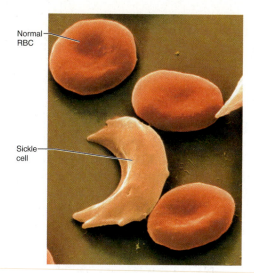

Normal RBC

Sickle cell

figure 11.1 Sickle Cell Anemia

D54

Note that there is no category D54.

D55–D59 Hemolytic Anemias

Codes in this range of ICD-10-CM codes correspond with those in categories 282–283 in ICD-9-CM. Categories D55–D59 are assigned to report hemolytic anemias, conditions that are the result of red blood cells being destroyed. These anemias can be caused by enzyme disorders, thalassemia, **sickle cell anemia** (see Figure 11.1), hereditary conditions, and acquired conditions. When reporting sickle cell disorders, an additional code should be reported to identify an associated fever, if it is documented.

sickle cell anemia Anemic condition caused by insufficient amount of hemoglobin in the blood cells with sickle cell disease.

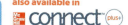

Think About It 11.1

also available in **McGraw Hill connect** (plus+)

Assign ICD-10-CM codes for the following situations, applying any appropriate sequencing guidelines.

1. Sickle cell thalassemia with splenic sequestration and associated fever   _____

2. Toxic hemolytic anemia   _____

3. Vegan anemia   _____

4. Hb S trait   _____

5. Pernicious anemia   _____

Beyond the Code: General coding guideline *I.B.6.* directs coders not to assign associated symptoms with a definitive diagnosis. However, the instructional note associated with category D57 guides the coder to assign an additional code to report any associated fever. Why is sickle cell disease an apparent exception to that rule?

11.2 Aplastic Anemias, Other Anemias, and Other Bone Marrow Failure Syndromes

aplastic anemias Condition in which bone marrow is unable to produce sufficient red blood cells, white blood cells, and platelets.

In contrast to hemolytic anemias, in which anemia results from the destruction of existing RBCs or a reduction in their capacity, **aplastic anemias** are characterized by an inability to produce new blood cells. In these cases, the source of new blood cells—bone marrow—is inhibited from producing all three kinds of blood cells by an underlying disorder or external agent. Aplastic anemias, together with other non-hemolytic anemias, are classified with additional bone marrow failure syndromes in the ICD-9-CM and ICD-10-CM coding manuals. In ICD-10-CM, they are coded from categories D60–D64.

In this section of ICD-10-CM, coders should be alert to the sequencing guidelines that are discussed. Some codes are specified as being for use only as secondary codes, with underlying conditions sequenced first.

D60–D64 Aplastic and Other Anemias and Other Bone Marrow Failure Syndromes

Codes in this subsection of ICD-10-CM correspond with those in categories 284–285 in ICD-9-CM. Many of the conditions classified in this subsection require the assignment of multiple codes to completely and accurately report anemia conditions. Documentation is a critical factor when coding acute posthemorrhagic anemia as a postoperative complication. Code assignment must be based on physician documentation, not on comparison of preoperative and postoperative hemoglobin levels or the amount of blood loss noted during a surgical procedure. Remember, the coder is not the physician. If clinical presentation of nonphysician documentation suggests acute posthemorrhagic anemia as a postoperative complication, it is appropriate to query the physician. Be sure to present your query without asking leading questions based on the documentation.

> **Spotlight on A&P**
>
> Several conditions in this subsection are associated with other disease processes. These connections require coders to understand the pathophysiology of the relationship between a given pair of conditions.

When reporting codes for aplastic anemia that is drug-induced or due to other external agents, a code to report the substance must be sequenced prior to the anemia code. Note, too, that myelophthisis is coded with a secondary code to identify the underlying disorder. Codes in category D63, anemia in chronic diseases classified elsewhere, are to be assigned only as secondary codes, following the code for the underlying disease. Codes D64.1 and D64.2 are also intended for assignment as secondary codes, following codes for the underlying disease, drug, or toxin.

Think About It 11.2

also available in **connect** plus+

Assign ICD-10-CM codes for the following situations, applying any appropriate sequencing guidelines.

1. Idiopathic aplastic anemia _____

2. Myelophthisic anemia associated with pulmonary tuberculosis _____

3. Pancytopenia _____

4. Erythropoietin resistant anemia in a dialysis-dependent patient with end-stage renal disease _____

5. Acute blood-loss anemia _____

Beyond the Code: What are some potential results of not reporting codes in the proper sequence in this section?

11.3 Coagulation Defects, Purpura, and Other Hemorrhagic Conditions

In ICD-10-CM, coagulation defects, **purpura,** and other hemorrhagic conditions, all of which are disorders of blood clotting, are reported with codes in categories D65–D69. In coding for hemorrhagic conditions, coders should be especially aware of pharmacological agents that impact coagulation, because the source of coagulation determines the code. Figure 11.2 provides an overview of the blood coagulation process.

purpura Skin hemorrhages that are red initially and then turn purple.

Spotlight on A&P

Pharmacology knowledge is one of the keys to accurate coding of coagulation defects, along with comprehension of the physiological functions related to coagulation.

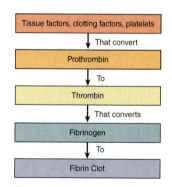

figure 11.2
Blood Coagulation

D65–D69 Coagulation Defects, Purpura, and Other Hemorrhagic Conditions

Codes in this subsection of ICD-10-CM correspond with those in categories 286–287 in ICD-9-CM. Coagulation defects are often a source of confusion for coders, mainly due to a lack of understanding about **coagulopathy,** which refers to any disorder of blood clotting. Coagulopathy may be external, due to the adverse effects of anticoagulant medication therapy, or it may be due to an intrinsic impairment or a deficiency of plasma proteins, commonly referred

coagulopathy Describes any disorder of blood clotting.

Table 11.1 Commonly Prescribed Medication

Anticoagulant Medications	Thrombolytic Medications (Drug Names in Parentheses)
• Argatroban	• Urokinase (Abbokinase)
• Coumadin	• Alteplase (Activase)
• Heparin	• Anisoylated purified streptokinase activator complex (APSAC)
• Lepirudin	• Prourokinase (Saruplase)
• Warfarin (generic Coumadin)	• Reteplase (Retavase)
	• Streptokinase (Streptase)
	• Tissue plasminogen activator (t-PA)

Source: Hardman, Joel Griffith, Lee E. Limbird, and Alfred G. Gilman. *Goodman and Gilman's the Pharmacological Basis of Therapeutics,* 10th ed. New York: McGraw-Hill, 2001.

to as coagulation factors. Changes with ICD-10-CM have helped minimize this confusion for coders: Code D68.31 is assigned to report a hemorrhagic disorder due to **intrinsic circulating anticoagulants** (a disease process). On the other hand, if the problem is due to an anticoagulant medication, code D68.32, hemorrhagic disorder due to **extrinsic circulating anticoagulants,** preceded by a code from the T45.5- series and followed by code Z79.01, long-term (current) use of anticoagulants, is assigned. Table 11.1 provides a list of commonly prescribed anticoagulant medications, but coders should also keep abreast of newly developed pharmaceuticals as they are released. This is an example of the ongoing need for continuing education for coders.

intrinsic circulating anticoagulants Anticoagulants occurring naturally in the human body.

extrinsic circulating anticoagulants External agents or drugs that act as anticoagulants.

CODING TIP ▶

Intrinsic circulating anticoagulants are those naturally produced by the body, whereas extrinsic circulating anticoagulants are from medicinal substances.

Think About It 11.3

also available in **McGraw Hill connect** plus+

Assign ICD-10-CM codes for the following situations, applying any appropriate sequencing guidelines.

1. Idiopathic thrombocytopenic purpura _____

2. Relapsed multiple myeloma with secondary hemophilia _____

3. Disseminated intravascular coagulation _____

4. Hemorrhagic disorder caused by long-term use of warfarin taken as prescribed _____

5. Factor VIII deficiency with vascular defect _____

Beyond the Code: Make a list of medications that are classified as anticoagulants and that be reported as extrinsic circulating anticoagulants.

11.4 Other Disorders of Blood and Blood-Forming Organs and Intraoperative and Postprocedural Complications of Spleen

In ICD-10-CM, disorders of blood and blood-forming organs that are not addressed by the codes discussed earlier in this chapter are coded from categories D70–D78. These categories include codes for intraoperative and postprocedural complications related to the spleen. Sequencing guidelines are important for several conditions in this subsection.

D70–D77 Other Disorders of Blood and Blood-Forming Organs

Codes in this subsection of ICD-10-CM correspond with those in categories 288–289 in ICD-9-CM. Conditions include neutropenia, functional disorders of polymorphonuclear neutrophils, other white blood cell disorders, disease of the spleen, methemoglobinemia, other diseases of the blood and blood-forming organs, and other specified diseases with participation of lymphoreticular and reticulohistiocytic tissue. When reporting neutropenia, if there is documentation of associated fever or mucositis, an additional code should be reported as a secondary diagnosis. Agranulocytosis that is documented as drug-induced or due to cancer chemotherapy should be reported following a code to identify the drug. When it is due to cancer chemotherapy, the neoplasm should also be reported as a secondary diagnosis. Myelofibrosis also has a variety of associated instructional notes for the assignment of additional codes with sequencing guidance.

> **CODING TIP ▸**
>
> Both agranulocytosis and myelofibrosis have several instructional notes regarding coding and sequencing for codes that should be assigned before and after the condition.

If hemophagocytic syndrome is associated with an infectious process, a secondary code should be assigned to specify the infectious agent. Code D77, other disorders of blood and blood-forming organs in diseases classified elsewhere, is only for use as a secondary code, following a code for the underlying disease.

D78 Intraoperative and Postprocedural Complications of Spleen

This subsection is new in ICD-10-CM. It does not correspond to a specific category in ICD-9-CM. The previous classification of complications related to operative procedures in ICD-9-CM was less specific and was not classified within the specific body systems.

Codes in this category specify complications, including intraoperative or postoperative hemorrhage and hematoma of the spleen (Figure 11.3), accidental

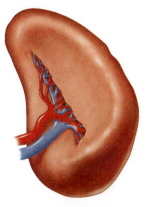

figure 11.3 Spleen

puncture and laceration of the spleen during a procedure, and other intraoperative or postoperative complications of the spleen. If D78.81, other intraoperative complications of spleen, or D78.89, postprocedural hemorrhage and hematoma of spleen following other procedure, is assigned, an additional code should be assigned to further specify the disorder.

D79

Note that there is no category D79.

Think About It 11.4
also available in McGraw Hill **connect** plus+

Assign ICD-10-CM codes for the following situations, applying any appropriate sequencing guidelines.

1. Splenic infarction _____

2. Benign polycythemia _____

3. Cyclic neutropenia with associated fever _____

4. Leukocytopenia _____

5. Progressive septic granulomatosis _____

Beyond the Code: Explain why disorders of the spleen are classified in this chapter and how these disorders may impact blood.

11.5 Certain Disorders Involving the Immune Mechanism

Disorders involving the immune mechanism are reported with codes in categories D80–D89. These disorders involve deficiencies of antibodies and other defects. Sarcoidosis and other disorders of immune mechanisms are also included in this category.

Spotlight on A&P

A&P knowledge helps coders recognize deviations from normal physiological function of immune mechanisms. Pathophysiology takes that knowledge one step further by providing details of disease processes that impact immune physiological function.

D80–D89 Certain Disorders Involving the Immune Mechanism

immunodeficiency Failure of the immune system to effectively fight disease and protect the body from harmful antigens.

Codes in this subsection of ICD-10-CM correspond with those in category 279, disorders involving the immune mechanism, in ICD-9-CM. Conditions classified in this section include **immunodeficiency** with predominantly antibody defects, combined immunodeficiencies, immunodeficiency associated with major defects, common variable immunodeficiency, sarcoidosis, and others. Immune reconstitution syndrome may be drug-induced and should have the causal agent identified by a code from T36–T50, followed by D89.3 if documented.

For codes in the D89.8- subclassification, graft versus host disease, there are a series of instructions regarding the assignment of codes both before and after the condition. If there is documentation of any complication of a transplanted organ or a blood transfusion, it should be coded and sequenced prior to a code from the D89.81- subclassification. If there are any associated manifestations of graft-versus-host disease, such as diarrhea, elevated bilirubin, or hair loss, these conditions should be coded and sequenced as additional diagnoses following the code from the D89.81- subclassification. For example, if a patient has an acute graft-versus-host reaction to a blood transfusion, which causes the patient to have elevated bilirubin, the appropriate code assignment and sequencing is as follows:

T80.89, Other complications following infusion, transfusion and therapeutic injection; D89.810, Acute graft-versus-host disease; R17, Unspecified jaundice

CODING TIP ▸

Codes in the D89.8- subclassification, graft-versus-host disease, have complex instructions for code sequencing.

Think About It 11.5

also available in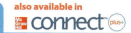

Assign ICD-10-CM codes for the following situations, applying any appropriate sequencing guidelines.

1. Sarcoid arthropathy _____

2. Acute graft-versus-host disease related liver transplant failure, manifested by jaundice _____

3. Immunodeficiency with thrombocytopenia and eczema _____

4. Selective deficiency of IgM _____

5. Common variable immunodeficiency with autoantibodies to B or T cells _____

Beyond the Code: What are some documentation obstacles that a coder might encounter with the codes in this subsection? How might you address these obstacles?

Chapter Summary

Learning Outcome	Key Concepts/Examples
11.1 Discuss aspects of coding for nutritional and hemolytic anemias. **(pages 154–155)**	• Coders must exercise caution when assigning codes for iron deficiency anemia secondary to blood loss, as reimbursement issues may arise if acute and chronic posthemorrhagic anemias are confused in the coding process. • When reporting sickle cell disorders, an additional code should be reported to identify associated fever, if documented.
11.2 Assign codes for aplastic and other anemias and other bone marrow failure syndromes in the appropriate sequence. **(pages 156–157)**	• Codes in category D63, anemia in chronic diseases classified elsewhere, are to be assigned only as secondary codes, following the code for the underlying disease.
11.3 Apply knowledge of pathophysiology related to coagulation defects, purpura, and other hemorrhagic conditions in order to correctly assign codes. **(pages 157–158)**	• Coagulation defects may be external, due to adverse effects of anticoagulant medication therapy, or they may be due to an intrinsic impairment or deficiency of plasma proteins, commonly referred to as coagulation factors. • Intrinsic circulating anticoagulants are those naturally produced by the body, whereas extrinsic circulating anticoagulants are from medicinal substances.
11.4 Explore documentation needs for coding other disorders of blood and blood-forming organs. **(pages 159–160)**	• Agranulocytosis and myelofibrosis have several instructional notes for coding, and sequencing codes that should be assigned both before and after the condition. • Code D77 is for use as a secondary code only, following a code for the underlying disease.
11.5 Assign codes for certain disorders involving the immune mechanism. **(pages 160–161)**	• Codes in the D89.8- subclassification, graft-versus-host disease, have complex instructions associated with it regarding the assignment of codes both before and after the condition.

Applying Your Skills

Assign codes for the following conditions using both ICD-9-CM and ICD-10-CM.

Condition	ICD-9-CM Codes	ICD-10-CM Codes
1. *[LO 11.1]* Sickle cell thalassemia with splenic sequestration	_____	_____
2. *[LO 11.3]* Multiple myeloma with secondary hemophilia	_____	_____
3. *[LO 11.3]* Coagulation disorder due to acquired vitamin K deficiency	_____	_____
4. *[LO 11.4]* Eosinophilic leukopenia	_____	_____
5. *[LO 11.2]* Chronic blood-loss anemia	_____	_____
6. *[LO 11.5]* Sarcoidosis of the lung	_____	_____
7. *[LO 11.1]* Beta thalassemia minor	_____	_____
8. *[LO 11.5]* Selective deficiency of immunoglobulin G (IgG)	_____	_____
9. *[LO 11.3]* Disseminated intravascular coagulation (DIC)	_____	_____
10. *[LO 11.1]* Pernicious anemia	_____	_____
11. *[LO 11.4]* Hemophagocytic lymphohistiocytosis (HLH) due to Epstein-Barr virus (EBV) infection	_____	_____
12. *[LO 11.1]* Abnormal hemoglobin	_____	_____
13. *[LO 11.4]* Leukemoid reaction	_____	_____
14. *[LO 11.3]* Intrinsic circulating anticoagulants	_____	_____
15. *[LO 11.2, 11.4]* Splenic infarction with acute blood-loss anemia	_____	_____
16. *[LO 11.1]* Chronic idiopathic hemolytic anemia	_____	_____
17. *[LO 11.3]* Idiopathic thrombocytopenic purpura	_____	_____
18. *[LO 11.2]* Pancytopenia	_____	_____
19. *[LO 11.3]* Presence of systemic lupus erythematosus (SLE) inhibitor	_____	_____
20. *[LO 11.5]* Severe combined immunodeficiency (SCID) with reticular dysgenesis	_____	_____

Checking Your Understanding

Select the letter that best answers the question or completes the sentence.

1. *[LO 11.2]* Which of the following codes is not intended for assignment as a secondary code?

   a. D64.1
   b. D61.82
   c. D63.1
   d. D630

2. *[LO 11.4]* What is the proper code assignment for agranulocytosis due to chemotherapy for cancer of the lower outer quadrant of the left breast in a female patient?

   a. C50.512, D70.1, T45.1x5   **b.** T45.1x5, C50.512, D70.1
   c. T45.1x5, D70.1, C50.512   **d.** D70.1, T45.1x5, C50.512

3. *[LO 11.1]* What is the correct code assignment for sickle cell disease with splenic sequestration and associated fever?

   a. D57.02   **b.** D57.02, R50.81
   c. R50.81, D57.02   **d.** D57.02, R50.9

4. *[LO 11.5]* What is the correct sequencing for a blood transfusion complication causing acute graft-versus-host disease with a manifestation of elevated bilirubin?

   a. T80.89, D89.810, R17   **b.** R17, T80.89, D89.810
   c. T80.89, R17, D89.810   **d.** D89.810, T80.89, R17

5. *[LO 11.4]* What is the correct code assignment for hemophagocytic syndrome associated with Epstein-Barr virus mononucleosis?

   a. D76.2   **b.** D76.2, B27.99
   c. B27.99   **d.** B27.99, D76.2

6. *[LO 11.2]* Which of the following codes represents a diagnosis that does not imply the presence of a causal condition?

   a. D64.1   **b.** D64.81
   c. D60.1   **d.** D63.0

7. *[LO 11.4]* What is the correct code assignment for postoperative splenic infarction?

   a. D73.5   **b.** D78.89
   c. D73.5, D78.89   **d.** D78.89, D73.5

8. *[LO 11.1]* Why must a coder be cautious when coding iron deficiency anemia secondary to blood loss?

   a. An incorrect code assignment may impact the patient's ability to qualify for insurance coverage in the future.
   b. Physicians do not know the correct way to document it.
   c. Reimbursement issues may arise if acute and chronic posthemorrhagic anemias are confused in the coding process.
   d. It is confusing to determine the correct code assignment.

9. *[LO 11.3]* Which code would be assigned if a patient had a coagulation disorder due to Coumadin?

   a. Z79.01, D68.32, T45.5-   **b.** D68.31, 79.01
   c. T45.5-, D68.32, Z79.01   **d.** T45.5-, D68.31, Z79.01

10. *[LO 11.5]* What is the correct code assignment for sarcoid pyelonephritis?

   a. N10   **b.** D86.84
   c. D86.84, N10   **d.** N10, D86.84

Online Activity

[LO 11.1] Search online for information about the reimbursement implications of incorrect coding of acute blood-loss anemia. Report your findings.

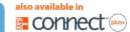
Assign ICD-10-CM codes for the following situations, applying any appropriate sequencing guidelines.

1. Kaposi's sarcoma of the skin in patient with AIDS _____

2. Carcinomatosis _____

3. Left lower lobe lung cancer with history of tobacco dependence _____

4. Thyroid cancer with iodine-deficiency-related nodular goiter _____

5. Lymphocyte-depleted classical Hodgkin lymphoma, intra-abdominal lymph nodes _____

Beyond the Code: What are the benefits of reporting laterality for neoplasm codes?

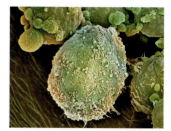

Lymphoma lymph cell. Lymphomas of various types are coded from categories C81–C96. Note that there are no categories C27–C29, C42, C59, or C97–C99.

9.3 In Situ Neoplasms

In situ neoplasms are neoplasms that are non-invasive. They are coded from ICD-10-CM categories D00–D09 and correspond with those in categories 230–234 in ICD-9-CM. The term **dysplasia,** which is literally abnormal formation of cells or tissue, is often used when documenting in situ neoplasms. Some anatomic sites, such as the skin, breast, cervix, and prostate, also have specific terms used for documenting in situ neoplasms. A pathology report is your best source of documentation when trying to identify the behavior of any neoplasm.

dysplasia Abnormal development of cells or tissue.

Examples of in Situ Neoplasms and Related Terminology

Bowen's disease is a specific type of in situ squamous cell carcinoma of the skin. Ductal carcinoma in situ (DCIS) is a form of in situ neoplasm of the breast. Cervical intraepithelial neoplasia (CIN) and cervical dysplasia are frequently documented terms for in situ neoplasms of the cervix. Similarly, prostatic intraepithelial neoplasia (PIN) is occasionally documented for in situ neoplasms of the prostate.

Many of these codes are accompanied by instructions similar to those in the subsection for malignant neoplasms, such as reporting exposure to tobacco. Codes in this subsection are generally straightforward to report, with minimal sequencing guidance.

Bowen's disease A type of in situ squamous cell carcinoma of the skin.

Spotlight on A&P

Identification of morphology for in situ neoplasms requires a thorough knowledge of pathophysiology.

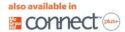
Assign ICD-10-CM codes for the following situations, applying any appropriate sequencing guidelines.

1. Papillary intraductal carcinoma of the left breast _____

2. Cervical intraepithelial neoplasia III _____

3. Carcinoma in situ of the anterior bladder wall _____

4. Severe prostatic dysplasia _____

5. Bowen's epithelioma of vulva _____

Beyond the Code: What is the significance of reporting in situ neoplasms separately from malignant neoplasms?

9.4 Benign Neoplasms

Benign neoplasms are non-cancerous. In ICD-10-CM, they are coded to categories D10–D36 and D3a, which correspond with ICD-9-CM categories 209–229. When reporting benign neoplasm of the pancreas, ovary, testis, thyroid, and other endocrine glands, an additional code should be assigned to identify functional activity. **Hemangioma, lymphangioma,** and **nevus** are some terms that may be used to document benign neoplasms.

Benign neuroendocrine tumors are reported in category D3a. When reporting, additional codes should be assigned to identify documentation of associated multiple endocrine neoplasia (MEN) or associated endocrine syndrome.

hemangioma Benign tumor composed of dilated blood vessels and often encapsulated within a fibrous shell.

lymphangioma Tumor composed of lymphatic vessels.

nevus Congenital discoloration of a circumscribed area of the skin due to pigmentation.

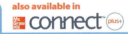
Assign ICD-10-CM codes for the following situations, applying any appropriate sequencing guidelines.

1. Intracranial nevus _____

2. Intra-abdominal hemangioma _____

3. Subserosal leiomyoma of the uterus _____

4. Cystic lymphangioma _____

5. Mammary myxoid fibroma of the right breast _____

Beyond the Code: Why is it pertinent to report an additional code to identify the functional activity of endocrine glands with benign neoplasm?

9.5 Neoplasms of Uncertain or Unspecified Behavior

Sometimes neoplasms cannot be determined to be either malignant or benign. If not, they are classified as being of uncertain or unspecified behavior. This section of the neoplasm chapter is not used as frequently as the malignant, benign, and in situ sections.

Codes in this subsection of ICD-10-CM are coded to categories D37–D49 and correspond with those in categories 235–239 in ICD-9-CM. Categories D37–D44 and D48 classify neoplasms of uncertain behavior by site. **Uncertain behavior** means that histologic confirmation regarding whether the neoplasm is malignant or benign cannot be made.

Similar to the instructions for in situ neoplasms, additional codes should be assigned to identify the functional activity for neoplasm of uncertain behavior of ovaries, adrenal glands, or pituitary glands. If a myelodysplastic syndrome is drug-induced, a code from T36–T50 should be assigned and sequenced prior to the code from category D46. When reporting post-transplant lymphoproliferative disorder (PTLD), a code from category T86 should be assigned to identify a complication of transplanted organs and tissue, followed by code D47.z1.

Note that a neoplasm can be examined thoroughly yet can be determined to be of uncertain behavior. However, codes for neoplasms of unspecified nature are rarely used. Because of the higher degree of specificity afforded by ICD-10-CM's more numerous codes and the necessary specificity in documentation for an encounter, neoplasms will almost always be identified to the degree necessary to avoid a code for "unspecified nature." When contemplating a code for a neoplasm of unspecified nature, examine the available documentation and query the provider if necessary.

Spotlight on A&P

A variety of names are used for neoplastic conditions classified as being of unspecified or uncertain behavior. Become familiar with these terms, so that you can recognize and code these conditions correctly.

uncertain behavior
Describes neoplasms for which histologic confirmation regarding whether the neoplasm is malignant or benign cannot be made.

CODING TIP ▶

Uncertain behavior means that histologic confirmation regarding whether the neoplasm is malignant or benign cannot be made.

Think About It 9.5

also available in

connect plus+

Assign ICD-10-CM codes for the following situations, applying any appropriate sequencing guidelines.

1. Polycythemia vera _____

2. Malignant hydatidiform mole _____

3. Post-transplant lymphoproliferative disorder following liver transplant _____

4. Retinal freckle _____

5. Myelodysplastic syndrome with 5q deletion _____

Beyond the Code: In your opinion, should a neoplasm of a transplanted organ always be considered a complication?

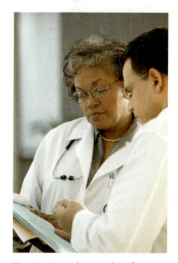

Use caution when coding for neoplasms of uncertain or unspecified behavior. Query the physician if an encounter's documentation does not provide enough specificity to code the encounter.

Chapter Summary

Learning Outcome	Key Concepts/Examples
9.1 Apply general neoplasm coding guidelines. (pages 125–128)	• Neoplasms are classified primarily by site or topography, within subsections to identify behavior as malignant, in situ, benign, uncertain, or unspecified. • If the reason for the encounter is solely for the administration of chemotherapy, immunotherapy, or radiation therapy, a code from the Z51 category should be assigned as the principal or first-listed diagnosis, with the malignancy assigned as an additional code.
9.2 Discuss aspects of coding malignant neoplasms. (pages 128–131)	• For malignant neoplasms, many of the categories have instructions to assign additional codes to identify any alcohol abuse and dependence, history of tobacco use, tobacco dependence, or tobacco use. • If Kaposi's sarcoma is associated with human immunodeficiency virus (HIV) disease, code B20 should be assigned prior to the code for Kaposi's sarcoma in category C46.
9.3 Identify terms used to document in situ neoplasms. (pages 131–132)	• In situ neoplasms are non-invasive. • The term *dysplasia* is often used when documenting in situ neoplasms.
9.4 Classify conditions related to benign neoplasms. (page 132)	• When reporting benign neoplasm of the pancreas, ovary, testis, thyroid, and other endocrine glands, an additional code should be assigned to identify functional activity.
9.5 Describe neoplasms of uncertain behavior and neoplasms of unspecified behavior. (page 133)	• Uncertain behavior means that histologic confirmation regarding whether the neoplasm is malignant or benign cannot be made. • When reporting post-transplant lymphoproliferative disorder (PTLD), a code from category T86 should be assigned to identify a complication of transplanted organs and tissue, followed by code D47.z1.

Applying Your Skills

For each condition, assign the appropriate code(s) using ICD-9-CM and ICD-10-CM.

Condition	ICD-9-CM	ICD-10-CM
1. [LO 9.2] Osteosarcoma of the left fibula	_____	_____
2. [LO 9.2.] Melanoma of the right forearm	_____	_____
3. [LO 9.2.] Adenocarcinoma of the distal esophagus	_____	_____
4. [LO 9.3.] Ductal carcinoma in situ (DCIS) of the left breast axillary tail in a female patient	_____	_____
5. [LO 9.1.] Multiple myeloma in remission	_____	_____
6. [LO 9.1.] Adenocarcinoma of the transverse colon	_____	_____
7. [LO 9.1.] Patient with large-cell undifferentiated carcinoma of the left lower lobe of the lung admitted for treatment focused on brain metastasis (two codes, must be sequenced properly)	_____	_____
8. [LO 9.1.] Patient with adenocarcinoma of the prostate seen for radiation therapy (two codes, must be sequenced properly)	_____	_____
9. [LO 9.1.] Burkitt's lymphoma of the facial nodes	_____	_____
10. [LO 9.1.] Chronic lymphocytic B-cell type leukemia in remission	_____	_____
11. [LO 9.1.] Infiltrating (invasive) lobular carcinoma (ILC) of the upper inner quadrant of the right breast in a male patient	_____	_____
12. [LO 9.1.] Malignant neoplasm of the anterior bladder wall	_____	_____
13. [LO 9.1.] Malignant lesion of contiguous sites in the esophagus	_____	_____
14. [LO 9.5.] Polycythemia vera	_____	_____
15. [LO 9.5.] Transitional cell papilloma of the right ureter	_____	_____
16. [LO 9.1.] Medullary carcinoma of the thyroid (MTC)	_____	_____
17. [LO 9.1.] Patient admitted for additional surgical treatment of site of previously excised microinvasive squamous cell carcinoma of the skin of the nose	_____	_____
18. [LO 9.1.] Primary adenocarcinoma of the uterine endocervix	_____	_____
19. [LO 9.1.] Malignant carcinoid tumor of the rectum	_____	_____
20. [LO 9.1.] Patient admitted for surgical treatment of squamous cell carcinoma of the parotid gland, which was determined to be metastatic from a skin lesion of the scalp, which was recently excised (two codes, must be sequenced properly)	_____	_____

Checking Your Understanding

Select the letter that best answers the question or completes the sentence.

1. *[LO 9.2]* What is the correct coding assignment for a patient with AIDS-related Kaposi's sarcoma of the skin of the right lower leg?

   a. B20, C44.71   **b.** C46.0
   c. C46.0, B20   **d.** B20, C46.0

2. *[LO 9.4]* What should be reported with an additional code when coding benign neoplasm of the pancreas, ovary, testis, thyroid, and other endocrine glands?

   a. risk factors   **b.** functional activity
   c. symptoms   **d.** sequelae

3. *[LO 9.1]* Which of the following is not a behavioral classification of neoplasms?

   a. benign   **b.** in situ
   c. malignant   **d.** transitional

4. *[LO 9.3]* *Dysplasia* is a term often used to document what kind of neoplasms?

   a. benign   **b.** in situ
   c. of uncertain behavior   **d.** unspecified

5. *[LO 9.2]* What is the appropriate code assignment for a patient with advanced metastatic disease and no known primary or secondary sites are specified?

   a. C80.0   **b.** C80.1
   c. C76.7   **d.** C79.9

6. *[LO 9.1]* What is the principal diagnosis if a patient is admitted for administration of chemotherapy for malignancy of a metastatic site?

   a. encounter for antineoplastic chemotherapy
   b. the primary neoplasm
   c. the secondary neoplasm
   d. A physician query must be performed to determine the principal diagnosis.

7. *[LO 9.3]* Non-invasive neoplasms are classified as

   a. benign.   **b.** in situ.
   c. of uncertain behavior.   **d.** unspecified.

8. *[LO 9.5]* What condition should be coded prior to assigning a code for post-transplant lymphoproliferative disorder?

   a. complication of transplanted organs and tissue
   b. abnormal CBC findings
   c. specific site of biopsy for diagnosis
   d. status post-transplant

9. *[LO 9.4]* Which of the following should be reported with an additional code when coding benign neuroendocrine tumors?

   a. functional activity   **b.** symptoms
   c. multiple endocrine neoplasia   **d.** residual effects

10. *[LO 9.1]* If a patient has had a malignancy surgically removed and no further treatment is needed, it is coded as

    a. a primary malignancy.   **b.** history.
    c. remission.   **d.** a secondary malignancy.

Real-World Application: Case Study

[LO 11.3] Assign ICD-10-CM codes for the following office visit note.

History of Present Illness: 53-year-old woman with a history of pancytopenia presented for follow-up after bone marrow biopsy.

Current Medications: Furosemide 80 mg b.i.d.

Allergies: No known medication allergies.

Review of Systems: As per the HPI, otherwise negative.

Past Medical History: Chronic renal disease.

Social History: Denies tobacco use. Occasional alcohol use. Married, lives with husband and two teenage children. Works part-time in office setting.

Family History: Unremarkable.

Physical Exam:

General: blood pressure 120/68, pulse 80, and temperature 98.8.

HEENT: PERRLA, no oropharyngeal lesions.

Lymphatic: No cervical or axillary lymphadenopathy.

Heart: Regular rate and rhythm; no murmurs, rubs, or gallops.

Lungs: Clear to auscultation bilaterally.

Abdomen: Nontender, no distention, active bowel sounds, no hepatosplenomegaly.

Extremities: No edema noted.

Assessment:

1. Erythropoietin resistant anemia
2. Stage IV chronic renal disease

Plan: CMP today to reassess kidney function. Add prednisone, Bactrim double strength 1 tablet b.i.d. CBC and follow up in one month.

12

MENTAL AND BEHAVIORAL DISORDERS

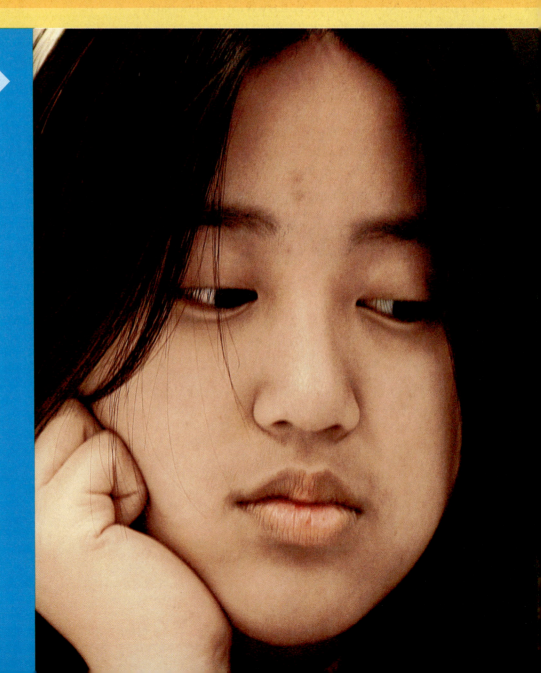

Learning Outcomes *After completing this chapter, students should be able to*

12.1 Explain coding for mental disorders due to physiological conditions and psychoactive substance use.

12.2 Classify schizophrenia and delusional, non-mood psychotic, and mood disorders.

12.3 Apply coding guidelines for anxiety, behavioral, and adult personality disorders.

12.4 Assign codes appropriately sequenced for mental retardation and pervasive and specific developmental disorders.

12.5 Determine appropriate code assignment for childhood and adolescent behavioral and emotional disorders.

Key Terms

abuse
delirium
dementia
dependence
developmental disorders
mental retardation
mood disorders
organic brain syndrome
pervasive developmental
  disorder
schizophrenia
somatoform disorders
use

Introduction

Mental and behavioral disorders are classified in a group for the purposes of both ICD-9-CM and ICD-10-CM. These disorders can be caused by genetic factors, issues during fetal development, chemical imbalances, environmental factors, physiological conditions, or psychoactive substance abuse. Conditions coded in this category include **schizophrenia,** delusional disorders, non-mood psychotic disorders, **mood disorders,** anxiety, behavioral disorders, adult personality disorders, mental retardation, **pervasive** and specific **developmental disorders,** childhood and adolescent behavioral disorders, and emotional disorders. ICD-9-CM classifies these conditions in Chapter 5, which includes code categories 290–319. ICD-10-CM classifies these conditions in Chapter 5, which includes code categories F01–F99.

Use extreme caution when assigning the codes in this chapter. Many of these disorders have serious implications for current and future insurance coverage if they are mistakenly reported for patients. If you have any questions about which codes to assign, ask for help or query the physician.

12.1 Mental Disorders Due to Physiological Conditions and Psychoactive Substance Use

This section addresses codes for mental disorders due to known physiological conditions and mental and behavioral disorders due to psychoactive substance use. When coding the mental disorders due to physiological conditions, you will note that most of the conditions require the assignment of multiple codes, one for the mental disorder and another code for the underlying physiological condition. Substance use codes are classified according to substance, then subclassified to specify if it is simply use or more serious abuse or dependence, along with the presence or absence of withdrawal, psychosis, or other manifestations. The conditions discussed are reported with codes in categories F01–F19.

> ### Spotlight on A&P
>
> Coding mental disorders due to known physiological conditions requires coders to be familiar with the physiological processes that can cause mental disorders when a variety of pathophysiological changes or deterioration of the anatomic structures in the brain or nervous system occur. Pharmacology knowledge is also important when coding substance use/abuse/dependence conditions.

F01–F09 Mental Disorders Due to Known Physiological Conditions

Codes in this subsection of ICD-10-CM correspond with those in categories 290, 293–294, 296, and 310 in ICD-9-CM. Conditions in this subsection include, but are not limited to, **organic brain syndrome, dementia** due to vascular disorders or other disease processes, and postconcussion

---

schizophrenia Disorder of perception, thought, emotion, and behavior.

mood disorders Mental disorders characterized by disturbance of mood including depression, mania, seasonal affective disorder (SAD), and cyclothymia.

pervasive developmental disorder Developmental disorder that involves many functions.

developmental disorders Impairments in cognitive, physical, social, or emotional growth.

organic brain syndrome Any of a group of mental disorders associated with impaired cerebral function, brain damage, or a non-psychiatric medical condition.

dementia Chronic, progressive, irreversible loss of the mind's cognitive and intellectual functions.

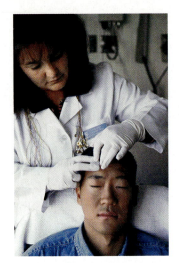

When coding for mental conditions due to physiological conditions, such as epilepsy, sequence the underlying physiological condition's code before the code for the mental disorder.

delirium Acute altered state of consciousness with agitation and disorientation; this condition is reversible.

use Intake of a substance in a non-abusive manner.

abuse Incorrect usage of substances such as drugs and alcohol, whether prescribed or not.

dependence Addiction to or reliance on a drug in order to function.

CODING TIP ▶

Classification of the use of, abuse of, and dependence on drugs and alcohol is done solely by the physician; if you ever have any doubt, query the physician for clarification.

syndrome. Most codes in this subsection include instructions for sequencing the underlying physiological condition prior to the code for the mental disorder. Some of the common physiological conditions that can cause mental disorders classified in this category are Alzheimer's disease, Lewy bodies, epilepsy, HIV, hypercalcemia, hypothyroidism, multiple sclerosis, Parkinson's disease, systemic lupus erythematosus, and vitamin B deficiency.

F10–F19 Mental and Behavioral Disorders Due to Psychoactive Substance Use

Codes in this subsection of ICD-10-CM correspond with those in categories 291, 303, and 305.0 in ICD-9-CM. Note that ICD-10-CM has introduced the classification F109 for alcohol use, which did not exist in ICD-9-CM. A major change from ICD-9-CM that was introduced in ICD-10-CM was the addition of codes to specify the use of alcohol and drugs. Previously, the only designations were for abuse and dependence of these substances, and simple use of the substances either was not reported or was classified as abuse. Another change from ICD-9-CM to ICD-10-CM that coders will notice is that, rather than referencing a list of fifth digits for unspecified, continuous, episodic, or in remission, these specifications are simply provided with each code. ICD-10-CM has also expanded the substance-related disorders. When coding for disorders related to drugs and alcohol, the new specifications in ICD-10-CM include options for uncomplicated, remission, current intoxication, the presence of **delirium,** mood disorders, psychotic disorders, delusions, hallucinations, amnestic disorders, perceptual disturbances, sexual dysfunction, sleep disorders, anxiety disorders, and withdrawal. An example of the variables that are specified for substance-related disorders is demonstrated by code F12.151, cannabis abuse with psychotic disorder with hallucinations. The classification of the **use** of, **abuse** of, and **dependence** on drugs and alcohol is done solely by the physician; if you ever have any doubt, query the physician for clarification.

Think About It 12.1

also available in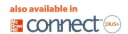

Assign ICD-10-CM codes for the following situations, applying any appropriate sequencing guidelines.

1. Early-onset Alzheimer's disease with aggressive behavior _____

2. Alcohol use with hallucinations, blood alcohol level of 250 mg/100 ml _____

3. Alprazolam dependence with withdrawal delirium _____

4. Postconcussion encephalopathy _____

5. Caffeine abuse _____

Beyond the Code: A major change from ICD-9-CM to ICD-10-CM was the addition of codes to specify the use of alcohol and drugs, in addition to reporting abuse and dependence. What are some examples of when this code may be assigned and what documentation obstacles might exist?

12.2 Schizophrenia and Delusional, Non-mood Psychotic, and Mood Disorders

Schizophrenia; schizotypal, delusional, and other non-mood psychotic disorders; and mood disorders are classified by codes in this section. When comparing ICD-9-CM and ICD-10-CM classifications for these disorders, note that remission is no longer specified in ICD-10-CM. The conditions discussed in this section are reported with codes in categories F20–F39.

F20–F29 Schizophrenia, Schizotypal, Delusional, and Other Non-mood Psychotic Disorders

Codes in this subsection of ICD-10-CM correspond with those in category 295 in ICD-9-CM. This is another subsection, which is presented differently in ICD-10-CM than it was in ICD-9-CM, as coders are no longer required to indicate the course of an illness, such as chronic, subchronic, acute exacerbation, or in remission; rather, schizophrenia and schizoaffective disorders are simply classified according to type in ICD-10-CM. The types of schizophrenia included in this section include paranoid, disorganized, catatonic, and residual. What was previously reported in ICD-9-CM as 295.22, chronic catatonic schizophrenia, is now just reported as F20.2, catatonic schizophrenia, in ICD-10-CM. This subsection also includes schizotypal disorder, delusional disorders, brief and shared psychotic disorders, and schizoaffective disorders.

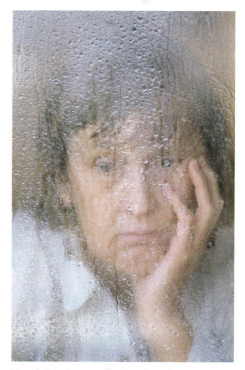

Mood disorders, or affective disorders, are classified by their symptoms and severity. ICD-10-CM provides specifications for severity with individual codes, rather than fifth digits in the same code.

F30–F39 Mood (Affective) Disorders

Codes in this subsection of ICD-10-CM correspond with those in category 296 in ICD-9-CM. These disorders are generally classified according to presentation of symptoms and severity. This is another subsection that experienced a change from ICD-9-CM to ICD-10-CM; coders will no longer reference a list of fifth digits for unspecified, mild, moderate, severe, with psychotic behavior, or in remission; rather, ICD-10-CM provides these specifications with each code. An example of a code from this subsection is F32.3, major depressive disorder, single episode, severe with psychotic features.

CODING TIP ▶

Mood (affective) disorders are generally classified according to presentation of their symptoms and their severity.

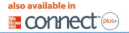
12.3 Anxiety, Behavioral, and Adult Personality Disorders

This section addresses codes for anxiety, dissociative, stress-related, somatoform, and non-psychotic disorders; behavioral syndromes associated with physiological disturbances and physical factors; and disorders of adult personality and behavior. The conditions discussed are reported with codes in categories F40–F69.

Spotlight on A&P

Many terms used to describe mental and behavioral disorders may appear to be confusing, but most are easily broken down with a thorough knowledge of basic medical terminology.

F40–F48 Anxiety, Dissociative, Stress-Related, Somatoform, and Other Non-psychotic Mental Disorders

somatoform disorders
Disorders characterized by physical symptoms without an identifiable physical cause.

Codes in this subsection of ICD-10-CM correspond with those in categories 300, 308, and 309 in ICD-9-CM. This subsection includes codes for phobias, panic disorders, anxiety disorders, stress disorders, adjustment disorders, dissociative and conversion disorders, and **somatoform disorders.**

If a patient has pain that is documented as being exclusively psychological, code F45.41 should be assigned. Acute or chronic pain that is documented as having a psychological component should be reported with a code from category G89, followed by F45.41. This instruction is supported by coding guideline *I.C.5.a. Pain disorders related to psychological factors.*

CODING TIP ▸

Assign code F45.41 for pain that is exclusively psychological.

F49

Note that there is no category F49.

F50–F59 Behavioral Syndromes Associated with Physiological Disturbances and Physical Factors

Codes in this subsection of ICD-10-CM correspond with those in categories 293, 302, and 307 in ICD-9-CM. This subsection includes codes for eating disorders, sleep disorders, sexual dysfunction not due to physiological conditions, puerperal psychoses, and abuse of non-psychoactive substances. If insomnia is due to a mental disorder, code F51.05 should be assigned, followed by a code to identify the specific mental disorder. For example, insomnia due to overanxious disorder is coded and sequenced as F51.05, insomnia due to other mental disorder, followed by F41.1, generalized anxiety disorder. Code F54, Psychological and behavioral factors associated with disorders or diseases classified elsewhere, is for use only as a secondary code, to be preceded by the code for the associated physical disorder causing the psychological or behavioral disorder.

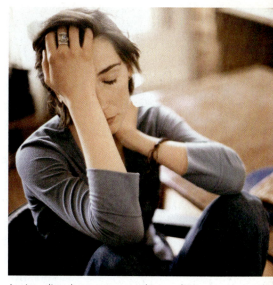
Anxiety disorders are among the conditions reported with codes in the F40–F48 range.

F60–F69 Disorders of Adult Personality and Behavior

Codes in this subsection of ICD-10-CM correspond with those in categories 297, 301, 302, and 312 in ICD-9-CM. This subsection includes codes for personality disorders, impulse disorders, gender identity disorders, and paraphilias. When reporting gender identity disorders of adolescence and adulthood with code F64.1, if the patient has had sex reassignment surgery, Z87.890, personal history of sex reassignment, should be used as a secondary code.

Think About It 12.3

also available in **McGraw Hill connect** plus+

Assign ICD-10-CM codes for the following situations, applying any appropriate sequencing guidelines.

1. Fear of injections and transfusions _____

2. Anorexia nervosa with binge eating and purging _____

3. Trichotillomania _____

4. Chronic post-traumatic stress disorder _____

5. Necrophilia _____

Beyond the Code: What are the potential implications of incorrectly reporting pain disorders with code F45.41 or F45.42?

12.4 Mental Retardation and Pervasive and Specific Developmental Disorders

mental retardation
Below-average intellectual functional level evident before age 18, associated with lack of the skills needed for daily living.

This section addresses the codes for **mental retardation** and pervasive and specific developmental disorders. These conditions are reported with codes in categories F70–F89.

F70–F79 Mental Retardation

Codes in this subsection of ICD-10-CM correspond with those in categories 317–319 in ICD-9-CM. Note that there is an instruction at the beginning of this subsection that directs the coder to sequence a code for an associated physical or developmental disorder prior to codes in this section. For example, atypical autism with mild mental retardation and IQ of 60 should be reported with code F84.9, pervasive developmental disorder, unspecified, sequenced first, followed by code F70, mild mental retardation, as a secondary code. Mental retardation codes are assigned according to the level of retardation that is based on IQ. The methods of documentation of mental retardation level may vary by provider.

> **CODING TIP ▸**
>
> Mental retardation codes are assigned according to the level of retardation that is based on IQ.

F80–F89 Pervasive and Specific Developmental Disorders

Codes in this subsection of ICD-10-CM correspond with those in categories 299 and 315 in ICD-9-CM. This subsection includes codes for speech and language developmental disorders, developmental disorders of scholastic skills, and pervasive developmental disorders. The type of hearing loss should be identified with a secondary code when assigning F80.4, speech and language development delay due to hearing loss. Coders should note that, when coding pervasive developmental disorders, such as autism, Rett's syndrome, or Asperger's syndrome, an additional code should be assigned to report any documented associated medical conditions and mental retardation.

Think About It 12.4   also available in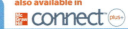

Assign ICD-10-CM codes for the following situations, applying any appropriate sequencing guidelines.

1. Developmental dyslexia with mild mental retardation and IQ of 60 _____

2. Clumsy child syndrome _____

3. Expressive language disorder with profound mental retardation and IQ of 15 _____

4. Autistic disorder with moderate mental retardation and IQ of 45 _____

5. Mathematics disorder _____

Beyond the Code: What is the significance of medical conditions, such as neurologic conditions, that are associated with pervasive developmental disorders?

12.5 Childhood and Adolescent Behavioral and Emotional Disorders

This section discusses the classification of behavioral and emotional disorders with an onset usually occurring in childhood and adolescence, along with unspecified mental illness. Aside from two codes in the section with instructional notes, coding of the conditions in this section is straightforward. The conditions discussed are reported with codes in categories F90–F99.

F90–F99 Behavioral and Emotional Disorders with Onset Usually Occurring in Childhood and Adolescence

Codes in this subsection of ICD-10-CM correspond with those in categories 307, 309, 312, and 314 in ICD-9-CM. This subsection includes codes for childhood and adolescent disorders including, but not limited to, attention deficit hyperactivity disorders, conduct disorders, childhood-specific emotional disorders, childhood and adolescent social functioning disorders, and tic disorders. These codes may be assigned for patients of any age. Although the onset of the disorders in this subsection is generally within the childhood or adolescent years, they may continue throughout life or not be diagnosed until adulthood. An additional code should be reported with F94.1, reactive attachment disorder of childhood, to identify associated failure to thrive or growth retardation. The cause of coexisting constipation should be specified through a secondary code when reporting psychogenic encopresis.

Category F99, unspecified mental disorder, is to be used only if the documentation is for a mental illness with no further specification. The use of this code should be rare, as specification should be attainable through physician query.

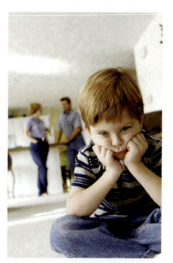

Although some behavioral and emotional conditions are classified as having an onset in childhood, the codes for these conditions may be assigned at any age.

> **CODING TIP ▸**
>
> Although the onset of the disorders in this subsection is generally within the childhood or adolescent years, they may continue throughout life or not be diagnosed until adulthood.

Think About It 12.5

also available in **connect** plus+

Assign ICD-10-CM codes for the following situations, applying any appropriate sequencing guidelines.

1. Psychogenic enuresis _____

2. Tourette's syndrome _____

3. Attention deficit hyperactivity disorder, predominantly inattentive _____

4. Oppositional defiant disorder _____

5. Nail biting _____

Beyond the Code: What are some reasons that some of the disorders in this subsection have an onset within the childhood or adolescent years but may not be diagnosed until adulthood?

Chapter Summary

Learning Outcome	Key Concepts/Examples
12.1 Explain coding for mental disorders due to physiological conditions and psychoactive substance use. **(pages 167–168)**	• A major change from ICD-9-CM to ICD-10-CM was the addition of codes to specify the use of alcohol and drugs, in addition to reporting abuse and dependence. • Classification of the use of, abuse of, and dependence on drugs and alcohol is done solely by the physician; if there is ever any doubt, the coder should query the physician for clarification.
12.2 Classify schizophrenia, delusional, non-mood psychotic, and mood disorders. **(pages 169–170)**	• Mood (affective) disorders are generally classified according to presentation of symptoms and severity.
12.3 Apply coding guidelines for anxiety, behavioral, and adult personality disorders. **(page 172)**	• Assign code F45.41 for pain that is exclusively psychological.
12.4 Assign codes appropriately sequenced for mental retardation and pervasive and specific developmental disorders. **(page 172)**	• Mental retardation codes are assigned according to the level of retardation that is based on IQ. • A code for an associated physical or developmental disorder is to be sequenced prior to codes for mental retardation.
12.5 Determine appropriate code assignment for childhood and adolescent behavioral and emotional disorders. **(page 173)**	• Although the onset of disorders in this subsection is generally within the childhood or adolescent years, they may continue throughout life or not be diagnosed until adulthood.

Applying Your Skills

Assign codes for the following conditions, using both ICD-9-CM and ICD-10-CM.

Condition	ICD-9-CM Codes	ICD-10-CM Codes
1. *[LO 12.4]* Asperger's syndrome		
2. *[LO 12.1]* Dementia with combative behavior due to vitamin B deficiency		
3. *[LO 12.3]* Laxative abuse		
4. *[LO 12.5]* Attention deficit hyperactivity disorder, predominantly hyperactive		
5. *[LO 12.1]* Late-onset Alzheimer's dementia with combativeness		
6. *[LO 12.5]* Nose picking		
7. *[LO 12.4]* Landau-Kleffner		
8. *[LO 12.3]* Münchhausen's syndrome		
9. *[LO 12.2]* Subchronic catatonic schizophrenia		
10. *[LO 12.3]* Antisocial personality disorder		
11. *[LO 12.3]* Postpartum depression		
12. *[LO 12.4]* Moderate mental retardation with IQ of 36		
13. *[LO 12.3]* Acute post-traumatic stress disorder		
14. *[LO 12.2]* Bipolar disorder with current severe depression without psychotic symptoms		
15. *[LO 12.1]* Hangover from alcohol		
16. *[LO 12.1]* Postconcussion syndrome		
17. *[LO 12.5]* Childhood separation anxiety		
18. *[LO 12.1]* Presenile dementia without complications		
19. *[LO 12.3]* Fear of blood		
20. *[LO 12.1]* Uncomplicated dependence on chewing tobacco		

Checking Your Understanding

Select the letter that best answers the question or completes the sentence.

1. *[LO 12.2]* Which of the following is a classification of schizophrenia in ICD-10-CM?

   a. disorganized
   b. subchronic
   c. acute exacerbation
   d. in remission

2. *[LO 12.4]* What condition should be sequenced prior to codes for mental retardation?

   a. confusion
   b. associated physical or developmental disorders
   c. decreased functional status
   d. social factors

3. *[LO 12.1]* Who is the source of documentation for the classification of the use of, abuse of, or dependence on drugs and alcohol?

   a. addiction counselor
   b. addiction counselor and physician
   c. physician
   d. statement by the patient at admission

4. *[LO 12.3]* What is the appropriate code assignment for the documentation of persistent somatoform pain disorder?

   a. F45.41
   b. R52
   c. F45.41, R52
   d. R52, F45.41

5. *[LO 12.1]* Why must coders be cautious about assigning codes from this chapter?

   a. Many codes in this chapter are very similar and easily confused with each other.
   b. Documentation for these conditions is frequently unclear.
   c. There are no guidelines for coding these conditions.
   d. There may be serious implications for current and future insurance coverage if they are mistakenly reported.

6. *[LO 12.5]* What type of patient records may have codes in the F90–F98 subsection assigned?

   a. adults only
   b. children only
   c. adolescents only
   d. patients of any age

7. *[LO 12.1]* Which of the following is not identified in ICD-10-CM when coding for alcohol and drugs?

   a. current intoxication
   b. episodic
   c. hallucinations
   d. withdrawal

8. *[LO 12.2]* Mood (affective) disorders are generally classified according to

   a. presence or absence of psychotic behavior.
   b. remission.
   c. exacerbation.
   d. presentation of symptoms and severity.

9. *[LO 12.1]* Which of the following is not part of a code assignment for alcohol and drugs in ICD-10-CM?

   a. abuse
   b. dependence
   c. episodic
   d. use

10. *[LO 12.4]* How are mental retardation codes classified?

   a. according to the level of retardation based on IQ
   b. according to associated developmental disorders
   c. according to the documented level of functioning
   d. according to associated physical disorders

Online Activity

[LO 12.1, LO 12.2, LO 12.3, LO 12.4, LO 12.5] Search online for information about reimbursement issues related to coding for mental and behavioral disorders. Outline your findings in a brief report.

Real-World Application: Case Study

[LO 12.2, LO 12.5] Assign ICD-10-CM codes for the following psychiatric hospitalization note.

Discharge Summary

Hospital Course: This 14-year-old patient was admitted with significant mood swings noted by parents. Initial presentation was depressed. Oppositional behavior was displayed toward staff on the unit. Therapist discussed family and school conflicts with the patient. Zoloft and Adderall were initiated with noted improvement during hospitalization.

Diagnostic Findings: Sleep-deprived EEG was performed and reported as normal. Basic metabolic panel, CBC, and TSH were reported within normal limits.

Final Diagnosis:

Axis I: Predominantly Inattentive Attention Deficit Hyperactivity Disorder, Bipolar Disorder currently with mild depression, and Oppositional Defiant Disorder.

Axis II: Deferred.

Axis III: Unremarkable.

Axis IV: Psychosocial stressors: Severe, peer, school, and family conflicts with educational problems.

Axis V: GAF: 45 to 50.

Discharge Disposition and Plan: The patient was discharged to home with appropriate mood, with denial of suicidal or homicidal ideation. Outpatient treatment to continue for patient with family sessions once a week. Parents instructed about medication regimen, importance of continuing treatment, and reporting side effects or significant behavioral changes immediately.

13

NERVOUS SYSTEM AND SENSE ORGANS

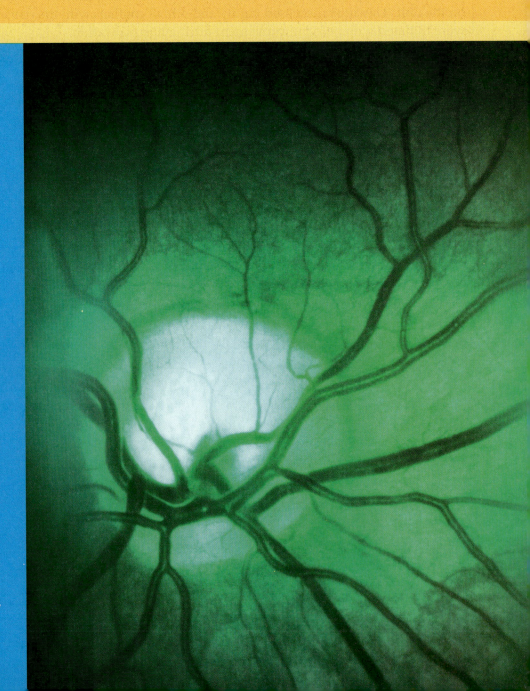

Learning Outcomes *After completing this chapter, students should be able to*

13.1 Explore documentation needs for diseases of the central nervous system and extrapyramidal movement disorders.

13.2 Analyze documentation and additional conditions to report with episodic and paroxysmal disorders, nerve disorders, polyneuropathies, and diseases of the myoneural junction and muscle.

13.3 Discuss coding guidelines for cerebral palsy, paralytic syndromes, and other disorders of the nervous system.

13.4 Assign codes for diseases of the eye and adnexa.

13.5 Identify terminology used for classification of diseases of the ear and mastoid process.

Key Terms

Alzheimer's dementia
Alzheimer's disease
aphakia
cataract
central nervous system
choroid
cranial nerves
demyelinating
encephalitis
encephalopathy
epilepsy
extrapyramidal
glaucoma
hemiparesis
hemiplegia
Huntington's disease
intractable
meningitis
migraine
multiple sclerosis
myoneural junction
neuropathy
palsy
paraplegia
Parkinson's disease
paroxysmal
plexus
quadriplegia
transient ischemic attacks

Introduction

This chapter is unique from the rest of the disease coding chapters in this text in that, instead of discussing only one chapter of the ICD-10-CM manual, it includes three chapters: diseases of the nervous system, the eye, and the ear. As the coding profession transitions from ICD-9-CM to ICD-10-CM, coders already familiar with ICD-9-CM can recognize and navigate this chapter's contents easily, whereas new coders will find it a helpful illustration of the new organization in ICD-10-CM.

Conditions in this chapter were previously reported in ICD-9-CM Chapter 6, "Diseases of the Nervous System and Sense Organs," which included categories 320–389. However, ICD-10-CM splits these conditions into three chapters. Chapter 6, "Diseases of the Nervous System," includes code categories G00–G99. Chapter 7, "Diseases of the Eye and Adnexa," includes categories H00–H59. Chapter 8, "Diseases of the Ear and Mastoid Process," includes categories H60–H95.

13.1 Diseases of the Central Nervous System and Extrapyramidal Movement Disorders

Central nervous system diseases and **extrapyramidal** movement disorders include inflammatory diseases, systemic atrophies, degenerative diseases, and **demyelinating** diseases. These conditions are classified by codes in categories G00–G37 in ICD-10-CM. Reporting of conditions in this section is sometimes complex, with the need to assign combination codes and multiple codes for complete and accurate identification of disease processes.

central nervous system Part of the nervous system composed of the brain and spinal cord.

extrapyramidal Related to the section of the brain that coordinates movement.

demyelinating Causing the loss of myelin from the nerve sheath, which slows conduction.

Spotlight on A&P

Many conditions reported in this section involve assignment for causative factors or manifestations. Pay attention to physiological processes that may be impacted between the central nervous system and other anatomic functions with disease processes identified. A diagram of the nervous system is provided in Figure 13.1.

G00–G09 Inflammatory Diseases of the Central Nervous System

Codes in this subsection of ICD-10-CM correspond with those in categories 320–326 in ICD-9-CM. Conditions classified to this subsection include **meningitis, encephalitis, encephalopathy,** intracranial and intraspinal abscesses and granulomas, intracranial and intraspinal phlebitis and thrombophlebitis, and sequelae of central nervous system inflammatory diseases. Note that all conditions in this subsection require coders

meningitis Inflammatory disease of the meninges, which are the membranes covering the brain and spinal cord

encephalitis Inflammation of brain cells and tissues.

encephalopathy Any disease of the brain.

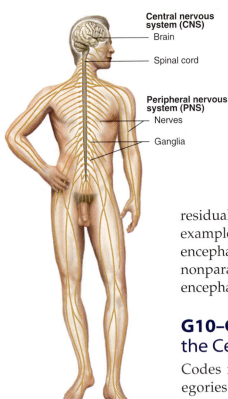

figure 13.1 The Nervous System

Central nervous
system (CNS)
— Brain
— Spinal cord

Peripheral nervous
system (PNS)
— Nerves
— Ganglia

Huntington's disease
Rare genetic disorder that appears at age 30–40, characterized by neurologic degeneration and usually resulting in death.

Parkinson's disease
Disease of the brain that causes muscular rigidity, tremors, and a masklike facial expression.

to assign an additional code for the purpose of reporting the infectious agent. One exception to this is in category G05, encephalitis, myelitis, and encephalomyelitis in diseases classified elsewhere, as both codes in this category are designated as being secondary codes to follow the code to report underlying diseases, such as poliovirus, suppurative otitis media, or trichinellosis. The other exception in this subsection is for code G09, sequelae of inflammatory diseases of central nervous system, which is used to report that there are residual effects from inflammatory diseases of the central nervous system. Code G09 is accompanied by instructions to first assign the code for the residual condition and then assign code G09 as a secondary code. For example, if a patient with acute nonparalytic poliomyelitis has associated encephalomyelitis, the appropriate code assignment is code A80.4, acute nonparalytic poliomyelitis, followed by code G05.3, encephalitis and encephalomyelitis in diseases classified elsewhere.

G10–G14 Systemic Atrophies Primarily Affecting the Central Nervous System

Codes in this subsection of ICD-10-CM correspond with those in categories 333–335 and 138 in ICD-9-CM. ICD-9-CM classifies postpolio myelitic syndrome with infectious diseases, whereas ICD-10-CM recognizes it as a neurologic condition. Conditions classified to this subsection in ICD-10-CM include **Huntington's disease,** hereditary ataxias, spinal muscular atrophies, related syndromes, and systemic atrophies primarily affecting the central nervous system in diseases classified elsewhere, and postpolio syndrome. Codes in category G13 are to be assigned as secondary codes, following assignment of underlying neoplasm or underlying diseases, such as hypothyroidism or myxedematous congenital iodine deficiency. For example, the appropriate code assignment for central nervous system atrophy caused by systemic atrophy from postinfectious hypothyroidism is, first, code E03.3, postinfectious hypothyroidism, followed by code G13.8, systemic atrophy primarily affecting central nervous system in other diseases classified elsewhere, as a secondary code.

G15–G19

Note that there are no categories G15–G19.

G20–G26 Extrapyramidal and Movement Disorders

Codes in this subsection of ICD-10-CM correspond with those in categories 332–333 in ICD-9-CM. This subsection includes codes for **Parkinson's disease,** degenerative diseases of the basal ganglia, dystonia, extrapyramidal disorders, and movement disorders. One instruction in this subsection that differs between ICD-9-CM and ICD-10-CM is the sequencing of codes for conditions caused by medications or other external agents. ICD-9-CM required the medication or external agent to be sequenced as a secondary code, but ICD-10-CM requires the causal agent to be sequenced prior to the codes in this subsection. For example, tardive dyskinesia caused by Haldol would appropriately be reported by first assigning code T43.4x5, adverse effect of butyrophenone and thiothixene neuroleptics, followed by G24.01, drug induced subacute dyskinesia, as a secondary code.

G27–G29

Note that there are no categories G27–G29.

G30–G32 Other Degenerative Diseases of the Nervous System

Codes in this subsection of ICD-10-CM correspond with those in categories 330, 331, and 336 in ICD-9-CM. Conditions reported by codes in this subsection include **Alzheimer's disease** and other degenerative diseases of the nervous system. Several instructional notes accompany the codes in this section regarding the assignment of other codes, either prior to or following the codes. A commonly reported condition in this subsection is late-onset **Alzheimer's dementia** with behavioral disturbance, which is appropriately reported by first assigning code G30.1, Alzheimer's disease with late onset, followed by the secondary code F02.81, dementia in other diseases classified elsewhere with behavioral disturbance.

G33–G34

Note that there are no categories G33 and G34.

G35–G37 Demyelinating Diseases of the Central Nervous System

Codes in this subsection of ICD-10-CM correspond with those in categories 323 and 340 in ICD-9-CM. This subsection contains codes for reporting **multiple sclerosis** and other demyelinating diseases of the central nervous system. Demyelinating diseases are those in which the myelin sheath covering the axon of nerve cells is destroyed. Figure 13.2 illustrates the structures involved. The myelin sheath facilitates quick transmission of nerve impulses. If the myelin is damaged, nerve impulses are slowed. Aside from three excludes1 notes, there are no significant instructions related to the coding of conditions in this subsection. Code assignment for a patient with multiple sclerosis is simply code G35, multiple sclerosis, without further specificity.

G38–G39

Note that there are no categories G38 and G39.

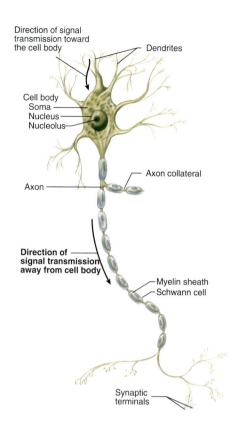

figure 13.2 Neuron

Alzheimer's disease Progressive neurologic disease of the brain that causes irreversible loss of neurons and eventual dementia.

Alzheimer's dementia Dementia characterized by loss of memory and impairment of judgment, decision making, language use, and awareness of surroundings.

multiple sclerosis Chronic demyelinating autoimmune disease of the nervous system that may cause partial paralysis, changes in speaking ability, and inability to walk.

Table 13.1 Cranial Nerves

Roman Numeral	Name	Description
I	Olfactory nerves	Sensory nerves for smell
II	Optic nerves	Sensory nerves for vision
III	Oculomotor nerves	Predominantly motor nerves for eye movement and pupil size
IV	Trochlear nerves	Predominantly motor nerves for eye movement
V	Trigeminal nerves	Sensory and motor nerves responsible for face, nose, and mouth sensations and for chewing
VI	Abducens nerves	Predominantly motor nerves responsible for eye movement
VII	Facial nerves	Mixed nerves associated with taste (sensory), facial expression (motor), and production of tears and saliva (parasympathetic fibers of motor nerves)
VIII	Vestibulocochlear (auditory) nerves	Predominantly sensory nerves associated with hearing and balance
IX	Glossopharyngeal nerves	Mixed nerves for sensation and swallowing in the pharynx
X	Vagus nerves	Mixed sensory and parasympathetic nerves supplying the pharynx, the larynx (speech), and the viscera of the thorax and abdomen
XI	Accessory nerves	Predominantly motor nerves supplying the neck muscles, pharynx, and larynx
XII	Hypoglossal nerves	Predominantly motor nerves that move the tongue in speaking, chewing, and swallowing

notes in this subsection regarding the assignment and sequencing of additional codes. Polyneuropathy in amyloidosis is reported with code E85.9, amyloidosis, unspecified, followed by code G63, polyneuropathy in diseases classified elsewhere.

G66–G69

Note that there are no categories G66–G69.

G70–G73 Diseases of Myoneural Junction and Muscle

Codes in this subsection of ICD-10-CM correspond with those in categories 358 and 359 in ICD-9-CM. Conditions reported by codes in this subsection include myesthenia gravis, myoneural disorders, primary muscle disorders, muscular dystrophy, myopathies, and disorders of myoneural junction and muscles in diseases classified elsewhere. Many codes in this subsection are designated for sequencing as secondary codes, following codes for medications, toxic agents, or other underlying diseases. Myasthenia in thyrotoxicosis with diffuse goiter and storm is coded E05.01, thyrotoxicosis with diffuse goiter with thyrotoxic crisis or storm, followed by code G73.3, myasthenic syndromes in other diseases classified elsewhere.

G74–G79

Note that there are no categories G74–G79.

Think About It 13.2

also available in McGraw Hill **connect** plus+

Assign ICD-10-CM codes for the following situations, applying any appropriate sequencing guidelines.

1. Obstructive sleep apnea _____

2. Intractable cyclical vomiting without status migrainosus _____

3. Grand mal seizure, intractable with status epilepticus _____

4. Guillain-Barré syndrome _____

5. Thoracic outlet syndrome _____

Beyond the Code: Discuss the difference between "intractable" and "status" as they pertain to migraines and epilepsy.

13.3 Cerebral Palsy, Paralytic Syndromes, and Other Disorders of the Nervous System

Coding guidelines for cerebral **palsy,** paralytic syndromes, and other disorders of the nervous system present a variety of sequencing instructions and requirements for multiple code assignment. In addition, documentation needs exist for conditions that have codes to identify laterality, along with dominance of the side impacted by these conditions.

palsy Paralysis that may be accompanied by uncontrolled tremors or loss of sensation.

hemiplegia Paralysis of one side of the body.

hemiparesis Weakness of part of one side of the body.

paraplegia Paralysis of both lower extremities.

quadriplegia Paralysis of all four limbs.

G80–G83 Cerebral Palsy and Other Paralytic Syndromes

Codes in this subsection of ICD-10-CM correspond with those in categories 342–344 in ICD-9-CM. These codes are used to report conditions that include cerebral palsies, **hemiplegia, hemiparesis, paraplegia, quadriplegia,** and other paralytic syndromes. When coding hemiplegia, hemiparesis, paraplegia, quadriplegia, and other paralytic syndromes, ICD-10-CM codes provide specificity for laterality and whether or not the dominant side is involved. If the documentation does not specify which side is dominant or if the patient is ambidextrous, the affected side is assumed to be dominant. This instruction is supported by coding guideline *I.C.6.a. Dominant/nondominant side.*

It is appropriate to assign these codes only when there is no further specification in the documentation regarding the cause, or if the paralytic condition is old or chronic in nature without specification of the initial cause. For example, if a patient experienced hemiplegia as a sequela of a cerebrovascular accident, a code from category G81, hemiplegia and hemiparesis, would not be assigned. However, if documentation reflected long-term flaccid hemiplegia of the left side in a right-handed patient, and no causal condition could be identified, it would be appropriate to report code G81.04, flaccid hemiplegia, affecting left nondominant side. The codes may be used in addition to causal codes for the purpose of identifying the type of paralytic condition.

G84–G88

Note that there are no categories G84–G88.

G89–G99 Other Disorders of the Nervous System

Codes in this subsection of ICD-10-CM correspond with those in categories 331, 336, 337, 338, 348, and 349 in ICD-9-CM. Conditions reported by codes in this subsection include pain, disorders of the autonomic nervous system, hydrocephalus, disorders of the brain, diseases of the spinal cord, other disorders of the central nervous system, and intraoperative or postprocedural complications and disorders of the nervous system that are not elsewhere classified. Code assignment for pain is generally based on the location of the pain, which is reflected in the excludes2 note in category G89, pain, not elsewhere classified. Some of these codes are located in Chapter 18 of ICD-10-CM, whereas others are classified in the chapters for the specific body systems. Sometimes it is appropriate to report a code from category G89 to provide greater detail about the pain condition. However, it is important for coders to remember the general coding guideline that prohibits the assignment of a symptom, such as pain, if a definitive diagnosis has been identified. The exception to this is if the reason for the episode of care is focused on managing the pain, rather than the underlying condition. One example of this is an admission for insertion of a neurostimulator for pain control. In this case, the appropriate code from category G89 should be reported first, followed by the code for the underlying condition as a secondary diagnosis.

If a code from category G89 provides additional information about the nature of the pain, it may be assigned in conjunction with a site-specific pain code, including codes from Chapter 18, in order to provide a complete picture of the condition. Regions of the body for referred pain are identified in Figure 13.4. Sequencing for these multiple pain-related code situations is dictated by the reasons for the episode of care. For example, an admission for the purpose of pain management in a patient with chronic low back pain due to trauma is reported with code G89.21, chronic pain due to trauma, sequenced first, followed by code M54.5, low back pain, as a secondary diagnosis code.

Additional pain codes are available to report postoperative pain, neoplasm-related pain, and chronic pain syndrome. Neoplasm-related pain is another condition that has sequencing guidelines dependent on the circumstances of admission. Greater detail about instructions for coding pain is located in coding guideline *I.C.6 b. Pain—Category G89.*

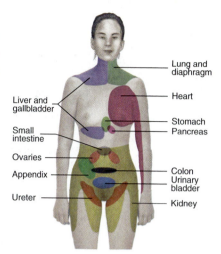

figure 13.4 Regions of Referred Pain

Think About It 13.3

also available in **connect** plus+

Assign ICD-10-CM codes for the following situations, applying any appropriate sequencing guidelines.

1. Fecal impaction causing autonomic dysreflexia

_____

2. Incomplete paraplegia

_____

3. Headache from lumbar puncture

_____

4. Benign intracranial hypertension

_____

5. Hydrocephalus due to congenital syphilitic encephalitis

_____

Beyond the Code: Symptom codes are not always reported when a definitive diagnosis is identified. What are the benefits of analysis of statistical data related to codes reported for pain? What are the shortcomings of this analysis?

13.4 Diseases of the Eye, Adnexa, Ear, and Mastoid Process

This section covers all of Chapter 7 in ICD-10-CM, which includes code categories H00–H59. However, ICD-9-CM classifies these conditions in a portion of Chapter 6— specifically, categories 360–379. Included in this section are specified disorders of the eyelid, lacrimal system, orbit, conjunctiva, sclera, cornea, iris, ciliary body, lens, **choroid,** retina, vitreous body, globe, optic nerve, visual pathways, and ocular muscles; binocular movement; accommodation; and refraction. In addition, it includes disorders such as **glaucoma,** visual disturbances and blindness, other disorders of the eye and adnexa, and intraoperative and postprocedural complications and disorders of the eye and adnexa, not elsewhere classified. Documentation for most conditions classified to this chapter of ICD-10-CM needs to specify laterality.

choroid Vascular layer between the retina and sclera.

glaucoma Common eye condition in which insufficient drainage of the fluid in the eye causes increased pressure and damage to the optic nerve, leading to impaired vision and eventual blindness.

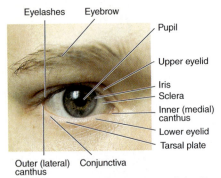

Eyelashes Eyebrow
Pupil
Upper eyelid
Iris
Sclera
Inner (medial) canthus
Lower eyelid
Tarsal plate
Outer (lateral) canthus Conjunctiva

figure 13.5 External Anatomy of the Eye

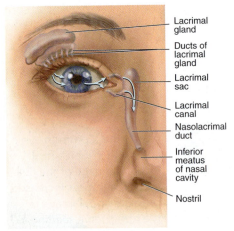

Lacrimal gland
Ducts of lacrimal gland
Lacrimal sac
Lacrimal canal
Nasolacrimal duct
Inferior meatus of nasal cavity
Nostril

figure 13.6 Lacrimal System

H00–H05 Disorders of Eyelid, Lacrimal System, and Orbit

Codes in this subsection of ICD-10-CM correspond with those in categories 373–376 in ICD-9-CM. Conditions reported include hordeolum and chalazion, other inflammation of the eyelid, other disorders of the eyelid, disorders of the lacrimal system, and disorders of the orbit. External anatomic structures of the eye are identified in Figure 13.5. Most codes in this subsection provide specificity not only for laterality but also for identification of upper versus lower eyelid. If deformity of the orbit is documented as being associated with a bone disease, the bone disease should be identified with an additional code. Note that there are no categories H03 and H06–H09.

H10–H11 Disorders of Conjunctiva

Codes in this subsection of ICD-10-CM correspond with those in category 372 in ICD-9-CM. Conjunctivitis, pterygium, conjunctival degenerations and deposits, conjunctival scars, conjunctival hemorrhage, pseudopterygium, and conjunctivochalasis are reported in this subsection. The medical diagnosis that represents the common term "pinkeye" is mucopurulent conjunctivitis, which is reported with code H10.02- (note the need for assignment of the appropriate sixth character to identify which eye is involved). The chemical and intent should be identified in the T51–T65 range, prior to the codes in subclassification H10.21 for acute toxic conjunctivitis. Structures in the lacrimal system are illustrated in 13.6.

H12–H14

Note that there are no categories H12–H14.

H15–H22 Disorders of Sclera, Cornea, Iris, and Ciliary Body

Codes in this subsection of ICD-10-CM correspond with those in categories 360, 364, 370, 371, and 379 in ICD-9-CM. Conditions reported in this subsection include disorders of the sclera, keratitis, corneal scars and opacities, other disorders of the cornea, iridocyclitis, other disorders of the iris and ciliary body, and disorders of the iris and ciliary body in diseases classified elsewhere. Anatomic structures impacted by these conditions are shown in Figure 13.7.

When reporting corneal deposits in metabolic disorders, the specific metabolic disorder should be identified with a secondary code. Kayser-Fleisher ring codes should be followed by a code for Wilson's disease, if documented. If documentation indicates that a cataract is associated with chronic iridocyclitis, an additional code should be assigned to identify the cataract. Code F21.81, floppy iris syndrome, should follow the code from

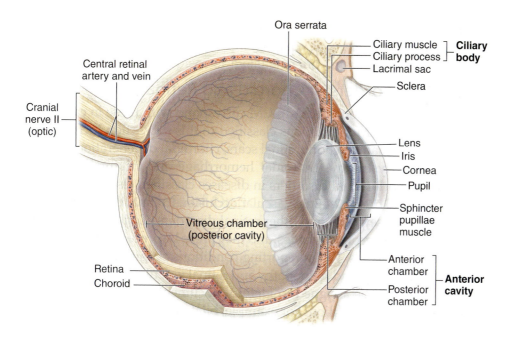

figure 13.7 Anatomy of the Eyeball

T36–T50, which specifies the causal agent. Code H22 is to be assigned only as a secondary code, following the code for the underlying disease. Note that there are no categories H19, H23, and H24.

H25–H28 Disorders of Lens

Codes in this subsection of ICD-10-CM correspond with those in categories 366 and 379 in ICD-9-CM. Age-related incipient **cataract,** other cataract, aphakia, dislocation of lens, and cataract in disease classified elsewhere are reported in this subsection. Age-related cataracts, which are often referred to as senile cataracts, are further specified by laterality and type. These types include cortical, anterior subcapsular polar, posterior subcapsular polar, nuclear, morgagnian, and combined forms of cataracts. Other cataracts also have specific codes to identify the type as infantile and juvenile, cortical, nuclear, anterior subcapsular polar, posterior subcapsular polar, or combined. Traumatic cataracts, including localized, partially resolved, total, and unspecified, require the assignment of an additional code from Chapter 20 to identify the external traumatic cause. An additional code is required for reporting drug-induced cataracts in order to identify the drug responsible for the condition.

When reporting **aphakia,** it is important for coders to know the cause and pay close attention to the excludes1 notes. For example, if a patient has previously lost the right lens due to a traumatic accident, the proper code assignment is H27.01, aphakia, right eye. However, if the patient has had the right lens surgically removed through cataract extraction, it should be reported as Z98.41, cataract extraction status, right eye.

Code H28, cataract in diseases classified elsewhere, is intended only for assignment as a secondary code. When reporting this code, the underlying disease should be identified and sequenced first.

cataract Clouding of the lens or lens capsule of the eye, which prevents incoming light from reaching the retina and can lead to impaired vision or blindness.

aphakia Absence or loss of the lens of the eye.

conditions that include paralytic strabismus, other strabismus, other disorders of binocular movement, and disorders of refraction and accommodation. Extrinsic muscles of the eye, which are involved in these disorders, are illustrated in Figured 13.9. When reporting Kearns-Sayre syndrome, an additional code should be reported to identify any other documented manifestations. For example, Kearns-Sayre syndrome of both eyes associated with heart block is coded as H49.813, Kearns-Sayre syndrome, bilateral, followed by I45.9, conduction disorder, unspecified.

H53–H54 Visual Disturbances and Blindness

Codes in this subsection of ICD-10-CM correspond with those in categories 368 and 369 in ICD-9-CM. Category H53, visual disturbances, includes codes to identify specific disorders that include amblyopia ex anopsia, subjective visual disturbances, diplopia, other and unspecified disorders of binocular vision, visual field defects, color vision deficiencies, night blindness, vision sensitivity deficiencies, and other visual disturbances. Category H54, blindness and low vision provides the ability to specify blindness of both eyes, blindness in one eye with low vision in the other eye, blindness in one eye, low vision in one eye, unqualified visual loss in one eye, unspecified visual loss, and legal blindness according to the

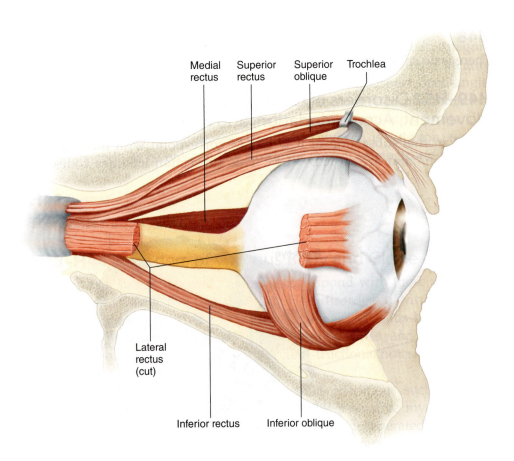

figure 13.9 Extrinsic Muscles of the Right Eye

United States of America definition. When reporting codes for blindness and low vision, the underlying cause of the blindness should be reported first, followed by a code from category H54.

H55 and H57 Other Disorders of Eye and Adnexa

Codes in this subsection of ICD-10-CM correspond with those in category 379 in ICD-9-CM. Category H55, nystagmus and other irregular eye movements, includes codes to specify types of nystagmus, such as congenital, latent, visual deprivation, and dissociated, and types of other irregular eye movements, including saccadic. Category H57, other disorders of eye and adnexa, provides the ability to identify anomalies of pupillary function, ocular pain, and other specified disorders of the eye and adnexa.

H56 and H58

There are no categories H56 and H58.

H59 Intraoperative and Postprocedural Complications and Disorders of Eye and Adnexa, Not Elsewhere Classified

Codes in this subsection of ICD-10-CM correspond with those in categories 996–998 in ICD-9-CM. The codes in this category identify variables, such as the type of disorder, the type of complication, and the type of procedure. An example of a code that identifies the type of surgery with the type of complication is code H59.021, cataract (lens) fragments in eye following cataract surgery, right eye. When selecting codes for intraoperative hemorrhage and hematoma of the eye and adnexa complicating a procedure or accidental puncture and laceration of eye and adnexa during a procedure, the type of procedure is specified as an ophthalmic procedure or other procedure.

Think About It 13.4

also available in **McGraw Hill connect** plus+

Assign ICD-10-CM codes for the following situations, applying any appropriate sequencing guidelines.

1. Bilateral age-related nuclear sclerotic cataracts _____

2. Secondary cataract, right eye _____

3. Stye of the left upper eyelid _____

4. Right eye cataract secondary to primary open angle glaucomatous flecks _____

5. Bilateral rubeosis iridis _____

Beyond the Code: In the healthcare field, who might benefit from the addition of specifying laterality in coding diseases of the eye and adnexa?

13.5 Diseases of the Ear and Mastoid Process

This section covers all of Chapter 8, "Diseases of the Ear and Mastoid Process," in ICD-10-CM, which includes code categories H60–H95. ICD-9-CM classifies these conditions in a portion of Chapter 6—specifically, categories 380–389. Conditions classified to codes in this section include diseases of the external ear, middle ear, mastoid, and inner ear.

> ## Spotlight on A&P
>
> Coding conditions of the external ear, middle ear, mastoid, and inner ear requires knowledge of anatomic structures in the ear and their physiological functions. Figure 13.10 provides an overview of the anatomic structures according to the region in which they are located.

H60–H62 Diseases of External Ear

Codes in this subsection of ICD-10-CM correspond with those in category 380 in ICD-9-CM. Conditions reported in this subsection include otitis externa, non-infectious disorders of the pinna, and disorders of the external ear in diseases classified elsewhere. Codes in category H62 are only for use as secondary codes, preceded by codes to identify an underlying disease.

Note that there are no categories H63 and H64.

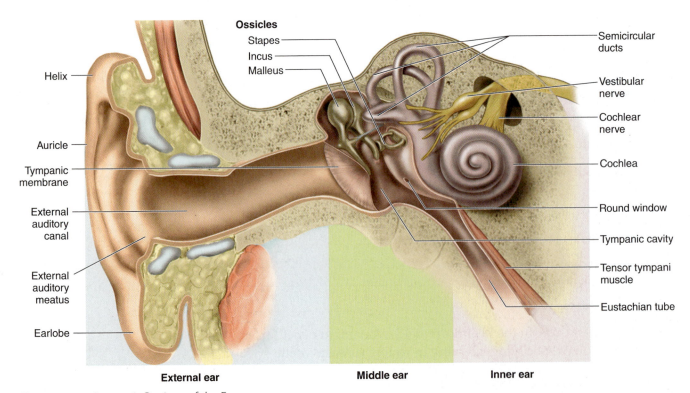

figure 13.10 Anatomic Regions of the Ear

H65–H75 Diseases of Middle Ear and Mastoid

Codes in this subsection of ICD-10-CM correspond with those in categories 381–385 in ICD-9-CM. This subsection includes codes for reporting non-suppurative otitis media, suppurative otitis media, otitis media in diseases classified elsewhere, eustachian salpingitis and obstruction, other disorders of the eustachian tube, mastoiditis and related conditions, cholesteatoma of the middle ear, perforation of the tympanic membrane, other disorders of the tympanic membrane, other disorders of the middle ear, mastoid, and other disorders of the middle ear and mastoid in diseases classified elsewhere. Figure 13.11 provides a diagram of anatomic structures in the middle ear.

Category H67 and H75 codes are only for assignment as secondary codes, to be assigned following the code to identify the underlying disease. When reporting codes in category H66, an additional code should be assigned to report any documented exposure to environmental tobacco smoke, a history of tobacco use, occupational exposure to environmental tobacco smoke, tobacco dependence, or tobacco use. Documentation of associated perforated tympanic membrane should be reported as a secondary code with categories H65–H69. This instruction is also reinforced by the note with category H72, directing the coder to code first any associated otitis media. Note that there are no categories H76–H79.

H80–H83 Diseases of Inner Ear

Codes in this subsection of ICD-10-CM correspond with those in categories 386–387 in ICD-9-CM. Conditions reported include otosclerosis, vestibular function disorders, vertiginous syndromes in diseases classified

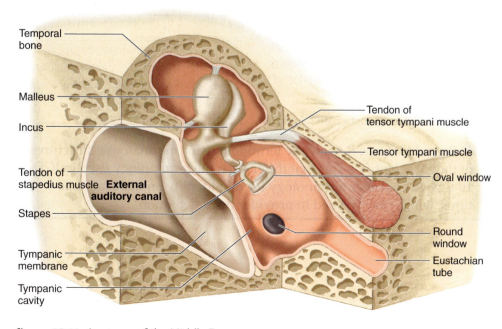

figure 13.11 Anatomy of the Middle Ear

Applying Your Skills

Assign codes for the following conditions, using both ICD-9-CM and ICD-10-CM.

Condition	ICD-9-CM Codes	ICD-10-CM Codes
1. *[LO 13.2]* Intractable generalized idiopathic epilepsy with status epilepticus	_____	_____
2. *[LO 13.1]* Cerebellar ataxia in patient with myxedematous congenital iodine deficiency	_____	_____
3. *[LO 13.1]* Dana-Putnam syndrome with pernicious anemia	_____	_____
4. *[LO 13.5]* Acute serous otitis media of the left ear	_____	_____
5. *[LO 13.1]* Postpolio myelitic syndrome	_____	_____
6. *[LO 13.3]* Cerebrospinal fluid leak from lumbar puncture	_____	_____
7. *[LO 13.1]* Early-onset Alzheimer's disease	_____	_____
8. *[LO 13.2]* Polyneuropathy in amyloid Portuguese polyneuropathy	_____	_____
9. *[LO 13.1]* Huntington's chorea	_____	_____
10. *[LO 13.2]* Transient ischemic attack	_____	_____
11. *[LO 13.3]* Incomplete paraplegia	_____	_____
12. *[LO 13.1]* Dementia in Parkinsonism	_____	_____
13. *[LO 13.2]* Intractable hemiplegic migraine with status migrainosus	_____	_____
14. *[LO 13.5]* Postauricular fistula of the right ear	_____	_____
15. *[LO 13.1]* Subacute necrotizing encephalopathy	_____	_____
16. *[LO 13.4]* Bilateral age-related nuclear sclerotic cataracts	_____	_____
17. *[LO 13.4]* Secondary cataract, right eye	_____	_____
18. *[LO 13.4]* Bilateral rubeosis iridis	_____	_____
19. *[LO 13.4]* Trichiasis of right lower eyelid	_____	_____
20. *[LO 13.5]* Central auditory processing disorder	_____	_____

Checking Your Understanding

Select the letter that best answers the question or completes the sentence.

1. *[LO 13.2]* Which of the following is not a basis for the coding of epilepsy?

    a. type of epilepsy
    b. intractable vs. non-intractable
    c. medication administered to treat epilepsy
    d. presence or absence of status epilepticus

2. *[LO 13.1]* Which of the following categories is designated as being assigned as secondarycodes?

    a. G01   b. G02
    c. G05   d. G06

3. *[LO 13.5]* What does the sixth character specify in the codes for noise effects on the inner ear?

    a. laterality
    b. source of noise
    c. presence or absence of tympanic membrane perforation
    d. presence or absence of hearing loss

4. **[LO 13.3]** What is the appropriate action related to the coding of hemiplegia if the documentation identifies laterality but does not specify which side is dominant?

    a. Code as unspecified side.   **b.** Code as dominant side.

    c. Code as nondominant side.   **d.** Do not code.

5. **[LO 13.4]** Which term is used to identify an age-related cataract?

    a. cortical   **b.** elderly   **c.** polar   **d.** senile

6. **[LO 13.5]** Which of the following is not a risk factor associated with conditions classified to category H66?

    a. tobacco dependence or use

    b. alcohol dependence or use

    c. history of tobacco use

    d. occupational exposure to environmental tobacco smoke

7. **[LO 13.1]** What is the appropriate code assignment and sequencing for a patient with tardive dyskinesia caused by Haldol?

    a. G24.01   **b.** T43.4x5

    c. G24.01, T43.4x5   **d.** T43.4x5, G24.01

8. **[LO 13.3]** A patient with chronic lumbar pain from trauma is admitted for insertion of a neurostimulator for pain control. What is the appropriate code assignment?

    a. G89.21   **b.** M54.5   **c.** G89.21, M54.5   **d.** M54.5, G89.21

9. **[LO 13.2]** Which of the cranial nerves is responsible for Bell's palsy?

    a. V   **b.** VII   **c.** IX,   **d.** X

10. **[LO 13.4]** Which of the following terms is the medical diagnosis referred to by the common term "pinkeye"?

    a. mucopurulent conjunctivitis   **b.** conjunctival hemorrhage

    c. blepharoconjunctivitis   **d.** conjunctival edema

Online Activity

[LO 13.2] Search online to find information about reimbursement issues related to episodic and paroxysmal neurologic conditions. Write a brief summary of your findings.

Real-World Application: Case Study

[LO 13.4] Assign ICD-10-CM codes for the following office visit progress note.

OFFICE VISIT PROGRESS NOTE

SUBJECTIVE: This 85-year-old female presented for evaluation of cataracts. Past ocular history is significant for atrophic age-related macular degeneration.

OBJECTIVE: Visual acuity with correction measures 20/400 OU without improvement by manifest refraction. No afferent pupillary defect noted. Intraocular pressure measures 16 mm OU. Slit-lamp examination demonstrates clear corneas OU. Nuclear sclerosis with 2+ posterior subcapsular cataract identified OU.

ASSESSMENT: Senile nuclear sclerotic cataracts OU with advanced atrophic age-related macular degeneration OU.

PLAN: Schedule for cataract extraction.

McGraw Hill **connect** plus+   **Enhance your learning by completing these exercises and more at mcgrawhillconnect.com**

CHAPTER 13 NERVOUS SYSTEM **199**

14

CIRCULATORY SYSTEM

Learning Outcomes *After completing this chapter, students should be able to:*

14.1 Understand the relationships between heart valve disorders and other conditions related to acute, chronic, rheumatic, and non-rheumatic heart disease.

14.2 Identify the various types of hypertension and associated conditions that impact code assignment and sequencing considerations.

14.3 Explain guidelines for code assignment and code sequencing of ischemic, pulmonary, and other forms of heart disease.

14.4 Describe risk factors, causal conditions, manifestations, and late effects of cerebrovascular diseases, in addition to specific arteries and sites to code for these conditions.

14.5 Apply knowledge of causal conditions and manifestations to code other circulatory and vascular diseases.

Key Terms

aneurysm

angina pectoris

arteriole

arteriovenous fistula

artery

atherosclerosis

capillary

cardiomyopathy

coronary artery bypass graft (CABG)

dissection

embolism

endocarditis

hypertension

hypertensive

infarction

intracerebral

ischemic

myocarditis

myocardial infarction (MI)

pericarditis

rheumatic

subarachnoid

subdural

thrombosis

vein

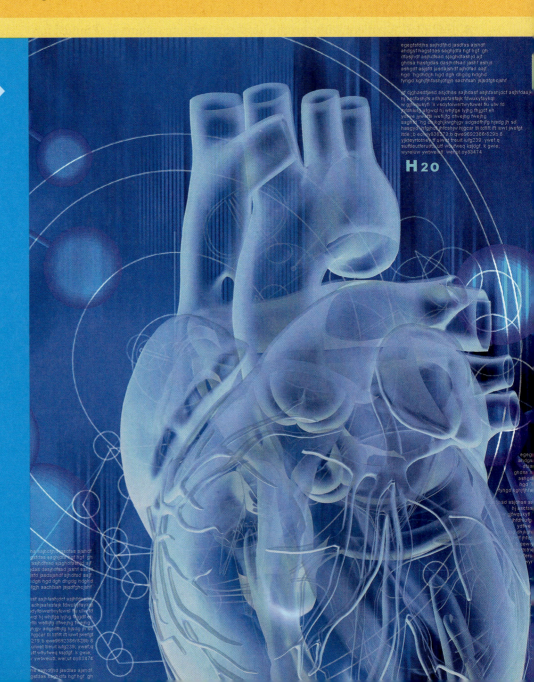

Introduction

A variety of diseases, such as rheumatic heart disease, hypertension, and ischemic heart disease, affect the heart and systemic circulation. These diseases are categorized in both the ICD-9-CM and the ICD-10-CM code systems. In ICD-9-CM, diseases of the circulatory system are classified in Chapter 7 under category codes 390–459. By comparison, ICD-10-CM classifies these conditions in Chapter 9, which includes category codes I00–I99. When coding circulatory conditions, in order to fully explain the diagnostic scenario as presented in the patient's medical record, the coder must be aware of any conditions or diseases that have underlying causes and/or secondary manifestations. For example, a patient may manifest paralysis secondary to a cerebral vascular accident (CVA), or stroke. Or the patient may have a primary condition of hypertension that leads to secondary chronic kidney disease. The coding guidelines in the ICD-10-CM manual provide instruction for sequencing these conditions.

Spotlight on A&P

Coding of conditions in this chapter requires the coder to apply knowledge of physiological interactions among cardiac function, circulatory function, pulmonary circulation, and renal function, as well as the resulting pathophysiological processes that occur when there is a deviation from normal functioning. An overview of the anatomic structures of the heart is provided in Figure 14.1.

14.1 Rheumatic Heart Diseases

Rheumatic heart diseases fall into two categories. They either occur with acute onset, requiring immediate medical attention, or are a chronic condition with associated remissions and exacerbations over an extended period of time. In ICD-10-CM, the codes in categories I00–I09 are used to report all rheumatic heart conditions.

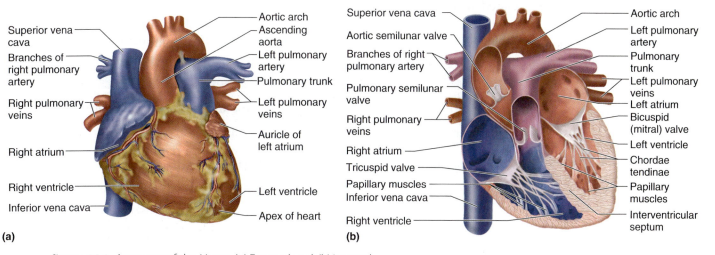

figure 14.1 Anatomy of the Heart: *(a)* External and *(b)* Internal

Online Activity

[LO 14.1, LO 14.2, LO 14.3, LO 14.4, LO 14.5] Search online to find information about reimbursement of circulatory system disorders in the inpatient setting. Describe your findings in a brief report.

Real-World Application: Case Study

[LO 14.2, LO 14.3] Assign ICD-10-CM codes for the following case, in the proper sequence.

A patient is admitted with complaints of fatigue and swelling. Initial documentation reflects ventricular dilation and contractile dysfunction, with orders for a reduced sodium diet and Lasix. The discharge summary provides diagnoses of congestive cardiomyopathy, hypertension, stage 4 chronic renal disease, and acute renal failure with acute cortical necrosis.

15

RESPIRATORY SYSTEM

Learning Outcomes *After completing this chapter, students should be able to*

15.1 Assign codes for conditions associated with respiratory infections to ensure complete and accurate reporting.

15.2 Apply coding guidelines for diseases and conditions of specified parts of the respiratory system.

15.3 Identify conditions that require additional codes assigned related to specified diseases of the lung and pleura.

15.4 Discuss coding and sequencing guidelines for respiratory failure and other diseases of the respiratory system.

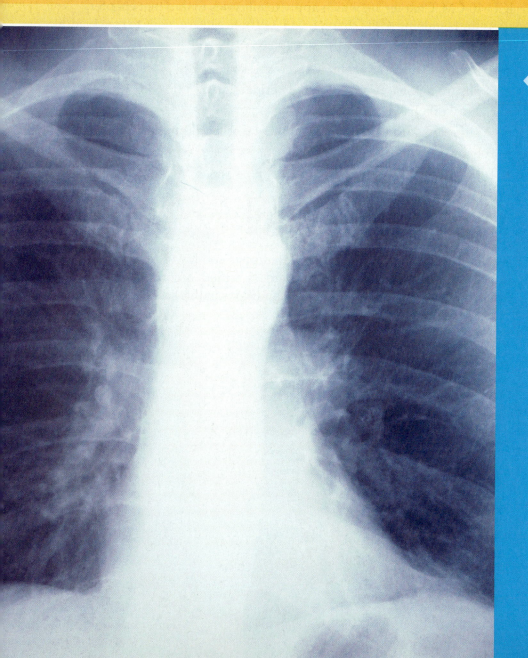

Key Terms

atelectasis

bronchiectasis

chronic obstructive pulmonary disease (COPD)

emphysema

laryngitis

pharyngitis

pneumoconiosis

pneumonia

pneumonitis

rhinitis

sinusitis

tonsillitis

tracheitis

Introduction

The major structures of the respiratory system include the nose, nasal cavities, mouth, larynx (voice box), trachea (windpipe), bronchi, and lungs. These, and other structures in the respiratory system, are identified in Figure 15.1. There are also accessory structures, such as diaphragmatic muscles and capillary vessels. These structures support the process of breathing and exchange of gases such as carbon dioxide (CO_2) and oxygen (O_2) across the smaller alveoli (air sacs) of the lungs. Respiratory diseases can result from a flaw in either the anatomy of the lungs or the physiological process of breathing. Other causes could be due to infection, allergens, or damage by smoke and pollutants. ICD-9-CM classifies these conditions in Chapter 8, "Diseases of the Respiratory System," which includes code categories 460–519. ICD-10-CM classifies these conditions in Chapter 10, "Diseases of the Respiratory System," which includes code categories J00–J99. It is important to note that there are instructions at the beginning *of* ICD-10-CM, Chapter 10, which apply to all codes within that chapter.

At the beginning of the chapter, you will notice instructions to assign additional codes, as may be necessary, when reporting the following conditions:

- Exposure to environmental tobacco smoke (Z77.22)
- Exposure to tobacco smoke in the perinatal period (P96.81)
- History of tobacco use (Z87.891)
- Occupational exposure to environmental tobacco smoke (Z57.31)
- Tobacco dependence (F17.-)
- Tobacco use (Z72.0)

15.1 Respiratory Infections

Respiratory infections, including acute upper and lower respiratory infections, influenza, and pneumonia, are classified according to site and organism. When assigning codes for conditions in this section, coders must

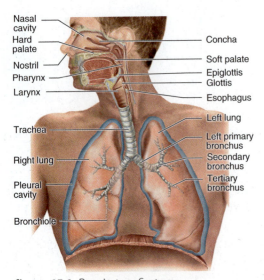

figure 15.1 Respiratory System

exercise caution so as to not make assumptions based upon laboratory findings. Physician documentation should otherwise substantiate diagnosis for appropriate code selection.

J00–J06 Acute Upper Respiratory Infections

Codes in this subsection of ICD-10-CM correspond with those in categories 460–465 in ICD-9-CM. Conditions reported with codes in this subsection include the common cold, acute **sinusitis**, acute **pharyngitis**, acute **tonsillitis**, acute **laryngitis**, acute **tracheitis**, and acute upper respiratory infections. Many of the anatomic structures involved in conditions coded in this subsection are illustrated in Figures 15.2 and 15.3. Note that ICD-9-CM had classified pharyngitis due to specific organisms, such as *Streptococcus*, in the chapter for infectious and parasitic diseases. Several codes in this subsection have instructional notes for the coder to assign an additional code to report the infectious agent by using codes from Chapter 1.

J09–J18 Influenza and Pneumonia

Codes in this subsection of ICD-10-CM correspond with those in categories 480–488 in ICD-9-CM. Conditions reported with codes in this subsection include avian influenza, H1N1 influenza, influenza due to other viruses, viral **pneumonia**, bacterial pneumonia, and pneumonia due to other infectious organisms. Instructional notes appear with various codes in this subsection to direct the coder to assign additional codes, along with sequencing instructions for associated conditions, including pneumonia, lung abscess, specification of virus, Q fever, rheumatic fever, and schistosomiasis.

Certain types of influenza are an exception to the inpatient coding guidelines regarding uncertain diagnoses. Avian influenza and novel H1N1 (swine flu) are coded only if they are confirmed. For coding purposes, the confirmation can be documented in a statement by the provider. Laboratory testing is not required. However, if avian influenza or novel H1N1 is documented as "possible," "probable," or in another uncertain manner, the appropriate code assignment is J10, Influenza due to other influenza virus. The official instruction for this is in coding guideline *10.c.1. Influenza due to certain identified influenza viruses.*

sinusitis Inflammation of the sinuses.

pharyngitis Inflammation of the pharynx; medical term for sore throat.

tonsillitis Inflammation of the tonsils.

laryngitis Inflammation of the larynx, often causing hoarse voice.

tracheitis Inflammation of the trachea.

pneumonia Inflammation of the lungs, with congestion, usually caused by a bacterial or viral infection.

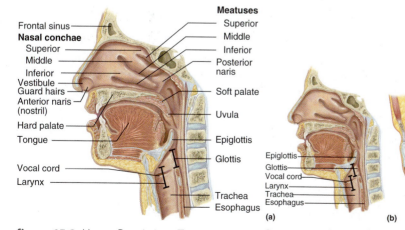

figure 15.2 Upper Respiratory Tract

figure 15.3 Larynx: *(a)* Location; *(b)* Structure

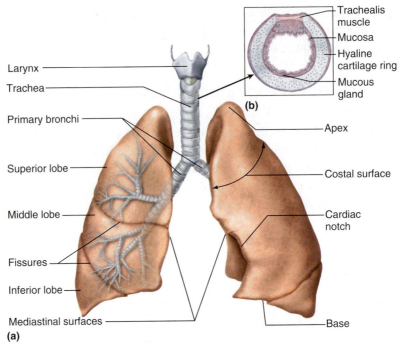

figure 15.4 Lower Respiratory Tract: *(a)* Gross Anatomy; *(b)* C-shaped Tracheal Cartilage

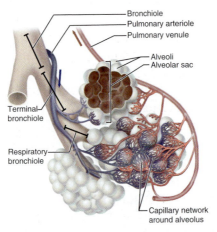

figure 15.5 Bronchioles and Alvioli

J20–J22 Other Acute Lower Respiratory Infections

Codes in this subsection of ICD-10-CM correspond with those in category 466 in ICD-9-CM. Conditions reported with codes in this subsection include acute bronchitis and acute bronchiolitis. These categories expanded in ICD-10-CM to provide specificity regarding infectious organisms, eliminating the need for two codes, as was required in ICD-9-CM. Lower respiratory anatomic structures are identified in Figures 15.4 and 15.5.

J23–J29

Note that there are no categories J23–J29.

Assign ICD-10-CM codes for the following situations, applying any appropriate sequencing guidelines.

1. Acute streptococcal bronchitis _____

2. SARS pneumonia _____

3. Influenzal gastroenteritis _____

4. Acute recurrent frontal sinusitis _____

5. Acute obstructive laryngitis _____

Beyond the Code: What benefits or drawbacks may be associated with the change from ICD-9-CM to ICD-10-CM, with the codes providing specificity regarding infectious organisms, eliminating the need for two codes?

15.2 Diseases of the Upper Respiratory System

Commonly coded conditions of the upper respiratory system include **chronic obstructive pulmonary disease (COPD),** sinusitis, rhinitis, and asthma. Due to the nature of the conditions reported with the codes in this subsection, many reminders appear throughout these subsections regarding the instructions that appear at the beginning of the chapter. Assignment of these additional codes provides valuable statistical information regarding the risk factors for respiratory conditions. Coders often forget that their job impacts more than billing and reimbursement. A variety of healthcare organizations, researchers, insurance analyst, legislators, and other interest groups also use the information that coders report.

chronic obstructive pulmonary disease (COPD) Chronic progressive lung disorder with persistent airflow obstruction.

J30–J39 Other Diseases of Upper Respiratory Tract

Codes in this subsection of ICD-10-CM correspond with those in categories 470–478 in ICD-9-CM. Conditions reported with codes in this subsection include vasomotor **rhinitis,** allergic rhinitis, chronic rhinitis, chronic nasopharyngitis, chronic pharyngitis, chronic sinusitis, nasal polyps, nasal cellulitis, nasal cyst, deviated nasal septum, nasal turbinate hypertrophy, chronic tonsillitis, chronic adenoiditis, peritonsillar abscess, chronic laryngitis, chronic laryngotracheitis, vocal cord and larynx paralysis, laryngeal spasm, and other upper respiratory diseases.

rhinitis Inflammation of the mucous membrane of the nose.

Risk factors should be identified by reporting additional codes for any documented tobacco use and exposure when reporting conditions classified to categories J31, J33, J35, J37, and J39. When reporting nasal mucositis, additional codes should be assigned for any associated antineoplastic or radiological therapy. For peritonsillar abscess, the infectious agent, if known and documented, should be identified with an additional code.

J40–J47 Chronic Lower Respiratory Diseases

emphysema Condition in which there is an increased accumulation of air in the organs and tissues, especially in the lungs, resulting in loss of lung elasticity and decreased gas exchange.

bronchiectasis Chronic dilation of the bronchi following inflammatory disease and obstruction.

Codes in this subsection of ICD-10-CM correspond with those in categories 490–494 and 496 in ICD-9-CM. Conditions reported with codes in this subsection include bronchitis, simple chronic bronchitis, mucopurulent chronic bronchitis, chronic bronchitis, **emphysema,** COPD, asthma, and **bronchiectasis.** When reporting conditions classified to categories in this subsection, risk factors should be identified by assigning additional codes for any documented tobacco use and exposure. For example, documentation of an acute exacerbation of bronchiectasis in a patient with a past history of smoking would be reported by first assigning code J47.1, bronchiectasis with (acute) exacerbation, followed by a secondary code of Z87.891, personal history of nicotine dependence.

COPD and asthma codes identify the difference between complicated cases and those with acute exacerbation. The coding guidelines define acute exacerbation as a worsening or a decompensation of a chronic condition. This should not be confused with a chronic condition with a superimposed infection, which may be a causal factor for an acute exacerbation. Official instructions are located in coding guideline *10.a.1. acute exacerbation of chronic obstructive bronchitis and asthma.*

J46 and J48–J59

Note that there are no categories J46 and J48–J59.

Think About It 15.2   also available in **McGraw Hill connect** plus+

Assign ICD-10-CM codes for the following situations, applying any appropriate sequencing guidelines.

1. Acute lower respiratory infection with bronchiectasis _____

2. Simple chronic bronchitis _____

3. Chronic tonsillitis and adenoiditis _____

4. Acute exacerbation of moderate persistent asthma _____

5. Left vocal cord and larynx paralysis _____

Beyond the Code: What are some of the uses of risk factor reporting, aside from research? Could the identification of risk factors affect reimbursement?

15.3 Specified Diseases of the Lung and Pleura

A significant number of the conditions classified as specified diseases of the lung and pleura occur due to other causal factors. Some of these causes include inhalation or aspiration of various substances, radiation, and medications. Anatomic structures in Figure 15.6 are involved in conditions reported with codes in this subsection. Because of this, coders should be aware of instructional notes throughout this section, which provide guidance about additional codes for risk factors, infectious agents, and underlying diseases. Some codes must be assigned prior to the code for the respiratory condition, whereas others must follow the code for the respiratory condition.

J60–J70 Lung Diseases Due to External Agents

Codes in this subsection of ICD-10-CM correspond with those in categories 495 and 500–508 in ICD-9-CM. Conditions reported with codes in this subsection include **pneumoconiosis** due to a variety of specified organic and inorganic agents, airway disease due to organic dust, hypersensitivity **pneumonitis** due to organic dust, respiratory conditions caused by inhalation of chemicals, gases, fumes and vapors, aspiration pneumonia, and respiratory conditions caused by other external agents such as radiation and drugs. Additional codes may be required for some codes in this subsection to report causal agents, such as drugs, chemicals, foreign bodies, and other external causes.

J71–J79

There are no categories J71–J79.

J80–J84 Other Respiratory Diseases Principally Affecting the Interstitium

Codes in this subsection of ICD-10-CM correspond with those in categories 514 and 518 in ICD-9-CM. Conditions reported with codes in this subsection include acute respiratory distress syndrome, pulmonary edema, pulmonary eosinophilia, and other interstitial pulmonary diseases. Codes in category J81, pulmonary edema, should be followed by additional codes for any documented tobacco use and exposure to identify these risk factors.

J85–J86 Suppurative and Necrotic Conditions of the Lower Respiratory Tract

Codes in this subsection of ICD-10-CM correspond with those in categories 510 and 513 in ICD-9-CM. Conditions reported with codes in this subsection include gangrene of the lung, lung abscess, and pyothorax. Additional codes may be required to report associated infectious agents or the type of pneumonia. For example, pneumococcal abscess of the lung with pneumonia should be reported by first assigning the code J85.1, abscess of lung with pneumonia, with secondary code J13, pneumonia due to streptococcus pneumoniae.

J87–J89

Note that there are no categories J87–J89.

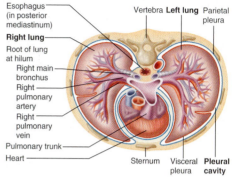

figure 15.6 Pleural Cavity and Membranes: Superior View

pneumoconiosis Chronic lung disease, such as asbestosis and silicosis, caused by long-term inhalation of particulate matter, such as coal dust.

pneumonitis Inflammation of the lungs.

J90–J94 Other Diseases of the Pleura

Codes in this subsection of ICD-10-CM correspond with those in categories 511 and 512 in ICD-9-CM. Conditions reported with codes in this subsection include pleural effusion, pleural plaque, pneumothorax, hemothorax, hydropneumothorax, and other pleural conditions. Note that pleurisy was previously classified to this area in ICD-9-CM; however, ICD-10-CM classifies it as symptoms and signs. Pleural effusion codes in category J91 are to be reported only as secondary codes, with the principal or first-listed code assigned to report neoplasm or underlying disease, such as filariasis.

J95 Intraoperative and Postprocedural Complications and Disorders of Respiratory System, Not Elsewhere Classified

Codes in this subsection of ICD-10-CM correspond with some codes in category 519 in ICD-9-CM. Conditions reported with codes in this subsection include intraoperative and postprocedural complications and disorders of the respiratory system. Additional codes may be required to report type of infection, poisoning by adverse effects of anesthesia (using category T41), or type of pneumonia. For example, chemical pneumonitis due to an adverse effect of general anesthesia is reported by first assigning code T41.205, adverse effect of unspecified general anesthetics, followed by code J95.4, chemical pneumonitis due to anesthesia (Mendelson syndrome), as a secondary code.

Think About It 15.3

also available in **McGraw Hill connect** plus+

Assign ICD-10-CM codes for the following situations, applying any appropriate sequencing guidelines.

1. *Staphylococcus aureus* cellulitis of the neck associated with infected tracheostomy stoma _____

2. Radiation pneumonitis from exposure to radioactive isotopes _____

3. Initial treatment for aspiration pneumonia due to aspiration of vomit _____

4. Acute pulmonary edema in a patient who is a nonsmoker but is exposed to smoke while working as a bartender _____

5. Iron-miner's lung _____

Beyond the Code: Many of the conditions classified in these subsections are caused by the presence of risk factors or exposure to a variety of substances. Discuss how the presence of risk factors or exposure to other substances might affect insurance coverage for these conditions.

15.4 Respiratory Failure and Other Diseases of the Respiratory System

Although the word "other" in the phrase "other diseases" may give the impression that this section is simply a collection of miscellaneous conditions that do not fit other classifications in the chapter, there are actually some significant, and very common, conditions in this section. Just because the conditions are classified as "other" does not mean that they are any less important or less common than conditions in the rest of the chapter. Some examples of important and very common conditions included in this section are respiratory failure, **atelectasis,** and bronchospasm. In particular, respiratory failure has associated coding guidelines with which coders must become familiar, in addition to developing an understanding of the relationship with other conditions that may coexist with respiratory failure.

atelectasis Collapse of part of a lung.

J96–J99 Other Diseases of the Respiratory System

Codes in this subsection of ICD-10-CM correspond with those in categories 517 and 518 in ICD-9-CM. Conditions reported with codes in this subsection include acute respiratory failure, chronic respiratory failure, acute bronchospasm, pulmonary collapse (atelectasis), interstitial emphysema, and other respiratory disorders in diseases classified elsewhere. Note that code J99 is to be assigned only as a secondary code, with the principal or first-listed code assigned to report underlying diseases, such as amyloidosis, ankylosing spondylitis, congenital syphilis, cryoglobulinemia, early congenital syphilis, hemosiderosis, or schistosomiasis.

Acute respiratory failure may be listed as the principal diagnosis if it meets the general guideline definition of a principal diagnosis. However, if chapter-specific guidelines provide other direction, those must be followed, and respiratory failure should be reported as a secondary diagnosis. This is according to directions in coding guideline *10.b.1. acute respiratory failure as principal diagnosis*. For example, a patient is admitted for acute respiratory failure associated with a disease related to acquired immune deficiency syndrome (AIDS); code B20, Human immunodeficiency virus (HIV) disease, must be reported prior to any code for acute respiratory failure.

According to coding guideline *10.b.2. acute respiratory failure as secondary diagnosis*, if respiratory failure occurs after admission or if it is present on admission without meeting the definition of principal diagnosis, it should be listed as a secondary diagnosis.

Coding guideline *10.b.3. sequencing of acute respiratory failure and another acute condition* addresses situations in which admission is for respiratory failure and another acute condition. Determination of the principal diagnosis depends on the circumstances of admission. It does not matter if the nature of the acute condition is respiratory or nonrespiratory, and each situation is unique. Sometimes the acute condition and respiratory failure equally meet the definition of principal diagnosis. In these cases, if no chapter-specific guidelines exist, the guidelines in Section II C should be applied. Whenever the documentation lacks clarity regarding which condition is responsible for occasioning the admission, the physician should be queried.

For example, a patient is admitted with documentation of acute respiratory failure and an acute myocardial infarction. The coder carefully reviews the record and determines that the patient presented to the emergency room with complaints of chest pain. The electrocardiogram demonstrates an acute nontransmural myocardial infarction, which was also clearly documented as the reason for admission. In this case, the appropriate code assignment is code I21.4, non-ST elevation myocardial infarction (NSTEMI) sequenced as the principal diagnosis, followed by code J96.00, acute respiratory failure, unspecified whether with hypoxia or hypercapnia, assigned as a secondary diagnosis.

Think About It 15.4

also available in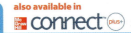

Assign ICD-10-CM codes for the following situations, applying any appropriate sequencing guidelines.

1. Patient admitted for lobar pneumonia and developed acute respiratory failure on third day of admission _____

2. Hemochromatosis with pulmonary manifestations _____

3. Patient admitted for treatment of acute respiratory failure, put on ventilator, and developed ventilator-associated bronchopneumonia _____

4. Calcification of lung _____

5. Acute chronic respiratory failure _____

Beyond the Code: Sequencing of acute respiratory failure is often associated with significant differences in reimbursement in the inpatient setting. What is the importance of focusing on objective information without allowing reimbursement to drive a physician query for unclear documentation of the principal diagnosis?

Chapter Summary

Learning Outcome	Key Concepts/Examples
15.1 Assign codes for conditions associated with respiratory infections to ensure complete and accurate reporting. **(pages 218–221)**	• Instructional notes appear with various codes in this subsection to direct the coder to assign additional codes, along with sequencing instructions for associated conditions.
15.2 Apply coding guidelines for diseases and conditions of specified parts of the respiratory system. **(pages 221–222)**	• Due to the nature of the conditions reported with the codes in this subsection, many reminders appear throughout these subsections regarding the instructions that appeared at the beginning of the chapter, since the assignment of these additional codes provides valuable statistical information regarding the risk factors for respiratory conditions.
15.3 Identify conditions that require additional codes assigned related to specified diseases of the lung and pleura. **(pages 222–224)**	• Coders should be aware of instructional notes throughout this section, which provide guidance about additional codes for risk factors, infectious agents, and underlying diseases.
15.4 Discuss coding and sequencing guidelines for respiratory failure and other diseases of the respiratory system. **(pages 225–226)**	• Acute respiratory failure may be listed as the principal diagnosis if it meets the general guideline definition of a principal diagnosis, unless chapter-specific guidelines provide other direction.

Applying Your Skills

For each condition, assign the corresponding code(s) for ICD-9-CM and ICD-10-CM.

Condition	ICD-9-CM Codes	ICD-10-CM Codes
1. *[LO 15.3]* Aspiration pneumonia		
2. *[LO 15.4]* Atelectasis		
3. *[LO 15.3]* Empyema with fistula		
4. *[LO 15.1]* H1N1 influenza with gastrointestinal enteritis manifestation		
5. *[LO 15.2]* Acute exacerbation of bronchiectasis		
6. *[LO 15.3]* Pneumoconiosis due to graphite fibrosis		
7. *[LO 15.3]* Hemorrhage from tracheostomy stoma		
8. *[LO 15.2]* Strep throat		
9. *[LO 15.1]* Pleurisy		
10. *[LO 15.1]* Acute *Haemophilus influenzae* bronchitis		
11. *[LO 15.3]* Acute pulmonary edema		
12. *[LO 15.2]* Mild intermittent asthma with acute exacerbation		
13. *[LO 15.2]* Hypertrophy of tonsils and adenoids		
14. *[LO 15.2]* Hay fever due to pollen		
15. *[LO 15.2]* Chronic antritis		
16. *[LO 15.1]* Acute epiglottitis with obstruction		
17. *[LO 15.1]* Avian flu with respiratory manifestations		
18. *[LO 15.2]* Panlobular emphysema		
19. *[LO 15.3]* Air conditioner and humidifier lung		
20. *[LO 15.3]* Decompensated COPD		

Checking Your Understanding

Select the letter that best answers the question or completes the sentence.

1. *[LO 15.3]* Which of the following statements is true regarding pleural effusion?

   a. All pleural effusion codes are limited to use as secondary codes.
   b. ICD-10-CM classifies pleural effusion in symptoms and signs, rather than a condition of the respiratory system.
   c. Pleural effusion codes in category J91 are to be reported only as secondary codes.
   d. ICD-10-CM classifies pleural effusion in the cardiovascular system.

2. *[LO 15.4]* A patient is admitted for acute respiratory failure and acute exacerbation of COPD, and the documentation does not clearly present evidence to suggest that either condition better fits the definition of a principal diagnosis. Which diagnosis should be sequenced as the principal diagnosis?

   a. Acute exacerbation of COPD.
   b. Acute respiratory failure.

   c. Either may be assigned as the principal diagnosis.

   d. A physician query should be performed for clarification.

3. *[LO 15.1]* What is the appropriate action related to documentation of "probable H1N1 respiratory influenza"?

   a. Assign code J10.1.

   b. Assign code J09.11.

   c. Code only the symptoms.

   d. Assign code J10 with symptom codes.

4. *[LO 15.3]* What is the correct code assignment for septic pleurisy?

   a. J86.9

   b. R09.1

   c. R09.1, A41.9

   d. A41.9, R09.1

5. *[LO 15.2]* Which of the following should be reported with peritonsillar abscess?

   a. associated antineoplastic or radiological therapy

   b. infectious agent

   c. risk factors

   d. family history

6. *[LO 15.1]* What is the correct code assignment for acute parainfluenza virus bronchitis?

   a. J20.8

   b. J20.4

   c. J20.4, B34.8

   d. J20.8, B34.8

7. *[LO 15.1]* Which additional step is the coder instructed to perform when reporting acute recurrent pansinusitis?

   a. First code the underlying condition.

   b. Code any associated foreign body in the respiratory tract.

   c. Use an additional code, if applicable, to further specify the disorder.

   d. Use an additional code (B95–B97) to identify an infectious agent.

8. *[LO 15.2]* Which of the following statements best describes an acute exacerbation?

   a. a chronic condition with a superimposed infection

   b. the initial episode of a disease

   c. a worsening or a decompensation of a chronic condition

   d. a complication that cannot be controlled with medication

9. *[LO 15.4]* If a patient with AIDS is admitted for treatment of acute respiratory failure, how is the principal diagnosis established?

   a. Acute respiratory failure should be sequenced first.

   b. AIDS should be sequenced first.

   c. A physician query should be performed.

   d. Either diagnosis may be sequenced first.

10. *[LO 15.3]* Which of the following should be identified when reporting chemical pneumonitis due to anesthesia?

   a. poisoning and adverse effects of anesthetic agents

   b. tobacco use and history of tobacco use

   c. infectious agent

   d. sepsis

McGraw Hill **connect** ™ plus+ **Enhance your learning by completing these exercises and more at mcgrawhillconnect.com**

CHAPTER 15   RESPIRATORY SYSTEM   229

Online Activity

[LO 15.1, LO 15.2, LO 15.3, LO 15.4] Search online for information about what potential coding issues an auditor looks for related to pneumonia. Describe your findings in a brief report.

Real-World Application: Case Study

[LO 15.2, LO 15.4] Assign ICD-10-CM codes for the following scenario.

An 82-year-old female with decompensated COPD and a history of tobacco use was admitted to the ICU on presentation to the ER with a five-day onset of respiratory distress and rapid deterioration. The patient developed acute respiratory failure, which was the documented reason for admission. After a three-day hospitalization, the patient was discharged in stable condition.

16 DIGESTIVE SYSTEM

Learning Outcome *After completing this chapter, students should be able to*

16.1 Identify anatomic structures pertinent to coding for conditions of dental, oral, and salivary gland sites.

16.2 Assign and sequence additional codes related to diseases of the esophagus, stomach, duodenum, and appendix.

16.3 Determine the details necessary for complete and accurate reporting of hernias and diseases of the intestines.

16.4 Classify other diseases of the digestive system.

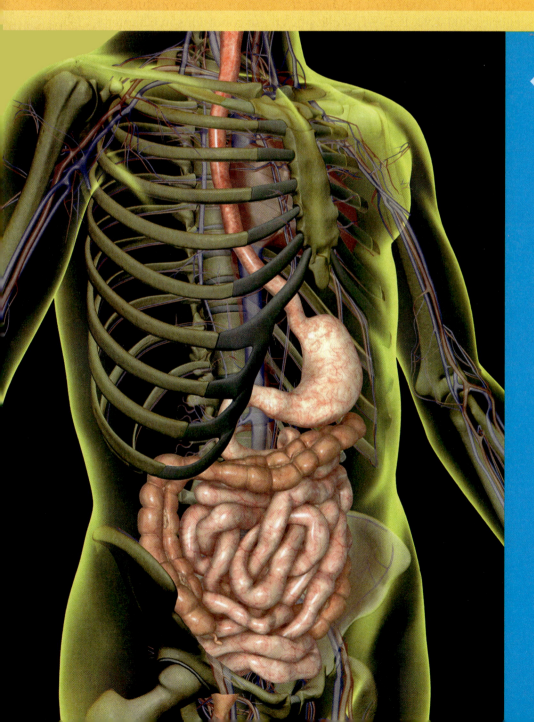

Key Terms

ascites
celiac disease
cholestasis
cirrhosis
Crohn's disease
diaphragmatic hernia
dyspepsia
enteritis
enterocele
femoral hernia
fibrosis
fissure
fistula
gastroenteritis
gastroesophageal reflux
    disease (GERD)
hemoperitoneum
hernia
ileitis
inguinal hernia
intussusception
jejunitis
malabsorption
peritonitis
polyp
portal hypertension
prolapse
retroperitoneum
sclerosis
sigmoiditis
steatorrhea
ulcerative colitis
umbilical hernia
ventral hernia

Introduction

The digestive system, also known as the alimentary canal, is comprised of the oral cavity and teeth, salivary glands, esophagus, stomach, small intestine (duodenum, jejunum, and ileum), large intestine (ascending colon, transverse colon, descending colon, and terminal sigmoid colon), rectum, and anus. Figure 16.1 provides an overview of the alimentary canal, and Figure 16.2 identifies specific structures in the digestive system. When coding conditions of the digestive system, coders need to take note of any associated signs and symptoms or related diseases that may complicate the patient's care and delivery of healthcare services. Coders must then determine whether the signs, symptoms, or related diseases should be coded in addition to the primary disease. ICD-10-CM classifies these conditions in Chapter 11, "Diseases of the Digestive System," which includes code categories K00–K94. ICD-9-CM classifies these conditions in Chapter 9, "Diseases of the Digestive System," which includes code categories 520–579.

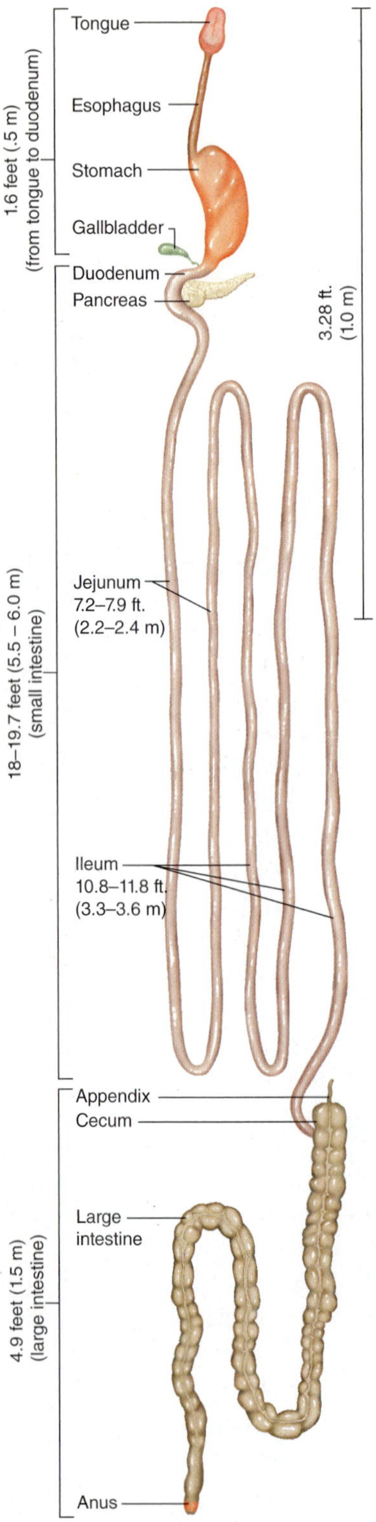

16.1 Conditions of Dental, Oral, and Salivary Gland Sites

The teeth, oral mucosa, and salivary glands are a part of many digestive processes that occur throughout the alimentary canal. With salivation, enzymes are released in response to the foods we eat. Food is broken down before it enters the highly acidic environment of the stomach where

figure 16.1 Alimentary Canal

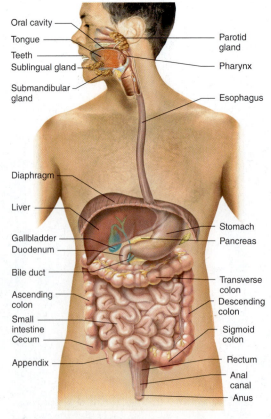

figure 16.2 Digestive System

further digestion will take place. Teeth grind food matter with the overall goal of eventually breaking it down into chemicals that can transverse cell membranes and flow throughout the bloodstream to target tissues for their maintenance and repair. Absorption in this way is dependent on these initial digestive processes. This section addresses the codes for conditions of dental, oral, and salivary gland sites, which are reported with codes in categories K00–K14. The use of dental codes is not limited to dental offices, as occasionally patients present to physician offices or hospital settings for the treatment of dental disorders. Additionally, coders should not rule out dental office settings as potential career opportunities.

K00–K14 Diseases of Oral Cavity and Salivary Glands

Codes in this subsection of ICD-10-CM correspond with those in categories 520–529 in ICD-9-CM. Coders should be able to identify a variety of structural and physiological conditions that can occur with a variety of pulp, gingival, and tooth abnormalities. These conditions can impair one's ability to chew (mastication). These conditions can impair one's ability to chew. While some diseases of the oral cavity may be due to poor hygiene or a lack of flossing such as is seen with gingivitis. Other disorders such as anorexia and bulimia may lead to dental problems. These conditions involve self-induced vomiting after a meal, which exposes the teeth to the corrosive effects of the stomach's hydrochloric acid and bile. These conditions may lead to secondary nutritional deficiencies and ultimately damage to tissue and vital organs. Therefore, complicated co-morbid disease processes may a consideration for coding diseases in this category.

When coding gingivitis and periodontal diseases, stomatitis, lip diseases, diseases of the oral mucosa, and diseases of the tongue, additional codes should be assigned to report any documented exposure to environmental tobacco smoke, exposure to tobacco smoke in the perinatal period, a history of tobacco use, occupational exposure to environmental tobacco smoke, tobacco dependence, or tobacco use, as these underlying causes (etiologies) and risk factors may influence the onset of disease or impact its progression. This also has the potential to complicate the level of care provided and the use of services over time if these conditions become chronic, which impacts healthcare costs. Tracking disease trends and risk factors through coding allows the Centers for Disease Control and Prevention (CDC) and other public health professionals to develop programs for the prevention of disease.

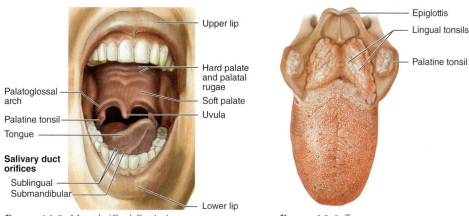

figure 16.3 Mouth (Oral Cavity)

figure 16.4 Tongue

Coding conditions of dental, oral, and salivary gland sites requires knowledge of dental structures, which may or may not be covered in anatomy and physiology or medical terminology courses, so this is an area that may require additional references or review. Many of these structures are diagramed in Figures 16.5 and 16.6.

K15–K19

Note that there are no code categories K15–K19.

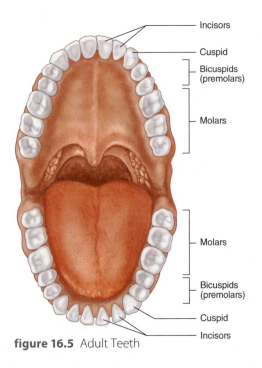

figure 16.5 Adult Teeth

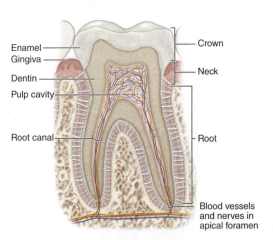

figure 16.6 Anatomy of a Molar

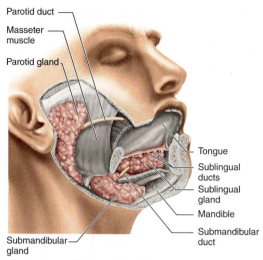

Parotid duct
Masseter muscle
Parotid gland
Tongue
Sublingual ducts
Sublingual gland
Mandible
Submandibular duct
Submandibular gland

figure 16.7 Salivary Glands

Assign ICD-10-CM codes for the following situations, applying any appropriate sequencing guidelines.

1. Calculus of the salivary gland _____

2. Dentoalveolar abscess without sinus _____

3. Dental caries on pit and fissure surface penetrating into dentin _____

4. Peg-shaped tooth _____

5. Gingival recession _____

Beyond the Code: Most medical coding students consider the potential career paths of working in a physician office or hospital after graduation. However, many end up working in dental settings. What types of additional education or training might be necessary to be well prepared as a coder in a dental setting?

16.2 Conditions of the Esophagus, Stomach, Duodenum, and Appendix

Once food has been chewed and swallowed, it passes through the esophagus via wringing and squeezing peristaltic action until the food bolus reaches the stomach. There it can be further digested by highly caustic hydrochloric (HCL) acid before entering the first segment of the small intestine, called the duodenum. The duodenum works with other accessory organs, such as the pancreas, gallbladder, and liver, which are responsible for the secretion of digestive enzymes and bile to break down fats, proteins, and carbohydrates and neutralize or detoxify any metals or other harmful substances that have been ingested. Conditions of the esophagus, stomach, duodenum, and appendix are reported with categories K20–K39 in ICD-10-CM. Most disorders classified to these categories are fairly common and become well known to coders. Coding of conditions in this subsection is relatively straightforward, aside from the need to identify relationships with alcohol use/abuse for some of the conditions.

K20–K31 Diseases of Esophagus, Stomach, and Duodenum

Codes in this subsection of ICD-10-CM correspond to those in categories 530–538 in ICD-9-CM. Conditions coded in this subsection include a variety of esophageal ulcers, strictures, perforations, spasms, diverticular disease, **gastroesophageal reflux disease (GERD),** inflammation of the gastric mucosa (gastritis), **dyspepsia,** pyloric stenosis, and a variety of ulcerations occurring at various anatomic sites in the gastrointestinal tract. Figures 16.8 and 16.9 highlight some of the anatomic structures impacted by conditions coded in this subsection.

gastroesophageal reflux disease (GERD) Disease in which there is recurrent backward flow of stomach acids into the esophagus, causing burning pain and discomfort and sometimes ulcers, neoplastic changes, and stricture.

dyspepsia Medical term for indigestion.

> **CODING TIP ▶**
>
> With repeat ingestion, alcohol may impair the functioning of the gastrointestinal tract. If documented, alcohol abuse or dependence should be assigned as a secondary code from categories K20 and K25–K29. For example, documentation of an acute bleeding peptic ulcer related to alcohol abuse is reported by first assigning K27.0, acute peptic ulcer, site unspecified, with hemorrhage, followed by the secondary code, F10.188, alcohol abuse with other alcohol-induced disorder.

Spotlight on A&P

Eosinophilic esophagitis is a more prevalent disease today than in the past, and it is thought to be due to the repeat ingestion or inhalation of some allergen or antigen that affects the tissue. Food allergies and environmental exposure to pollutants and chemicals are a consideration for the coding of this disease, which may warrant the use of an additional code to fully explain the reason for the changes seen in the esophagus when the patient undergoes an esophagogastroduodenoscopy (EGD).

If a drug or chemical is specified as the causative agent for an esophageal ulcer, the code to identify the causal agent should be assigned and sequenced prior to one of the codes in subclassification K22.1-, ulcer of esophagus. Note that code K23, disorders of esophagus in diseases classified elsewhere, is designated for use only as a secondary code. It should be preceded by a code for the underlying disease, such as congenital syphilis.

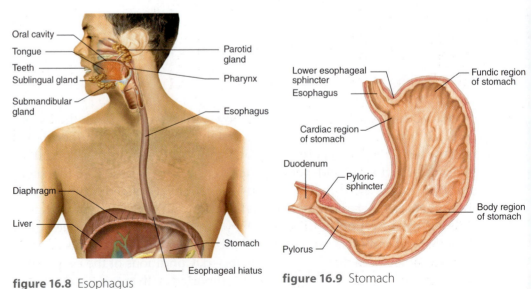

figure 16.8 Esophagus

figure 16.9 Stomach

K24 and K32–K34

No codes are available for categories K24 and K32–K34.

K35–K38 Diseases of Appendix

The appendix is a small pouch attached to the beginning of the large intestine. Controversy continues over what the appendix is used for in the digestive tract. Some speculate that it harbors useful intestinal bacteria, whereas evolutionary biologists might say that humans have evolved as a species to the point of no longer needing this anatomic structure to serve any physiological function. Nonetheless, the appendix does exist regardless of its function, and it can become infected and rupture, causing a potentially painful, life-threatening condition. Although abdominal surgery can lead to complications with the appendix, other known and unknown factors can also cause appendicitis. It usually occurs when the appendix becomes blocked by feces, a foreign object, or rarely a tumor. The patient may present to a health care facility with a chief complaint of lower abdominal pain. If the appendix ruptures, peritonitis can develop, thereby complicating matters. Coders may need to code for more than one condition and any related conditions or associated signs and symptoms not integral to the primary condition itself. Other reasons for appendicitis are structural abnormalities, postoperative abscesses, and surgical wound infections.

Codes in this subsection of ICD-10-CM correspond with those in categories 540–543 in ICD-9-CM. Conditions coded in this subsection include acute appendicitis, chronic/recurrent appendicitis, hyperplasia of appendix, appendicular concretions, diverticulum of appendix, **fistula** of appendix, and **intussusception** of appendix.

fistula Abnormal passage between two anatomic structures.

intussusception Slippage of one part of the bowel inside another to cause obstruction.

K39

There are no codes for category K39.

Think About It 16.2   also available in McGraw Hill CONNECT plus+

Assign ICD-10-CM codes for the following situations, applying any appropriate sequencing guidelines.

1. Barrett's esophagus with high-grade dysplasia _____

2. Duodenitis with hemorrhage _____

3. Acute appendicitis with rupture _____

4. GERD with esophagitis _____

5. Esophageal spasm _____

Beyond the Code: What is the relationship of alcohol abuse or dependence with the conditions coded from categories K20, K25, K26, K28, and K29?

hernia Protrusion through a weak spot of tissue due to increased pressure on the anatomic structure from pregnancy, obesity, heavy lifting, or aging.

inguinal hernia Herniation of abdominal contents through the inguinal canal in the inner groin.

femoral hernia Hernia in which a portion of the intestine pushes through the fascia enclosing the femoral vessels and into the groin.

umbilical hernia Abdominal hernia of newborns in which a section of the intestine bulges up through an opening between the abdominal muscles beneath or near the umbilicus.

ventral hernia Hernia in the midline of the abdomen, often resulting from a surgical incision or scar.

diaphragmatic hernia Hernia in which the contents of the abdomen protrude into the chest through a weak spot in the diaphragm.

enterocele Hernia sac containing a portion of the small intestine.

Crohn's disease Inflammatory bowel disease with narrowing and thickening of the terminal small bowel.

ulcerative colitis Serious inflammatory disease of the colon and rectum marked by ulcers of the intestinal lining and continual attacks of abdominal pain, diarrhea, and rectal bleeding.

polyp Stalk-like tissue growth on mucous membrane.

enteritis Inflammation of the small intestine.

gastroenteritis Acute inflammation of the lining of the stomach and intestines.

16.3 Hernia and Diseases of the Intestines

A **hernia** is a protrusion through a weak spot of tissue due to increased pressure on the anatomic structure from pregnancy, obesity, heavy lifting, or aging. The most common type of hernia is the **inguinal hernia** in the inner groin. Other hernias can appear near the outer groin, the belly-button, or the upper stomach (hiatal hernia). Enteritis is inflammation of the small intestine due to irritants, poisons, or viral or bacterial infections. Colitis is an inflammation of the colon of the large intestine. Hernias, enteritis, colitis, and other diseases of the intestines are coded from categories K40–K63 in ICD-10-CM. When reviewing the codes for both hernias and intestinal disorders, coders should consider all the additional details that are identified by the codes, such as the presence or absence of hemorrhage, gangrene, obstruction, and other complications. The ability to code to the fullest level of accuracy is dependent not only on the coder's recognition of each of these details but also on the provider's documentation.

K40–K46 Hernia

Codes in this subsection of ICD-10-CM correspond with those in categories 550–553 in ICD-9-CM. Conditions coded in this subsection include inguinal hernia, **femoral hernia**, **umbilical hernia**, **ventral hernia**, **diaphragmatic hernia,** and **enterocele**. Organs that are prone to herniation include, but are not limited to, the intestines and the esophagus. However, other organs, such as the stomach, liver, spleen, and kidney, can also become herniated.

> ### Spotlight on A&P
>
> Coders must understand the anatomic structures involved with hernias, along with having the ability to relate physiological processes impacted by hernias, including obstruction and gangrene.

K47–K49

There are no codes for categories K47–K49.

K50–K52 Non-infective Enteritis and Colitis

Codes in this subsection of ICD-10-CM correspond with those in categories 555, 556, and 558 in ICD-9-CM. Conditions coded in this subsection include **Crohn's disease, ulcerative colitis,** inflammatory **polyps** of colon, colitis, **enteritis, gastroenteritis, ileitis, jejunitis,** and **sigmoiditis.** There is an excludes1 note associated with K51.4-, which refers the coder to category D12 for polyps that are categorized as neoplasms. ICD-10-CM provides the ability to code significantly greater detail for Crohn's disease, colon polyps, and ulcerative colitis. This is accompanied by the need for documentation regarding complications of rectal bleeding, intestinal obstruction, fistula, abscess, and other complications. If a patient record has documentation of Crohn's disease and obstruction of the ileum, the appropriate code assignment is K50.012, Crohn's disease of small intestine with intestinal obstruction.

K55–K63 Other Diseases of Intestines

Codes in this subsection of ICD-10-CM correspond to those in categories 557, 560–565, and 568 in ICD-9-CM. Conditions coded in this subsection include intestinal impactions, adhesions, and obstructions; constipation and diarrhea; irritable bowel syndrome; anal and rectal spasms; fistulas; **fissures;** abscesses; stenosis; **prolapse;** polyps; perforations; and diverticular disease. Structures addressed in codes presented in this subsection are identified in Figures 16.10, 16.11, 16.12, and 16.13.

One difference between ICD-9-CM and ICD-10-CM in this subsection is the provision of codes to report perforation or abscess in conjunction with diverticular disease. Another change is that ICD-10-CM classifies anal and rectal fissures and fistulae separately and provides specification of acute versus chronic for anal fissures. ICD-10-CM also has site-specific codes for abscesses, polyps, and prolapse of the anus and rectum.

ileitis Inflammation of the ileum.

jejunitis Inflammation of the jejunum.

sigmoiditis Inflammation of the sigmoid colon.

fissure Deep furrow or cleft.

prolapse Falling or slippage of a body part from its normal position.

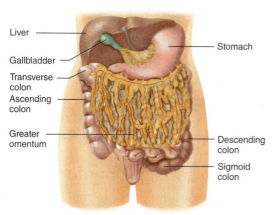

figure 16.10 Greater Omentum

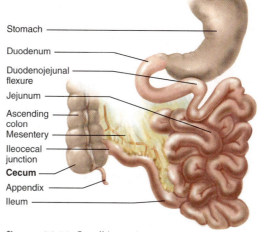

figure 16.11 Small Intestine

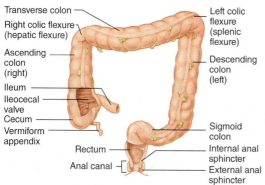

figure 16.12 Large Intestine

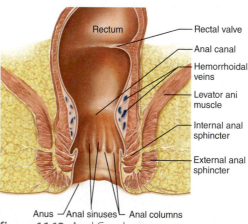

figure 16.13 Anal Canal

Think About It 16.3

also available in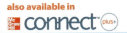

Assign ICD-10-CM codes for the following situations, applying any appropriate sequencing guidelines.

1. Hiatal hernia with gangrene _____

2. Diverticulosis of the colon with perforation, abscess, and hemorrhage _____

3. Nontraumatic tear of anal sphincter with fecal incontinence _____

4. Left hemicolitis with fistula _____

5. Gangrenous incisional hernia _____

Beyond the Code: Consider the changed documentation needs with the increased level of specificity associated with the transition from ICD-9-CM to ICD-10-CM in these subsections. How might you approach the task of addressing physicians about the documentation needs related to this increased specificity? How might you ensure that the physicians are cooperative with coders' need for increased specificity in documentation of these conditions?

16.4 Conditions of Other Digestive System Sites

For the conditions of the digestive system, the coder must identify the site that is being affected by the disease or condition. Conditions of the peritoneum, retroperitoneum, liver, gallbladder, biliary tract, and pancreas are addressed in this subsection, along with the codes for miscellaneous diseases of the digestive system in general, included in categories K65–K94 in ICD-10-CM.

K65–K68 Diseases of Peritoneum and Retroperitoneum

Codes in this subsection of ICD-10-CM correspond to those in categories 567 and 568 in ICD-9-CM. Conditions coded in this subsection include **peritonitis,** peritoneal adhesions, **hemoperitoneum,** disorders of the peritoneum in infectious diseases classified elsewhere, and disorders of the **retroperitoneum.**

peritonitis Inflammation of the membrane that lines the abdominal cavity.

hemoperitoneum Blood in the peritoneal cavity.

retroperitoneum Space behind the peritoneum.

Spotlight on A&P

The peritoneum is a membrane lining around the abdominal and pelvic cavities, and it can become infected or inflamed. The liver, gallbladder, biliary tract, and pancreas are accessory organs of the digestive system; they aid in the digestive processes. The pancreas secretes the hormone insulin, which causes sugar from ingested carbohydrates. The liver detoxifies the blood and breaks down or neutralizes drugs and chemicals for absorption or elimination. The gallbladder stores denatured red blood cells, which form bile, the substance responsible for the breakdown of dietary lipids. The pancreas secretes the hormone insulin, which causes sugar from ingested carbohydrates to leave the bloodstream and enter the mitochondria of the cells, so that the cells are able to go through the process of glycolysis. This biochemical process produces the cellular energy necessary for life-sustaining metabolic functions.

The liver detoxifies the blood and breaks down or neutralizes drugs and chemicals for absorption or elimination. The gallbladder stores denatured red blood cells, which form bile, the substance responsible for the breakdown of dietary lipids. The pancreas secretes the hormone insulin, which causes sugar from ingested carbohydrates to leave the bloodstream and enter the mitochondria of the cells, so that the cells are able to go through the process of glycolysis. This biochemical process produces the cellular energy necessary for life-sustaining metabolic functions.

CODING TIP ▸

Coding for peritoneal effusion is one point of difference between ICD-9-CM and ICD-10-CM. Rather than being coded from category 568, peritoneal effusion is now reported with the same code as ascites (from Chapter 18 in ICD-10-CM).

There is an extensive list of conditions in the excludes1 note with category K65, along with instructions to assign an additional code to report an infectious agent, if documented. Code K67, disorders of the peritoneum in infectious diseases classified elsewhere, is appropriate to report only as a secondary code, following the code for the underlying infectious disease. This subsection is impacted by one condition, peritoneal effusion, which was coded to a greater level of specificity in ICD-9-CM than it is in ICD-10-CM. Whereas ICD-9-CM had a code that was specific to category 568 for peritoneal effusion, ICD-10-CM classifies it in Chapter 18 with signs and symptoms and assigns the same code as for **ascites.**

K70–K77 Diseases of Liver

Codes in this subsection of ICD-10-CM correspond to those in categories 570–573 in ICD-9-CM. Conditions coded in this subsection include alcoholic liver disease, toxic liver disease, hepatic failure, chronic hepatitis, **fibrosis** and **cirrhosis** of the liver, liver abscess, inflammatory liver diseases, fatty liver, **portal hypertension,** cyst of liver, and liver disorders in diseases classified elsewhere. Figure 16.14 identifies the location of the liver. When reporting alcoholic liver disease, if documentation is present, a secondary code should be assigned to report alcohol abuse or dependence. Alcoholic liver disease is further specified with codes for alcoholic fatty liver, hepatitis, fibrosis, **sclerosis,** cirrhosis with or without ascites, and hepatic failure. An example of this is documented chronic alcoholic liver failure (without documentation of coma) in a patient with chronic alcohol dependence. The appropriate code assignment is K70.40, alcoholic hepatic failure without coma, followed by a secondary code, F10.288, alcohol dependence with other alcohol-induced disorder.

Toxic liver disease should be reported following the code(s) for the causative drug or toxic agent. Similar to alcoholic liver disease, toxic liver disease is also further specified with codes to report it with **cholestasis,** hepatic necrosis, hepatitis, fibrosis, and cirrhosis. One change may be confusing for coders transitioning from ICD-9-CM to the increased specificity of ICD-10-CM; hepatic fibrosis was coded as cirrhosis in ICD-9-CM. Note that there are no code categories K78–K79.

K80–K87 Disorders of Gallbladder, Biliary Tract, and Pancreas

Codes in this subsection of ICD-10-CM correspond to those in categories 574–577 in ICD-9-CM. Conditions coded in this subsection include cholelithiasis (see Figure 16.15 for an image of cholelithiasis or gallstones), cholecystitis,

fibrosis Formation of extra fibrous tissue as a reactive process or in repair of something, rather than as part of normal tissue building.

cirrhosis Degenerative liver disease, often resulting from alcoholism or hepatitis.

portal hypertension Increased blood pressure in the portal vein, which carries blood to the liver from the stomach, intestine, pancreas, and spleen.

sclerosis Thickening or hardening of a tissue.

cholestasis Cessation of the flow of bile, usually resulting in jaundice.

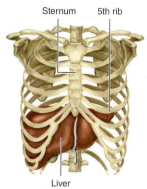

figure 16.14 Location of the Liver

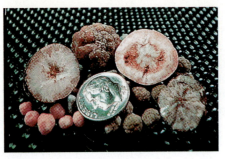

figure 16.15 Gallstones

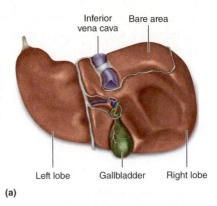

Inferior
vena cava   Bare area

Left lobe   Gallbladder   Right lobe

(a)

gallbladder and bile duct obstructions, cholangitis, ruptures, fistulas, spasms, pancreatitis, cysts, and other disorders. Structures of the biliary tract are identified in Figures 16.16, 16.17, and 16.18.

ICD-9-CM listed fifth-digit subclassifications for the presence or absence of obstruction at the beginning of the cholelithiasis category, but ICD-10-CM has the details built into each code, eliminating the need for the list at the start of the category. This subsection

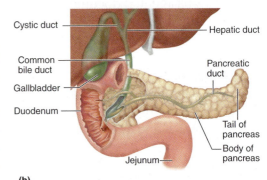

Cystic duct   Hepatic duct

Common
bile duct   Pancreatic
                                duct
Gallbladder

Duodenum
                                Tail of
                                pancreas
                                Body of
Jejunum   pancreas

(b)

figure 16.16 Gallbladder and Biliary Tract. *(a)* Underside of the Liver. *(b)* Anatomy of the Gallbladder, Pancreas, and Biliary Tract.

also gives coders the ability to report a greater level of specificity in ICD-10-CM than in ICD-9-CM. For example, a documented calculus of the bile duct with acute cholecystitis and obstruction is reported by assigning code K80.43, calculus of bile duct with acute cholecystitis with obstruction.

K88–K89

Note that there are no subsections K88–K89.

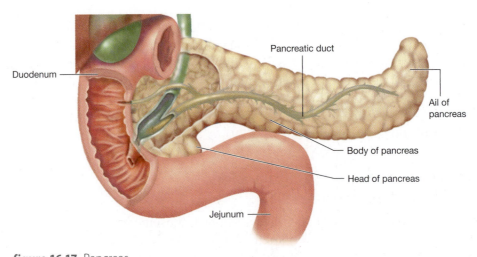

Duodenum   Pancreatic duct

                                                            Ail of
                                                            pancreas

                                            Body of pancreas

                                            Head of pancreas

Jejunum

figure 16.17 Pancreas

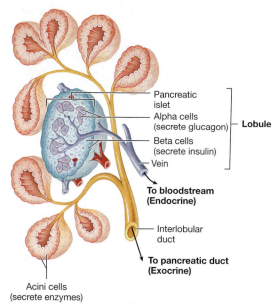

figure 16.18 Exocrine and Endocrine Aspects of the Pancreas

K90–K94 Other Diseases of the Digestive System

Codes in this subsection of ICD-10-CM correspond to those in categories 578 and 579, as well as several other codes scattered throughout other parts of the chapter in ICD-9-CM. Conditions coded in this subsection include **celiac disease**, pancreatic **steatorrhea**, Whipple's disease, **malabsorption** disorders, punctures, lacerations, structural abnormalities, intra-operative and postsurgical complications, hematemesis, melena, and gastrointestinal hemorrhage.

celiac disease Disease causing damage to small intestine lining, caused by sensitivity to gluten.

steatorrhea Excessive discharge of undigested fat in the feces.

malabsorption Inadequate gastrointestinal absorption of nutrients.

Think About It 16.4

also available in McGraw Hill **connect** plus+

Assign ICD-10-CM codes for the following situations, applying any appropriate sequencing guidelines.

1. Acute and chronic cholecystitis _____

2. Dumping syndrome following gastric bypass _____

3. Mixed liver cirrhosis _____

4. Toxic liver disease with cholestasis due to adverse effect of Naprosyn _____

5. Acute and subacute liver failure with coma _____

Beyond the Code: When performing a query regarding the relationship of alcohol use to conditions reported in this subsection, what potential HIPAA implications exist? What do you consider to be the most appropriate method of addressing physician queries of this nature?

Chapter Summary

Learning Outcome	Key Concepts/Examples
16.1 Identify anatomic structures pertinent to coding for conditions of dental, oral, and salivary gland sites. **(pages 232–235)**	• When coding gingivitis and periodontal diseases, stomatitis, lip diseases, diseases of the oral mucosa, and diseases of the tongue, additional codes should be assigned to report any documented exposure to environmental tobacco smoke, exposure to tobacco smoke in the perinatal period, a history of tobacco use, occupational exposure to environmental tobacco smoke, tobacco dependence, or tobacco use.
16.2 Assign and sequence additional codes related to diseases of the esophagus, stomach, duodenum, and appendix. **(pages 235–237)**	• Coding of conditions in this subsection is relatively straightforward, aside from the need to identify relationships with alcohol use/abuse for some of the conditions.
16.3 Determine the details necessary for complete and accurate reporting of hernias and diseases of the intestines. **(pages 238–240)**	• Coding of hernias requires documentation about laterality, the presence of obstruction or gangrene, and recurrent nature. • ICD-10-CM provides the ability to code significantly greater detail for Crohn's disease, colon polyps, and ulcerative colitis.
16.4 Classify other diseases of the digestive system. **(pages 240–243)**	• Conditions of the peritoneum, retroperitoneum, liver, gallbladder, biliary tract, and pancreas are addressed in this subsection, along with codes for other miscellaneous diseases of the digestive system in general.

Applying Your Skills

For each condition, assign the corresponding code(s) for ICD-9-CM and ICD-10-CM.

Condition	ICD-9-CM Codes	ICD-10-CM Codes
1. *[LO 16.2]* Reflux esophagitis		
2. *[LO 16.3]* Ulcerative pancolitis with intestinal obstruction		
3. *[LO 16.1]* Peritoneal effusion		
4. *[LO 16.4]* Acute hepatic failure without coma		
5. *[LO 16.4]* Choledocholithiasis with acute cholangitis and obstruction		
6. *[LO 16.4]* Pseudocyst of pancreas		
7. *[LO 16.4]* Malabsorption due to gluten sensitivity		
8. *[LO 16.3]* Inflammatory colon polyp with fistula		
9. *[LO 16.4]* Hepatic fibrosis		
10. *[LO 16.2]* Barrett's esophagus with low-grade dysplasia		
11. *[LO 16.1]* Occult blood in stool		
12. *[LO 16.3]* Irritable bowel syndrome with diarrhea		
13. *[LO 16.4]* Acute cholecystitis with cholelithiasis without obstruction		
14. *[LO 16.3]* Enteroptosis		
15. *[LO 16.4]* Melena		
16. *[LO 16.2]* Acute pyloric ulcer with hemorrhage, perforation, and obstruction		
17. *[LO 16.3]* Left-sided colitis with rectal bleeding		
18. *[LO 16.4]* Dumping syndrome following gastrectomy		
19. *[LO 16.4]* Biliary cyst		
20. *[LO 16.3]* Chronic anal fissure		

Checking Your Understanding

Select the letter that best answers the question or completes the sentence.

1. *[LO 16.4]* Which term is introduced in ICD-10-CM to identify cirrhosis?

   a. fibrotic cirrhosis
   b. fibrotic liver
   c. hepatic fibrosis
   d. hepatofibrosis

2. *[LO 16.2]* What should be reported with secondary codes from categories K20 and K25–K29?

    a. the drug or chemical that caused the disorder
    b. alcohol abuse or dependence
    c. underlying disease
    d. an infectious organism

3. *[LO 16.3]* All of the following organs in the digestive system may become herniated except for the

    a. large intestine.
    b. small intestine.
    c. tongue.
    d. esophagus.

4. *[LO 16.1]* Which healthcare settings report dental diagnoses?

    a. only dental offices
    b. physician offices and hospitals
    c. dental offices and hospitals
    d. dental offices, physician offices, and hospitals

5. *[LO 16.3]* Which of the following is not pertinent to the coding of hernias?

    a. gangrene
    b. obstruction
    c. infection
    d. recurrence

6. *[LO 16.4]* Which of the following may be reported as a principal diagnosis code?

    a. K67   b. K74.4

    c. K77   d. K87

7. *[LO 16. 2]* What should be coded prior to the code for an esophageal ulcer?

    a. the drug or chemical that caused the disorder
    b. alcohol abuse or dependence
    c. underlying disease
    d. an infectious organism

8. *[LO 16. 4]* Which of the following conditions is not specified for additional code assignment with liver disorders?

    a. alcohol use and dependence
    b. viral hepatitis
    c. tobacco use
    d. drug or toxic agent

9. *[LO 16.1]* Which of the following should be reported as risk factors for diseases of the salivary glands?

    a. tobacco dependence, tobacco use, and history of tobacco use
    b. tobacco dependence, tobacco use, history of tobacco use, alcohol use or dependence, and exposure to tobacco smoke in the environment or during the perinatal period
    c. tobacco dependence, tobacco use, history of tobacco use, and exposure to tobacco smoke in the environment or during the perinatal period
    d. Tobacco dependence, tobacco use, history of tobacco use, and alcohol use or dependence

10. *[LO 16.3]* Which of the following items does not impact the coding for Crohn's disease?

    a. abscess   b. fistula
    c. incontinence   d. obstruction

Online Activity

[LO 16.1] Search online for information about reimbursement and documentation issues related to the coding of dental diagnoses. Summarize your findings in a brief report.

Real-World Application: Case Study

[LO 16.4] Assign ICD-10-CM diagnosis codes for the following discharge summary.

Discharge Summary

Admission Date: June 14, 20xx

Discharge Date: June 17, 20xx

Admission Diagnoses: Acute cholecystitis, NIDDM, OSA, and HTN.

Discharge Diagnoses: Acute cholecystitis with cholelithiasis, NIDDM requiring insulin, OSA, and HTN.

Procedure: Laparoscopic cholecystectomy.

History of Present Illness: Frances Anderson is a 44-year-old, morbidly obese woman with a long history of non-insulin-dependent diabetes mellitus and obstructive sleep apnea. She presented to the emergency department with sudden onset of severe right upper quadrant abdominal pain and fever.

Hospital Course: Ms. Anderson was admitted to the hospital. General surgical consult was obtained and, on the second day of admission, she underwent her laparoscopic cholecystectomy, which she tolerated without difficulty. Postoperative blood sugar was noted 450, and she was started on a sliding scale insulin, to which she responded well. Recovery was uneventful and she was discharged home.

Discharge Instructions: Follow up in two weeks. She may shower, but no tub bath. Keep wounds clean and dry. No heavy lifting. No driving until after postoperative follow-up visit. Continue with her CPAP machine and continue to monitor her sugars.

17

GENITOURINARY SYSTEM

Learning Outcomes *After completing this chapter, students should be able to*

17.1 Interpret guidelines for coding glomerular and renal tubulo-interstitial diseases.

17.2 Apply coding guidelines for acute kidney failure, chronic kidney disease, urolithiasis, and other disorders of the urinary system.

17.3 Identify additional codes required with disorders of male genital organs.

17.4 Describe terminology used to document conditions of the breast and female genitourinary organs.

17.5 Assign codes for intra-operative and postprocedural complications of the genitourinary system.

Key Terms

calculus
cystitis
cystocele
dysmenorrhea
endometriosis
gynecomastia
hydrocele
hydronephrosis
lower urinary tract
    symptoms (LUTS)
nephrolithiasis
nephropathy
nocturnal enuresis
obstructive uropathy
pyelonephritis
pyonephrosis
rectocele
spermatocele
stress incontinence
tubulo-interstitial
    nephritis

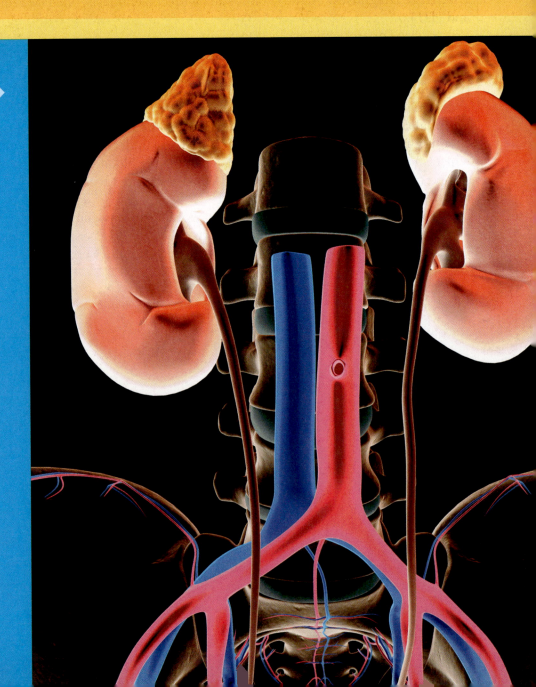

Introduction

The genitourinary system is comprised of the kidneys, kidney tubules, urinary bladder, and genitals. The kidneys contain a glomerulus, which acts as a filter. This filter separates blood and nutrients from the toxic by-products of metabolism. These toxins constitute urine needing to be eliminated by the body. The coder should understand the various anatomic structures and the functioning of each in order to describe the terminology used in documenting these conditions. Interpretation of the coding guidelines is needed in order to properly sequence codes for the diseases of this system. At times, additional codes may be required to more fully explain the diagnostic scenario and any associated complications that occur.

This chapter includes guidelines for coding glomerular and renal tubulo-interstitial diseases, acute kidney failure, chronic kidney disease, urolithiasis, other disorders of the urinary system, disorders of the male genital organs, disorders of the breast and female genitourinary organs, and intra-operative and postprocedural complications of the genitourinary system. ICD-9-CM classifies these conditions in Chapter 10, "Diseases of the Genitourinary System," which includes code categories 580–629. ICD-10-CM classifies these conditions in Chapter 14, "Diseases of the Genitourinary System," which includes code categories N00–N99. Structures in the urinary system are illustrated in Figure 17.1.

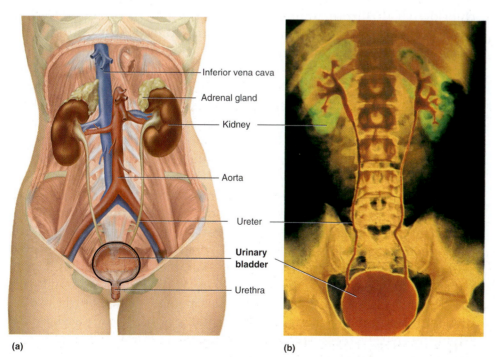

(a) (b)

figure 17.1 Urinary System: *(a)* Major Organs; *(b)* Structures Shown in a Colored Intravenous Pyelogram.

17.1 Glomerular and Renal Tubulo-Interstitial Diseases

There are about 500,000 tiny balls of capillaries, called glomeruli, within the cortex of each kidney. These structures are responsible for filtering blood at a normal rate of about 100 ml/minute. Following glomerular filtration, urine is transported in a tubule to the renal pelvis. Diseases of these structures are classified as nephritis or nephrotic syndromes, depending on the clinical presentation, and can be either infectious or non-infectious in etiology. Coders should be alert to the many instructional notes associated with these codes for conditions to be assigned and sequenced either before or after the codes in this section. ICD-9-CM classifies these conditions in Chapter 10, "Diseases of Genitourinary System," which includes codes from categories 580–589. ICD-10-CM classifies these conditions in Chapter 14, "Diseases of the Genitourinary System," which includes code categories N00–N16.

N00–N08 Glomerular Diseases

ICD-9-CM classifies glomerular diseases in Chapter 10, "Diseases of the Genitourinary System," which includes code categories 580–629. Similarly, ICD-10-CM classifies these conditions in Chapter 14, "Diseases of the Genitourinary System," which includes code categories N00–N99. The conditions coded in the subsection include disorders in the nephrons of the kidneys which contain glomerular filtration units that act under pressure to make urine. Elemental sodium (Na^+), potassium (K^+), chloride (Cl^-), glucose, amino acids, hydrogen (H^+), ammonia (NH_4^+), and water are spared in varying degrees and collected back through the kidney's collecting tubules and returned to systemic circulation. The kidneys regulate blood pressure, blood volume, and the pH (hydrogen ion concentration), which correlates with acidity in an organism's environment. A variety of nephritic and glomerular diseases, such as nephritis, glomerulonephritis, **nephropathy,** and lesions can occur in the diseased malfunctioning kidney. Other conditions associated with these conditions are blood and protein in the urine, known as hematuria and proteinuria, respectively.

Note that any associated kidney failure should be coded using codes from the N17–N19 range, if documented. Category N02, recurrent and persistent hematuria, is not used for reporting hematuria as a symptom, but rather for reporting recurrent and persistent hematuria associated with specific glomerular diseases. For example, if a patient is simply experiencing hematuria, the appropriate code is R31.9, hematuria, unspecified. However, if the patient has persistent hematuria associated with a minimally changing glomerular lesion, the code assignment should be N02.0, recurrent and persistent hematuria with minor glomerular abnormality.

Codes from category R31 in Chapter 18 are assigned when it is appropriate to report hematuria as a symptom. Similarly, category N06, isolated proteinuria associated with specified morphological lesions, is not

nephropathy Any disease of the kidney.

Spotlight on A&P

In order to accurately report codes for glomerular disorders, the coder must fully understand the details of the normal physiological function of the urinary system. Coders must also be familiar with the impact of pathophysiological processes, so that they can recognize abnormal functions, such as hematuria or proteinuria.

appropriate to report for proteinuria as a symptom; instead a code from category R80, proteinuria, in Chapter 18 should be assigned. Note that code N08, glomerular disorders in diseases classified elsewhere, is appropriate to assign only as a secondary code, following the code for the underlying disease.

N09

Note that there is no category N09.

N10–N16 Renal Tubulo-Interstitial Diseases

Codes in this subsection of ICD-10-CM correspond with those in code categories 590–593 in ICD-9-CM. Conditions coded in this subsection include **pyelonephritis,** interstitial nephritis of the tubules (or **tubulo-interstitial nephritis**), pyelitis, tubular necrosis, **obstructive uropathy, hydronephrosis,** hydroureter, **pyonephrosis,** vesicoureteral reflux, and tubular disorders due to drugs and heavy metals. Figure 17.2 illustrates renal tubule structures

Codes from category N11, chronic tubulo-interstitial nephritis, and code N13.6, pyonephrosis, require the assignment of an additional code from the B95–B97 range if the infectious agent is documented. For example, documented nonobstructive chronic pyelonephritis due to *E. coli* is reported with code N11.8, other chronic tubulo-interstitial nephritis, followed by code B96.2, *Escherichia coli (E. coli)*, as the cause of diseases classified elsewhere.

Code N16, Renal tubulo-interstitial disorders in diseases classified elsewhere, is for use as a secondary code, following a code for the underlying disease, such as leukemia or lymphoma.

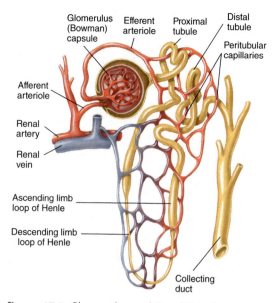

figure 17.2 Glomerulus and Renal Tubule

pyelonephritis Inflammation of the kidney and renal pelvis.

tubulo-interstitial nephritis Inflammation of the spaces between kidney tubules.

obstructive uropathy Disease of the urinary tract in which the flow of urine is blocked, causing it to back up and injure a kidney.

hydronephrosis Accumulation of excess urine in the kidneys due to obstruction in urine outflow.

pyonephrosis Collection of pus in the kidney, usually caused by obstruction.

Think About It 17.1

also available in **McGraw Hill connect** plus+

Assign ICD-10-CM codes for the following situations, applying any appropriate sequencing guidelines.

1. Hydronephrosis due to ureteral stricture _____

2. Glomerulonephritis associated with idiopathic gout of the vertebrae _____

3. Isolated proteinuria with diffuse membranous glomerulonephritis _____

4. Pyelonephritis due to Wilson's disease _____

5. Left-side vesicoureteral reflux with reflux nephropathy and hydroureter _____

Beyond the Code: Why do you think that hematuria was classified in Chapter 10, "Diseases of the Genitourinary System," in ICD-9-CM but was moved to Chapter 18, "Symptoms, Signs and Abnormal Clinical and Laboratory Findings, Not Elsewhere Classified," in ICD-10-CM? Which do you think is a more appropriate classification? Explain your answer.

17.2 Acute Kidney Failure, Chronic Kidney Disease, Urolithiasis, and Other Urinary System Disorders

Acute kidney failure, chronic kidney disease, urolithiasis, and other disorders of the urinary system are discussed in this section, along with corresponding coding guidelines. Kidney failure can occur for a variety of reasons, such as hypertension, heart disease, liver failure, obstruction in blood flow, kidney stones, cancer, neurologic disorders, immune system disorders, infections, and a variety of circulatory diseases. Pathophysiological processes are sometimes complex, especially with chronic kidney disease, which often requires the assignment of additional codes from other chapters to completely report the conditions.

Coders should be able to distinguish between acute and chronic conditions. Acute conditions occur immediately and spontaneously without other warning and usually require immediate medical attention. Chronic conditions are more longstanding and progressive over time. Chronic conditions may remit or worsen over time; they require regular and routine medical intervention to prevent exacerbations in the conditions. Acute conditions are sequenced before chronic conditions if both conditions exist at the same time and if both are to be coded. ICD-9-CM classifies these conditions in Chapter 10, "Diseases of the Genitourinary System," which includes categories 584–586. ICD-10-CM classifies these conditions in Chapter 14, "Diseases of the Genitourinary System," with codes N17–N39.

N17–N19 Acute Kidney Failure and Chronic Kidney Disease

Codes in this subsection of ICD-10-CM correspond with those in code categories 584–586 in ICD-9-CM. Conditions coded in this subsection include acute renal failure, chronic kidney disease (CKD), and unspecified kidney failure. Stages of chronic kidney disease are outlined in coding guideline *I.14.a.1) Stages of chronic kidney disease (CKD)*. These are also illustrated in Table 17.1, which identifies the ICD-10-CM code that corresponds with each stage of CKD. Secondary codes should

Table 17.1 Stages of Chronic Kidney Disease and Related ICD-10-CM Codes

Stage of CKD	ICD-10-CM Code
Stage I	N18.1
Stage II (mild)	N18.2
Stage III (moderate)	N18.3
Stage IV (severe)	N18.4
Stage V	N18.5
End-stage (note that patients on chronic renal dialysis should be coded as end-stage renal disease)	N18.6
Unspecified	N18.9

be assigned with codes for category N17 for any documented underlying conditions.

If both a stage of CKD and end-stage renal disease (ESRD) are documented, only code N18.6 should be assigned. Before assigning a code for CKD, first code either of the following associated conditions:

- Diabetic chronic kidney disease (E08.22, E09.22, E10.22, E11.22, E13.22)
- Hypertensive chronic kidney disease (I12.-, I13.-)

Use an additional code (Z94.0) to identify kidney transplant status, if applicable.

In the event that kidney disease progresses to end-stage renal disease, renal transplantation may be the best option. Although a renal transplant is beneficial to patients with chronic kidney disease, the transplant may not result in complete restoration of renal function. If a kidney transplant recipient has chronic kidney disease, a code from category N18, chronic kidney disease (CKD), should be assigned, followed by Z94.0, kidney transplant status as a secondary code. This is supported by coding guideline *I.14.1.2) Chronic Kidney Disease and Kidney Transplant Status*. However, coding for documentation of failure or rejection of a kidney transplant is directed through coding guideline *I.C.19.g.3) (b) Chronic kidney disease and kidney transplant complications*. Of course, any time there is a need for clarification regarding the issue of complication, it is appropriate to query the provider. For example, a patient has had a kidney transplant yet still has stage II chronic kidney disease. This patient's condition should be coded by first assigning code N18.2, chronic kidney disease, stage II (mild), followed by code Z94.0, kidney transplant status.

Other conditions are often present in patients with chronic kidney disease. Some of the most common coexisting conditions are hypertension and diabetes mellitus. Coders should pay close attention to instructional notes in the tabular list for sequencing. The instructions supporting this direction are found in coding guideline *I.14.1.3) Chronic Kidney Disease with Other Conditions*. For instructions specific to chronic kidney disease with hypertension, see coding guideline *I.C.9. Hypertensive chronic kidney disease*.

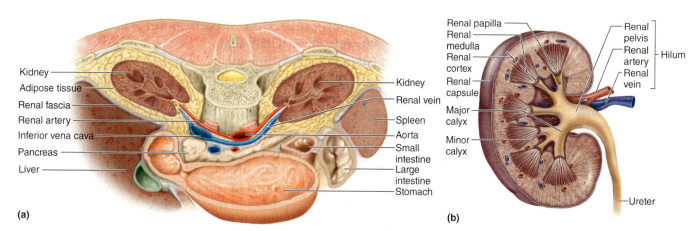

figure 17.3 Kidney: *(a)* Transverse Section of Abdomen; *(b)* Longitudinal Section of Kidney

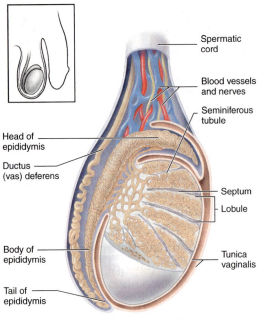

Spermatic cord

Blood vessels and nerves

Seminiferous tubule

Head of epididymis

Ductus (vas) deferens

Septum

Lobule

Body of epididymis

Tunica vaginalis

Tail of epididymis

figure 17.7 Testis and Associated Structures

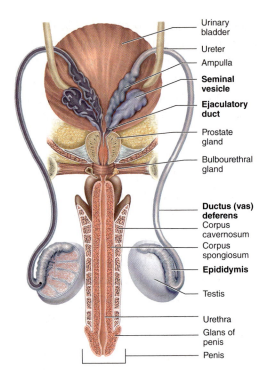

Urinary bladder

Ureter

Ampulla

Seminal vesicle

Ejaculatory duct

Prostate gland

Bulbourethral gland

Ductus (vas) deferens

Corpus cavernosum

Corpus spongiosum

Epididymis

Testis

Urethra

Glans of penis

Penis

figure 17.8 Components of Male Reproductive Ducts

Think About It 17.3

also available in connect plus+

Assign ICD-10-CM codes for the following situations, applying any appropriate sequencing guidelines.

1. Torsion of spermatic cord   _____

2. An ejaculatory orgasm   _____

3. Prostatic stone   _____

4. Benign prostatic hypertrophy with urinary frequency   _____

5. Paraphimosis   _____

Beyond the Code: General coding guidelines normally direct the coder not to report symptom codes when reporting definitive diagnoses. However, coding guidelines for reporting enlarged prostate require the coder to assign symptom codes as secondary codes for LUTS. What is the significance of LUTS, and who may benefit from the codes being reported?

17.4 Breast Disorders and Conditions of the Female Genital System

The breast and female genitourinary system are largely responsible for sexual and reproductive cycles that ensure the preservation of the human species. The breasts produce milk to nourish a growing baby. The genitourinary system contains the ovaries, fallopian tubes, uterus, cervix, vagina, and vulva, which are the anatomic structures responsible for carrying out the complex mechanisms of conception, pregnancy, and childbirth. When structural and physiological mechanisms go wrong, both inflammatory and noninflammatory disorders can affect the female breasts and genitourinary organs. In ICD-10-CM under this category of codes are a variety of disorders of the breast, such as dysplasias, fibrocystic disease, fibroadenosis and sclerosis, ectasia, abscesses, inflammatory disorders, hypertrophy, fissures, fistula, atrophy, nipple disorders, ptosis, and structural deformities, which impede normal functioning. Disorders of the female genitalia involve the ovaries, fallopian tubes, cervix, endometrium, uterus, pelvic region, vagina, and vulva.

Coding guidelines for this section of ICD-10-CM are relatively straightforward, with the greatest need for knowledge focused on terminology for the conditions reported. Several conditions of the female genitourinary organs are often documented by physicians using terms other than the boldfaced terms in the tabular list, so it may be helpful to review the alternate terminology listed with the codes. ICD-9-CM classifies these conditions in Chapter 10, "Diseases of the Genitourinary System," which includes code categories 610–612. ICD-10-CM classifies these conditions in Chapter 14, "Diseases of the Genitourinary System," which includes code categories N60–N65.

N60–N65 Disorders of Breast

Codes in this subsection of ICD-10-CM correspond with those in categories 610–612 in ICD-9-CM. Conditions coded in this subsection include cysts, fibroadenosis and sclerosis, ectasia, mammary duct disorders, abscesses, hypertrophy, **gynecomastia,** lumps, nodules, fissures, fistulas, fat necrosis, galactorrhea, galactocele, mastodynia, ptosis, nipple discharge, indurations, and other deformities.

The overall layout of this subsection is nearly identical in ICD-9-CM and ICD-10-CM. The most significant change in this subsection is the addition of laterality to the codes. This requires greater detail in documentation, along with ensuring clarity in laterality if the physician documents using drawings, as illustrated in Figure 17.9. Figure 17.10 identifies specific structures in the breast.

> **Spotlight on A&P**
>
> Because physicians occasionally use a variety of terms to document conditions of the female genital system, coders should be familiar with pathophysiological terms related to the ovaries, fallopian tubes, cervix, endometrium, uterus, pelvic region, vagina, and vulva.

gynecomastia Enlargement of the male breast.

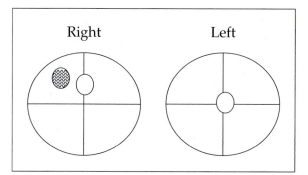

figure 17.9 Physician's Drawing of Solitary Cyst of Right Breast in Upper Outer Quadrant: Code N60.01, Solitary Cyst of Right Breast

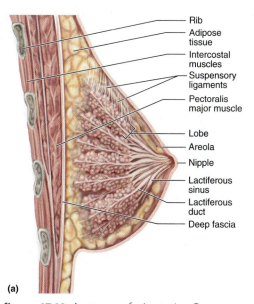

(a)

figure 17.10 Anatomy of a Lactating Breast

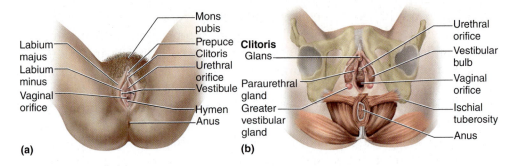

figure 17.11 Female Perineum and Vulva: *(a)* Surface Anatomy; *(b)* Subcutaneous Structures

N66–N69

Note that there are no code categories N66–N69.

N70–N77 Inflammatory Diseases of Female Pelvic Organs

Codes in this subsection of ICD-10-CM correspond with those in code categories 614–616 in ICD-9-CM. Conditions coded in this subsection include salpingitis, oophoritis, myometritis, cervicitis, pelvic inflammatory disease, ovarian and fallopian tube disorders, peritonitis, ulceration, inflammation, and vaginitis.

Codes for acute, chronic, and unspecified salpingitis and oophoritis have been expanded in ICD-10-CM to provide the ability to report salpingitis alone, oophoritis alone, or salpingitis and oophoritis together. When reporting conditions in categories N70–N73, if an infectious agent is documented, it should be reported with a secondary code from the B95–B97 range. Codes N74, N77.0, and N77.1 are for use only as secondary codes, following the code for the underlying disease.

N80–N98 Noninflammatory Disorders of Female Genital Tract

Codes in this subsection of ICD-10-CM correspond with those in code categories 617–629 in ICD-9-CM. Conditions coded in this subsection include **endometriosis,** urethrocele, **cystocele,** enterocele, **rectocele,** a variety of prolapses and fistulas, cysts, atrophy, adhesions, erosions, dysplasias and hypertrophies, strictures, stenosis, leukoplakia, hematocolpos, and menstrual and menopausal conditions such as **dysmenorrhea.** The subsection also includes codes for conditions related to fertility, infertility, and pregnancy, as well as complications that may arise from any female sexual or reproductive disorder. Structures affected by these disorders are presented in Figures 17.11 and 17.12.

The general layout of this subsection is relatively similar in ICD-9-CM and ICD-10-CM. Coding guidelines in this subsection are straightforward with no unusual situations, aside from instructional notes that specify the use of additional codes and sequencing.

endometriosis Presence of endometrial tissue in the abdomen outside the uterus.

cystocele Hernia of the bladder into the vagina.

rectocele Hernia of the rectum into the vagina.

dysmenorrhea Painful and difficult menstruation.

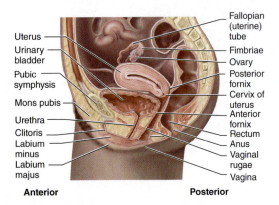

figure 17.12 Female Reproductive Organs

Assign ICD-10-CM codes for the following situations, applying any appropriate sequencing guidelines.

1. CIN II cervical dysplasia   _____

2. Endometriosis of the intestine   _____

3. Female infertility due to occlusion of fallopian tube   _____

4. Postcoital bleeding   _____

5. Rigid hymen   _____

Beyond the Code: Because physicians may use a variety of terms to document conditions of the female genitourinary system, terms that are different from the boldfaced terms in the tabular list, coders must become familiar with alternate terminology to describe the conditions. Review both the inflammatory and noninflammatory disorders of the female genitourinary system. List five conditions, along with at least one alternate way that each may be documented.

17.5 Intra-operative and Postprocedural Complications

Although medical and surgical treatments, procedures, and surgical interventions are intended to correct or cure diseases, occasionally complications occur. Complications can happen during a procedure or after it, and there is a wide variety of complications. Some are infectious; others involve hemorrhage or changes in the structure or function of an organ.

N99 Intra-operative and Postprocedural Complications and Disorders of Genitourinary System, Not Elsewhere Classified

Codes in this subsection of ICD-10-CM do not correspond with any code categories in the genitourinary system chapter in ICD-9-CM. Conditions coded in this subsection include postoperative kidney failure, postprocedural urethral stricture, postoperative vaginal adhesions, posthysterectomy vaginal vault prolapse, postoperative pelvic peritoneal adhesions, urinary tract stoma complications, intra-operative hemorrhage of a genitourinary system organ or structure complicating a procedure, and accidental puncture and laceration of a genitourinary system organ or structure during a procedure. When reporting postprocedural kidney failure, an additional code should be assigned to identify the type of kidney disease.

Postoperative complications are being minimized by the development of minimally invasive surgical techniques. It is now necessary for coders to identify conditions that are present on admission (POA) or acquired throughout the course of inpatient hospitalization. President George W. Bush signed the Deficit Reduction Act of 2005, which holds healthcare facilities accountable for hospital-acquired, or nosocomial, infections. Nosocomial infections are a risk for anyone who undergoes invasive surgical procedures that require extended surgical incisions and organ exposure. Outpatient laparoscopic procedures not only reduce the chances of postsurgical complications but also reduce the length of stay, utilization of supplies to treat the patient, and the costs associated with inpatient admission.

Spotlight on A&P

Nosocomial infections are a risk for anyone who undergoes invasive surgical procedures that require extended surgical incisions and organ exposure.

Think About It 17.5

also available in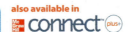

Assign ICD-10-CM codes for the following situations, applying any appropriate sequencing guidelines.

1. Acute renal failure with medullary necrosis documented as a postoperative complication   _____

2. Residual ovary syndrome   _____

3. Accidental puncture of the bladder during colon resection   _____

4. Posthysterectomy vaginal vault prolapse   _____

5. Cystostomy malfunction   _____

Beyond the Code: ICD-9-CM classified postprocedural complications for all systems in Chapter 17, "Injury and Poisoning." What are the pros and cons of classifying postprocedural complications in the respective chapters for the systems in which they occur, instead of classifying all complications in the same chapter?

Chapter Summary

Learning Outcome	Key Concepts/Examples
17.1 Interpret guidelines for coding glomerular and renal tubulo-interstitial diseases. **(pages 250–251)**	• Be aware of guidelines for reporting symptoms. • Watch for instructions to code underlying diseases or infectious agents.
17.2 Apply coding guidelines for acute kidney failure, chronic kidney disease, urolithiasis, and other disorders of the urinary system. **(pages 252–255)**	• Stages of CKD are classified by severity. • CKD may still be present following a kidney transplant. • Follow coding guidelines *I.C.9.* and *I.C.19* for additional guidance when hypertensive or complicating conditions are present.
17.3 Identify additional codes required with disorders of male genital organs. **(pages 256–258)**	• Codes for azoospermia and oligospermia have been expanded in ICD-10-CM to provide coders the ability to report causal factors. • Priapism, erectile dysfunction, and ejaculatory dysfunction codes have expanded in ICD-10-CM to report greater specificity.
17.4 Describe terminology used to document conditions of the breast and female genitourinary organs. **(pages 258–261)**	• Greater detail is needed in documentation to report laterality of breast diagnoses. • Several terms for conditions of the female genitourinary organs are often documented by physicians using terms other than the boldfaced terms in the tabular list
17.5 Assign codes for intra-operative and postprocedural complications of the genitourinary system. **(pages 261–262)**	• When reporting postprocedural kidney failure, an additional code should be assigned to identify the type of kidney disease.

Applying Your Skills

Assign codes for each of the following conditions, using ICD-9-CM and ICD-10-CM

Condition	ICD-9-CM Codes	ICD-10-CM Codes
1. *[LO 17.4]* Postural proteinuria		
2. *[LO 17.2]* Intrinsic sphincter deficiency causing stress incontinence		
3. *[LO 17.4]* Gynecomastia		
4. *[LO 17.2]* Calculus in diverticulum of bladder		
5. *[LO 17.3]* Acute prostatitis with hematuria		
6. *[LO 17.2]* Bilateral small kidneys		
7. *[LO 17.2]* Interstitial cystitis with hematuria		
8. *[LO 17.1]* Rapidly progressive nephritis with diffuse mesangiocapillary glomerulonephritis		
9. *[LO 17.3]* Multiple spermatoceles of epididymis		
10. *[LO 17.2]* ESRD		
11. *[LO 17.3]* Retarded ejaculation		
12. *[LO 17.1]* Chlamydial urethritis		
13. *[LO 17.4]* Subacute vulvitis		
14. *[LO 17.3]* Prostatic intraepithelial neoplasia II		
15. *[LO 17.2]* Gross hematuria		
16. *[LO 17.2]* Traumatic anterior urethral stricture in a male		
17. *[LO 17.2]* Female stress incontinence		
18. *[LO 17.2]* Megaloureter		
19. *[LO 17.1]* Left-sided vesicoureteral-reflux with reflux nephropathy and hydroureter		
20. *[LO 17.2]* Renal colic		

Checking Your Understanding

Select the letter that best answers the question or completes the sentence.

1. *[LO 17.2]* The physician documents that a patient has nephroureterolithiasis. What is the appropriate code assignment?

  a. N20.0   **b.** N20.1   **c.** N20.2   **d.** N20.0 and N20.1

2. *[LO 17.4]* What code(s) should be assigned for enterocele with second-degree uterine prolapse?

  a. N81.2   **b.** N81.5   **c.** N81.2 and N81.5   **d.** 81.3

3. *[LO 17.2]* What is the correct code assignment for a patient with stage V chronic kidney disease, dependent on dialysis?

  a. N18.5   **b.** N18.5 and Z99.2   **c.** N18.6   **d.** N18.6 and Z99.2

4. *[LO 17.3]* What is the appropriate code assignment for priapism caused by sickle cell anemia?

  a. D57.1, N48.32   **b.** N48.32, D57.1   **c.** N48.32   **d.** N48.39, D57.1

5. *[LO 17.4]* What is the appropriate code assignment for a patient experiencing flushing with menopause?

  a. N95.1   **b.** N95.1, R23.2   **c.** R23.2, N95.1   **d.** R23.2

6. **[LO 17.1]** Which of the following situations is appropriate for the assignment of a code from category N02?

   a. patient experiencing hematuria with bladder cancer
   b. patient experiencing gross hematuria
   c. patient with extracapillary glomerulonephritis having recurrent hematuria
   d. patient with benign essential hematuria

7. **[LO 17.5]** What is the appropriate code assignment for bladder hemorrhage as a complication during transurethral resection of a bladder tumor?

   a. N99.61   **b.** N99.61, N32.89   **c.** N32.89, N99.61   **d.** N32.89

8. **[LO 17.4]** What is the appropriate code assignment for chronic salpingitis and chronic oophoritis?

   a. N70.11, N70.12   **b.** N70.12, N70.11   **c.** N70.13   **d.** N70.93

9. **[LO 17.3]** What is the appropriate code assignment for benign prostatic hypertrophy with urinary frequency?

   a. N40.0   **b.** N40.1   **c.** N40.1, R35.0   **d.** R35.0, N40.1

10. **[LO 17.1]** What is the appropriate code assignment for isolated proteinuria with dense deposit disease?

   a. N05.6, R80.0   **b.** N06.6   **c.** N06.6, R80.0   **d.** R80.0, N06.6

Online Activity

[LO 17.1, LO 17.2, LO 17.3, LO 17.4, LO 17.5] Search online for information about how conditions of the genitourinary system can in turn cause problems such as retention of urine or incontinence. Summarize your findings in a brief report.

Real-World Application: Case Study

[LO 17.4] Assign ICD-10-CM diagnosis codes for the following discharge summary.

DISCHARGE SUMMARY

ADMISSION DIAGNOSES:
1. Menometrorrhagia.
2. Dysmenorrhea.

DISCHARGE DIAGNOSES:
1. Endometriosis of uterus and fallopian tube.
2. Menometrorrhagia.
3. Dysmenorrhea.

OPERATION PERFORMED: Total abdominal hysterectomy.

BRIEF HISTORY AND PHYSICAL: The patient is a 37-year-old white female, gravida 2, para 2, with two prior vaginal deliveries. She is having increasing menometrorrhagia and dysmenorrhea. Ultrasound shows endometriosis. She has failed oral contraceptives and surgical therapy is planned.

PAST HISTORY: Significant for reflux.

SURGICAL HISTORY: Appendectomy.

LABORATORY VALUES: Her discharge hemoglobin is 12.4.

HOSPITAL COURSE: The patient was admitted following a total abdominal hysterectomy, which was uneventful. Postoperatively, she has done well with bowel and bladder function returning to normal. She is ambulating well and tolerating a regular diet. On the second postoperative day, the patient was discharged home in good condition with routine postoperative instructions, Vicodin PRN for pain, and follow up in the office in four weeks.

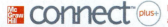

18

PREGNANCY, CHILDBIRTH, AND THE PUERPERIUM

Learning Outcomes *After completing this chapter, students should be able to*

18.1 Apply chapter-specific coding guidelines.

18.2 Classify pregnancy conditions with abortive outcomes.

18.3 Identify conditions that are considered high risk in pregnancy.

18.4 Describe coding requirements for maternal conditions impacting the management of pregnancy.

18.5 Determine appropriate codes and sequencing for conditions related to delivery.

18.6 Apply coding guidelines for conditions of the puerperium and other obstetric conditions.

Key Terms

active phase of labor
blighted ovum
cephalopelvic
    disproportion
deep transverse arrest
dystocia
eclampsia
ectopic pregnancy
fetopelvic disproportion
hydatidiform mole
latent phase of labor
malpresentation
miscarriage
missed abortion
molar pregnancy
primigravida
puerperium
rhesus isoimmunization
spontaneous abortion
uterine inertia

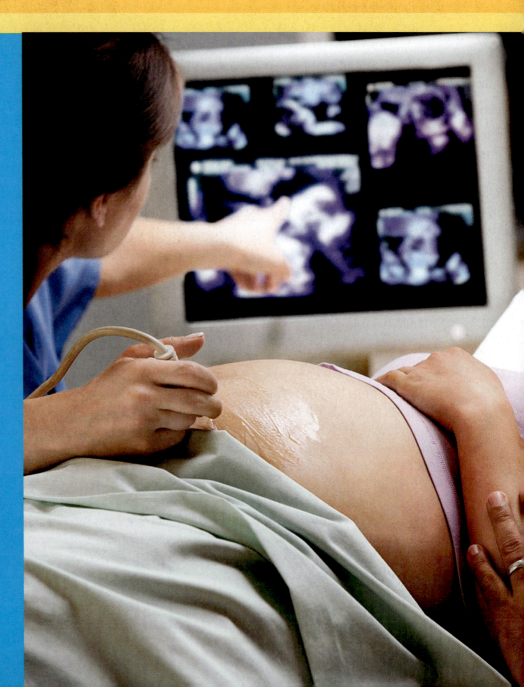

Introduction

There are many aspects to be considered when coding pregnancy, including high-risk pregnancy conditions and maternal conditions impacting the management of pregnancy. Coders must also be aware of conditions related to delivery and the **puerperium**, along with other obstetric conditions, including pregnancies with abortive outcomes. ICD-9-CM classifies all of these conditions in Chapter 11, "Complications of Pregnancy, Childbirth, and the Puerperium," which includes code categories 630–679. ICD-10-CM classifies these conditions in Chapter 15, "Pregnancy, Childbirth and the Puerperium," which includes code categories O00–O99.

puerperium Period of time beginning immediately after childbirth and continuing up to the time the uterus returns to its normal size, usually defined as 42 days.

> **Spotlight on A&P**
>
> ICD-10-CM codes for conditions in pregnancy, childbirth, and the puerperium require an understanding of the structures of the female reproductive system and the physiological changes that occur during specific trimesters of pregnancy.

18.1 Chapter-Specific Coding Guidelines

Many coding guidelines apply to the entire range of codes for pregnancy, childbirth, and the puerperium. Codes presented in this chapter are for assignment only on the maternal record, never on the newborn record. This is supported by coding guideline *I.C.15.a.2) Chapter 15 Codes Used Only on the Maternal Record*.

It is critical that coders are careful when entering codes from this section—they must be able to differentiate between the letter O and the number 0.

One significant difference between ICD-9-CM and ICD-10-CM regarding pregnancy and childbirth is that ICD-9-CM required the use of fifth digits to identify if an encounter was for delivery, antepartum care, or postpartum. ICD-10-CM no longer uses that approach for classification. However, ICD-10-CM classifies most conditions in this chapter according to trimester, using the final character in the code to designate the trimester. Details are outlined in coding guideline *I.C.15.a.3) Final Character for Trimester*. Table 18.1 defines trimesters according to weeks and days.

There are some exceptions, however, such as conditions that always occur during a specific trimester and conditions for which trimester is not considered to be a pertinent or applicable detail to be reported. Other conditions do not occur in all trimesters, so the codes for those conditions have

> **Spotlight on A&P**
>
> Calculation of trimester is based on the first day of the last menstrual period.

Table 18.1 Definitions of Trimesters

Trimester	Definition
1st trimester	0 days to 13 weeks 6 days
2nd trimester	14 weeks 0 days to 27 weeks 6 days
3rd trimester	28 weeks 0 days until delivery

final characters only to represent trimesters during which the conditions occur. Determining that final character for the trimester should be based on the dates of the current encounter being coded, and it should be consistent for both pre-existing conditions and those developing during or due to the pregnancy. If the patient delivers during the admission, the "in childbirth" option for the obstetric complication being coded should be assigned.

Coding guideline *I.C.15.a.4) Selection of Trimester for Inpatient Admissions That Encompass More Than One Trimester* addresses the question that coders may have about what to do if a patient is admitted to a hospital for complications of pregnancy during one trimester and remains in the hospital into a subsequent trimester. In these cases, the trimester character for the code should be assigned based on the trimester when the complication developed, rather than the trimester of the discharge. The trimester character for the trimester at the time of admission or the encounter should be assigned in cases of development of the condition prior to the admission or encounter or when the condition is considered to be a pre-existing condition.

Although codes are provided in each category for "unspecified trimester," these codes are available only for rare cases in which there is insufficient documentation to determine the trimester and it is not possible to obtain clarification, according to coding guideline *I.C.15.a.5) Unspecified Trimester*.

In the assignment of codes from this chapter for obstetric cases, the Chapter 15 codes in the range O00–O9A have priority for sequencing purposes. Additional codes from other chapters may be assigned as secondary codes to provide further specificity. However, if the reason for the episode of care is not obstetric and not related to the management of pregnancy, code Z33.1, Pregnant state, incidental, should be reported as an additional code. These instructions are supported by coding guideline *I.C.15.a.1) Codes from Chapter 15 and Sequencing Priority*.

Not every obstetric admission or encounter results in delivery. For cases that do not result in delivery, the principal diagnosis or first-listed code should be for the main complication of pregnancy that necessitated the encounter. If multiple complications meet the definition of principal diagnosis, codes for any of the complications may be sequenced first. This is supported by coding guidelines *I.C.15.b.3) Episodes When No Delivery Occurs*.

Whenever an admission results in delivery, the maternal record should have a code from category Z37, Outcome of delivery, assigned as a secondary code. This code is assigned only on the episode of care during which the delivery occurred, as supported by coding guideline *I.C.15.b.5) Outcome of Delivery*. The principal diagnosis for an admission in which a delivery occurs should be that which is the main circumstance of delivery or the complication that prompted delivery. If the delivery was via cesarean section, the principal diagnosis should be determined according to the Uniform Hospital Discharge Data Set (UHDDS) definition of principal diagnosis. If the admission was for a condition that resulted in a cesarean section, that condition should be sequenced as the principal diagnosis. However, if the reason for admission was not related to the reason for cesarean section, the code for the condition responsible for the admission should be assigned as the principal diagnosis. This instruction is supported by coding guideline *I.C.15.b.4) When a Delivery Occurs*.

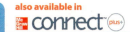
Identify the principal diagnosis in the following scenarios.

1. Patient with gestational diabetes develops severe pre-eclampsia admitted for an emergency cesarean section _____

2. Patient in the first trimester of pregnancy with twins with hyperemesis gravidarum admitted for IV fluids _____

3. Patient presenting to labor and delivery with premature rupture of membranes at 37 weeks' gestation; vaginal delivery resulting in single liveborn with nuchal cord _____

18.2 Pregnancy with Abortive Outcome

Not all pregnancies result in a live birth. When a pregnancy ends in an abortive outcome, it must be reported on the maternal record. This section presents the codes used to identify various types of abortive pregnancy outcomes, along with associated complications that can occur. ICD-10-CM categories O00–O08, which are similar to categories 630–639 in ICD-9-CM, are used to report pregnancies with abortive outcomes.

O00–O08 Pregnancy with Abortive Outcome

Codes in this subsection of ICD-10-CM correspond with those in categories 630–639 in ICD-9-CM. Conditions coded in this subsection include the following:

- **Ectopic pregnancy**
- Abdominal pregnancy
- Tubal pregnancy
- Ovarian pregnancy
- **Hydatidiform mole**
- **Blighted ovum**
- **Missed abortion**
- **Spontaneous abortion**
- **Miscarriage**
- Complications associated with spontaneous abortion
- Complications following termination of pregnancy
- Failed attempted termination of pregnancy
- Complications associated with failed attempted termination of pregnancy
- Complications following ectopic and **molar pregnancy**

ectopic pregnancy Pregnancy that occurs outside the cavity of the uterus, either in the fallopian tube or, rarely, in the abdomen.

hydatidiform mole Mass that forms inside the uterus at the beginning of pregnancy.

blighted ovum Pregnancy in which a fertilized egg becomes attached to the uterine wall but does not develop into an embryo.

missed abortion Early death of the fetus prior to 20 weeks gestation with retention of the deceased fetus.

spontaneous abortion Miscarriage.

miscarriage Spontaneous loss of the fetus before 20 weeks of gestation.

molar pregnancy Pregnancy in which the tissue, that would normally become a fetus, instead develops into an abnormal growth.

The term "young," when referring to pregnancy conditions, indicates a female who is less than 16 years of age at the expected date of delivery.

Think About It 18.3

also available in
McGraw Hill **connect** plus+

Assign ICD-10-CM codes for the following situations, applying any appropriate sequencing guidelines.

1. Office visit for routine prenatal care for uncomplicated first pregnancy in a 36-year-old patient at 13 weeks' gestation _____

2. Office visit for routine prenatal care of a 27-year-old patient at 18 weeks' gestation with history of pre-term labor in previous pregnancy _____

3. Office visit for routine prenatal care of uncomplicated first pregnancy in a 28-year-old patient at 27 weeks' gestation _____

4. Office visit for routine prenatal care of uncomplicated second pregnancy in a 15-year-old patient at 16 weeks' gestation _____

5. First prenatal care visit for a 17-year-old patient, who is at 34 weeks' gestation _____

Beyond the Code: For each of the following conditions, identify whether it is considered to be "high risk" for the purposes of coding pregnancy.

1. _____ In-vitro fertilization

2. _____ Elevated glucose tolerance test

3. _____ Patient age 37

4. _____ Social conditions, such as unemployment

5. _____ Patient age 17

6. _____ History of pre-term labor

18.4 Maternal Conditions Impacting the Management of Pregnancy

A pregnant woman may have a condition that existed prior to pregnancy, or that develops during pregnancy, that affects how the physician manages her care during the pregnancy. These conditions include edema, proteinuria, hypertension, diabetes, and other disorders. This section presents coding guidelines for these conditions, which are classified to categories O10–O29 in ICD-10-CM, which parallel categories 642, 642, 646, and 671 in ICD-9-CM.

O10–O16 Edema, Proteinuria, and Hypertensive Disorders in Pregnancy, Childbirth, and the Puerperium

Codes in this subsection of ICD-10-CM correspond with those in code category 642 and codes 646.1- and 646.2- in ICD-9-CM. Conditions coded in this subsection include pre-existing conditions of hypertension, hypertensive heart disease, and hypertensive chronic kidney disease, complicating pregnancy, childbirth, and the puerperium. Other conditions included in this subsection are pre-existing hypertension with pre-eclampsia, gestational edema and proteinuria without hypertension, gestational hypertension without significant proteinuria, pre-eclampsia, *HELLP* syndrome (combination of symptoms that include Hemolysis, Elevated Liver enzymes, and Low Platelet count), **eclampsia** in pregnancy, eclampsia in labor, and eclampsia in the puerperium. Note that there are no categories O17–O19.

Coding guideline *I.C.15.c. Pre-existing Conditions versus Conditions Due to the Pregnancy* stresses the importance of determining whether a condition existed prior to pregnancy or developed during the pregnancy. Some of the codes in this chapter do not differentiate conditions as being pre-existing or related to the pregnancy, so they may be used in either case. Codes specified as being for the puerperium may be assigned along with codes for complications of pregnancy and childbirth if a condition develops postpartum during the encounter for delivery.

Category O10, Pre-existing hypertension complicating pregnancy, childbirth, and the puerperium, provides codes to report hypertensive heart and hypertensive chronic kidney disease. Coding guideline *I.C.15.d. Pre-existing Hypertension in Pregnancy* directs the coder to add a secondary code from the appropriate hypertension category to specify the type of heart failure or chronic kidney disease when assigning one of the O10 codes including hypertensive heart disease or hypertensive chronic kidney disease.

eclampsia Convulsions or seizures associated with hypertension and proteinuria in pregnancy, not caused by epilepsy or other cerebral conditions, and potentially life-threatening to both mother and fetus.

O20–O29 Other Maternal Disorders Predominantly Related to Pregnancy

Codes in this subsection of ICD-10-CM correspond with those in code categories 640, 643, 646, and 671 and code 796.5 in ICD-9-CM. Conditions coded in this subsection include threatened abortion, other hemorrhage in early pregnancy, excessive vomiting, varicose veins of lower extremity, genital varices, superficial thrombophlebitis, deep phlebothrombosis, hemorrhoids, cerebral venous thrombosis, genitourinary tract infections, pre-existing diabetes mellitus, gestational diabetes mellitus, malnutrition, excessive weight gain, low weight gain, pregnancy care for patient with recurrent pregnancy loss, retained intrauterine contraceptive device,

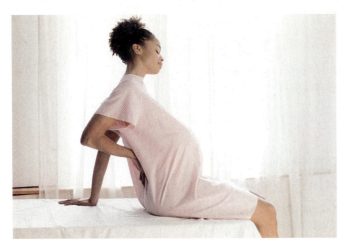

Complications can arise during a pregnancy if the mother has an existing condition. Maternal conditions can also arise as a result of pregnancy.

herpes gestationis, maternal hypotension syndrome liver disorders, subluxation of symphysis pubis, exhaustion and fatigue, peripheral neuritis, pregnancy-related renal disease, uterine size-date discrepancy, spotting, pruritic urticarial papules and plaques of pregnancy (PUPPP), cervical shortening, abnormal antenatal screening findings, and complications of anesthesia.

The code for genitourinary tract infections in pregnancy expanded significantly from ICD-9-CM to ICD-10-CM. ICD-10-CM allows for specification of the site of the infection, providing codes to report infections of the kidney, bladder, urethra, and other parts of the urinary tract. This specificity in codes has eliminated the need for the assignment of an additional code from Chapter 14, "Diseases of the Genitourinary System." However, an additional code is still necessary to report the organism responsible for the infection in category B95 or B96.

Any documented manifestations of diabetes mellitus require an additional code from categories E11, E08, E09, and E13. Also, code Z79.4, long-term (current) use of insulin, should be assigned as a secondary code if insulin is being used to treat diabetes mellitus, according to coding guideline *I.C.15.h. Long-Term Use of Insulin*. According to coding guideline *I.C.15.g. Diabetes Mellitus in Pregnancy*, the code O24, Diabetes mellitus in pregnancy, childbirth, and the puerperium, should be sequenced first for pregnant women who are diabetic, followed by the appropriate diabetes code(s) from Chapter 4 from the range E08–E13.

Gestational diabetes, or pregnancy-induced diabetes, may occur in the second or third trimester of pregnancy in non-diabetic women. Pregnancy complications of gestational diabetes are often similar to those caused by diabetes mellitus that existed prior to pregnancy. In addition, women who develop gestational diabetes are at an increased risk of developing diabetes mellitus following pregnancy. The condition is coded with specific combination codes in ICD-10-CM, which eliminates the need to assign an additional code for the presence of diabetes mellitus. Coding guideline *I.C.15 Gestational (Pregnancy-Induced) Diabetes* outlines the rules to be followed for coding gestational diabetes. Gestational diabetes is reported using codes in subcategory O24.4, gestational diabetes mellitus, which includes codes for diet-controlled and insulin-controlled gestational diabetes. It is not appropriate to assign any other codes from category O24, diabetes mellitus in pregnancy, childbirth, and the puerperium, with a code from this subcategory. It is also not appropriate to assign code Z79.4, long-term (current) use of insulin with codes from subcategory O24.4.

If a patient has an abnormal glucose tolerance test during pregnancy, it is reported using codes from subcategory O99.81, Abnormal glucose complicating pregnancy, childbirth, and the puerperium.

In ICD-9-CM, abnormal antenatal screening findings were classified with very general codes in Chapter 16, "Signs, Symptoms, and Ill-Defined

Conditions." However, in ICD-10-CM, they have very specific codes in Chapter 15, "Pregnancy, Childbirth, and the Puerperium." When assigning codes from category O29 for complications of anesthesia in pregnancy, an additional code should be used to report the specific complication.

Think About It 18.4

also available in **McGraw Hill connect** plus+

Assign ICD-10-CM codes for the following situations, applying any appropriate sequencing guidelines.

1. Female in second trimester of pregnancy with pre-existing hypertensive left heart failure _____

2. Gestational edema with proteinuria in the third trimester _____

3. Insulin-controlled gestational diabetes mellitus during pregnancy _____

4. *E. coli* pyelonephritis in the first trimester of pregnancy _____

5. Excessive vomiting in the third trimester of pregnancy _____

Beyond the Code: For each of the following conditions, identify how many codes are needed to report the condition.

1. _____ Gestational diabetes requiring insulin

2. _____ Cystitis in pregnancy

3. _____ Hypertensive heart disease in pregnancy

4. _____ Abnormal glucose tolerance in pregnancy

18.5 Conditions Related to Delivery

Another aspect of pregnancy that presents an opportunity for additional conditions and complications is the delivery process. These conditions are reported with codes in categories O30–O82 in ICD-10-CM, which are consistent with categories 645 and 650–669 in ICD-9-CM. Some of the conditions reported in this section are related to fetal issues that may contribute to potential delivery problems, whereas others are maternal in origin. There are also codes in this section to report reasons for various types of delivery.

Spotlight on A&P

When coding conditions related to delivery, coders should be aware of the physiological processes of each phase of labor. They should keep in mind the anatomic structures involved, along with potential complications of the delivery process.

7. *[LO 18.3]* A 42-year-old pregnant patient (first pregnancy), pregnant with twins, with diet-controlled gestational diabetes is seen in the office during the third trimester for a routine prenatal visit. What should be the first-listed diagnosis code?

    a. O09.513   **b.** O09.523   **c.** O24.410   **d.** O30.003

8. *[LO 18.1]* A pregnant patient with gestational diabetes is admitted for treatment of an infectious disease. While in the hospital, she develops eclampsia, for which an emergency cesarean delivery is performed. What should be assigned as the principal diagnosis?

    a. eclampsia   **b.** infection complicating pregnancy

    c. gestational diabetes   **d.** outcome of delivery

9. *[LO 18.4]* What is the appropriate code assignment for acute *E. coli* cystitis in the second trimester of pregnancy?

    a. O23.12, N30.00, B96.2   **b.** N30.00, O23.12, B96.2

    c. B96.2, O23.12   **d.** O23.12, B96.2

10. *[LO 18.6]* For coding purposes, how long is the postpartum period?

    e. four weeks   **f.** six weeks   **g.** eight weeks   **h.** five months

Online Activity

[LO 18.1] Search online for agencies that use obstetric codes for public health surveillance. Describe your findings in a brief report.

Real-World Application

[LO 18.1, LO 18.2, LO 18.3] Assign ICD-10-CM diagnosis codes for the following discharge summary.

Discharge Summary

Discharge Diagnosis: HELLP syndrome

History and Physical Examination: Susan Brown is a 37-year-old primigravida patient, who presented to the office at 32 weeks of gestation with complaints of blurred vision and severe headache. Review of systems was significant for scanty urination over previous 24 hours.

Admission Labs:

    Serum creatinine 1.6

    ALT: 24 U/L

    AST: 22 U/L

    Platelets: 50,000

Hospital Course: Patient was transported via ambulance from the office. Blood pressure at admission 220/120. IV hydralazine was administered in 10 mg bolus for control of blood pressure, and betamethasone was given to promote fetal lung maturity. A 42 cm, 3 pound 8 ounce male was delivered via emergency cesarean section, and the patient was transferred to ICU for monitoring. Magnesium sulfate was administered with a 4 g bolus postdelivery, followed by continuous infusion of 2 g/hr for the following 12 hours. Postdelivery course was uneventful and blood pressure at discharge was 140/88.

Discharge Condition: Patient was discharged to home in good condition with instructions to follow up in office next week, engage in pelvic rest, consume a low-sodium diet, and avoid caffeine. Discharge medications include continuing prenatal vitamins and metoprolol 50 mg PO bid.

19

CONDITIONS ORIGINATING IN THE NEWBORN (PERINATAL) PERIOD

Learning Outcomes *After completing this chapter, students should be able to*

19.1 Apply chapter-specific coding guidelines for conditions originating in the perinatal period.

19.2 Explain the maternal factors and complications of pregnancy, labor, and delivery that impact the newborn.

19.3 Interpret guidelines for coding newborn disorders related to length of gestation, fetal growth, abnormal neonatal screening findings, and birth trauma.

19.4 Apply coding guidelines for respiratory, cardiovascular, and infectious conditions specific to the perinatal period.

19.5 Classify hematological, endocrine, metabolic, and digestive disorders of the newborn.

19.6 Identify conditions of integument, temperature regulation, and other disorders originating in the perinatal period.

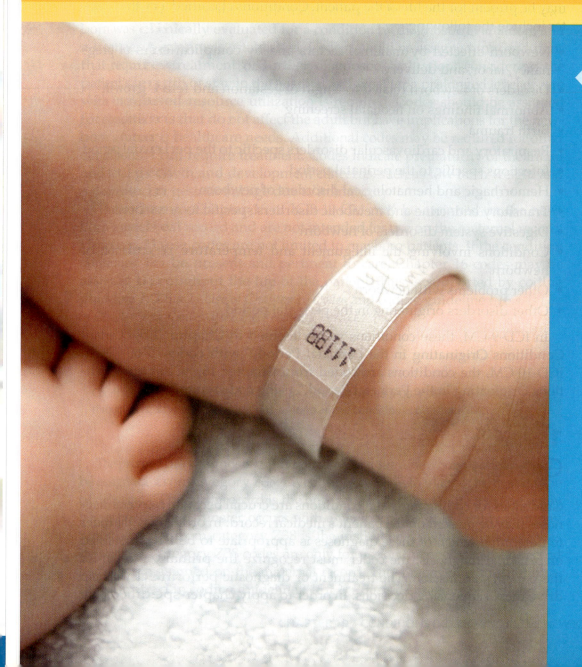

Key Terms

asphyxia

defibrination syndrome of newborn

disseminated intravascular coagulation

ductus arteriosus

ecchymosis

exchange transfusion

failure to thrive

hemolytic

hyaline membrane disease

hypercapnia

jaundice

meconium

neonatal

perinatal

petechia

stillbirth

transient tachypnea of newborn

wet lung syndrome

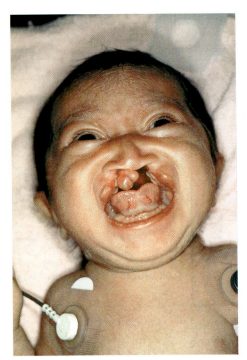

figure 20.4 Infant with Cleft Lip and Palate

Congenital malformations of the tongue, mouth, and larynx are further specified in category Q38 to report ankyloglossia, macroglossia, and other conditions. Category Q39 allows specific reporting for atresia of esophagus, tracheoesophageal fistula, congenital stenosis of stricture of esophagus, esophageal web, congenital dilation of esophagus, and congenital diverticulum of esophagus. Upper alimentary tract congenital malformations are reported according to the specific site in category Q40, including hypertrophic pyloric stenosis, hiatus hernia, and stomach malformations. Site specification is also the determining factor for code assignment in category Q41, which includes congenital absence, atresia, and stenosis of the small intestine, including specificity for the duodenum, jejunum, and ileum.

Congenital absence, atresia, and stenosis of the large intestine conditions are classified according to site and presence or absence of fistula in category Q42. Category Q43 reports other congenital malformations of the intestinal tract, including specific codes for Meckel's diverticulum, Hirschsprung disease, duplication of intestine, ectopic anus, congenital fistula of rectum and anus, and persistent cloaca. Congenital malformations of the gallbladder, bile ducts, and liver are further specified in category Q44, which includes codes for agenesis, aplasia, and hypoplasia of gallbladder; atresia of bile ducts; congenital stenosis and stricture of bile ducts; choledochal cyst; and cystic disease of the liver. Annular pancreas, congenital pancreatic cyst, and agenesis, aplasia, and hypoplasia of the pancreas are specified through codes in category Q45.

Think About It 20.4

also available in **McGraw Hill connect plus+**

There are several combination codes in this subsection, along with instructions for the assignment of additional codes. For each of the following scenarios, identify how many codes are required to report the condition.

1. _____ Cleft hard palate with cleft soft palate

2. _____ Median cleft lip with cleft nose

3. _____ Bilateral cleft lip with cleft hard and soft palate and cleft nose

4. _____ Cleft hard palate with unilateral cleft lip

Assign ICD-10-CM codes for the following situations, applying any appropriate sequencing guidelines.

1. Malrotation of the colon   _____

2. Accessory pancreas   _____

3. Congenital atresia of the salivary glands   _____

4. Fibrocystic disease of the liver   _____

5. Tongue tied   _____

20.5 Congenital Malformations of Genital Organs and Urinary System

Congenital malformations of the genital organs and urinary system present issues that may require surgical correction, whether the patient is an infant, a child, or an adult. These conditions are reported with categories Q50–Q64 in ICD-10-CM, which correlate with categories 752 and 753 in ICD-9-CM. Coders should note that some anatomic structures may overlap both the genital organ and urinary system classifications, which is why these two subsections were combined for this section of the chapter in ICD-10-CM.

Q50–Q56 Congenital Malformations of Genital Organs

Codes in this subsection of ICD-10-CM correspond with those in category 752 in ICD-9-CM. Conditions coded in this subsection include **ambiguous genitalia** and congenital malformations of ovaries, fallopian tubes, broad ligaments, uterus, cervix, vagina, hymen, labia, clitoris, vulva, testicles, penis, and vas deferens, and **ambiguous genitalia.**

Congenital malformations of ovaries, fallopian tubes, and broad ligaments are reported in category Q50 with codes to specify congenital absence of ovary, developmental ovarian cyst, congenital torsion of ovary, accessory ovary, ovarian streak, embryonic cyst of fallopian tube, and embryonic cyst of broad ligament. Note that laterality can be reported for congenital absence of ovary. Category Q51 specifies congenital malformations of the uterus and cervix, including agenesis and aplasia of uterus, doubling of uterus with doubling of cervix and vagina, **bicornuate** uterus, unicornuate uterus, agenesis and aplasia of cervix, **embryonic cyst** of cervix, congenital fistulae between uterus and digestive and urinary tracts, arcuate uterus, hypoplasia of uterus, cervical duplication, and hypoplasia of cervix. Other congenital malformations of female genitalia, which are reported in category Q52, include congenital absence of vagina, doubling of vagina, transverse vaginal septum, longitudinal vaginal septum, congenital rectovaginal fistula, imperforate hymen, fusion of labia, and congenital malformation of clitoris.

Undescended and ectopic testicles can be reported with specification of laterality, using codes in category Q53. Hypospadias is reported in category Q54, which provides codes to specify the condition as balanic, penile, penoscrotal, perineal, or congenital chordee. Other congenital malformations of male genital organs, which are reported in category Q55, may be specified as absence and aplasia of testis, hypoplasia of testis and scrotum, polyorchism, retractile testis, scrotal **transposition,** atresia of vas deferens, congenital absence and aplasia of penis, curvature of penis, hypoplasia of penis, and congenital vasocutaneous fistula. Category Q56 specifies conditions of indeterminate sex and pseudohermaphroditism, including ovotestis, male pseudohermaphroditism, female pseudohermaphroditism, and ambiguous genitalia.

Q57–Q59

Note that there are no categories Q57–Q59.

ambiguous genitalia
Appearing neither male nor female.

bicornuate Having two horns or two projections.

embryonic cyst Abnormal, fluid-containing sac that develops from embryonic tissue.

transposition Transfer of a DNA segment to a new site on the same or another chromosome or plasmid.

pes planus Flat foot with no plantar arch.

hallus varus, talipes calcaneovalgus, and **pes planus.** Category Q67 provides codes to classify congenital musculoskeletal deformities of head, face, spine, and chest, which include congenital facial asymmetry, compression facies, dolichocephaly, plagiocephaly, pectus excavatum, and pectus carinatum.

Q80–Q89 Other Congenital Malformations

Codes in this subsection of ICD-10-CM correspond with those in categories 757 and 759 in ICD-9-CM. Conditions coded in this subsection include congenital ichthyosis, epidermolysis bullosa, congenital malformations of the skin, congenital malformations of the breast, congenital malformations of the integument, phakomatoses, congenital malformation syndromes due to known exogenous causes, and congenital malformation syndromes affecting multiple systems.

Congenital ichthyosis, classified in category Q80, is further specified through codes for ichthyosis vulgaris, X-linked ichthyosis, lamellar ichthyosis, congenital bullous ichthyosiform erythroderma, and Harlequin fetus. Category Q81 provides specific classifications for epidermolysis bullosa simplex, epidermolysis bullosa letalis, and epidermolysis bullosa dystrophica. Other congenital skin malformations that are reported in category Q82 include hereditary lymphedema, xeroderma pigmentosum, mastocytosis, incontinentia pigmenti, ectodermal dysplasia, and congenital non-neoplastic nevus (which includes commonly known conditions, such as birthmarks, port-wine nevus, and strawberry nevus). Congenital malformations of the breast, reported in category Q83, include congenital absence of the breast with the absence of a nipple, accessory breast, absent nipple, and accessory nipple. Category Q84 classifies other congenital malformations of the integument, which include congenital alopecia, beaded hair, monilethrix, pili annulati, anonychia, congenital leukonychia, enlarged and hypertrophic nails, and other congenital malformations of nails and integument. Phakomatoses are further specified in category Q85 as type 1, type 2, schwannomatosis, and tuberous sclerosis. Congenital malformation syndromes due to known exogenous causes, classified in category Q86, include fetal alcohol syndrome, fetal hydantoin syndrome, and dysmorphism due to warfarin. When reporting codes from category Q87, it is necessary to assign additional codes to identify all associated documented manifestations. Conditions classified in this category include congenital malformation syndromes predominantly affecting facial appearance, congenital malformation syndromes predominantly associated with short stature, congenital malformation syndromes predominantly involving limbs, congenital malformation syndromes involving early overgrowth, Marfan syndrome, congenital malformation syndromes with other skeletal changes, Alport syndrome, asplenia, congenital malformations of the spleen, congenital malformations of the adrenal gland, congenital malformations of other endocrine glands, situs inversus, conjoined twins, and multiple congenital malformations. Note that there is no category Q88.

Q90–Q99 Chromosomal Abnormalities, Not Elsewhere Classified

Codes in this subsection of ICD-10-CM correspond with those in category 758 in ICD-9-CM. Conditions coded in this subsection include Down syndrome, **trisomy** 18, trisomy 13, whole chromosome trisomy, partial trisomy, duplications with other complex rearrangements, marker chromosomes, triploidy, polyploidy, monosomies and deletions from the autosomes, balanced rearrangements and structural markers, Turner syndrome, and sex chromosome abnormalities. Figure 20.5 demonstrates a normal set of male chromosomes. Chromosomal abnormalities are further classified as being nonmosaicism (meiotic nondisjunction), mosaicism (mitotic nondisjunction), or **translocation.**

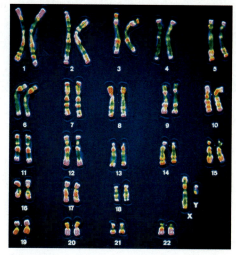

figure 20.5 Karyotype Showing the Complete Set of Chromosomes of a Normal Male

Q95

Note that there is no category Q95.

trisomy Presence of three chromosomes instead of two.

translocation Transfer of a part of a chromosome to a different location within the same chromosome, or the exchange of parts between two chromosomes.

Think About It 20.6

also available in **McGraw Hill connect** plus+

Assign ICD-10-CM codes for the following situations, applying any appropriate sequencing guidelines.

1. Accessory thumb _____

2. Trisomy 13 mosaicism _____

3. Webbed toes on the left foot _____

4. Congenital hallus varus _____

5. Supernumerary cervical rib _____

Beyond the Code: ICD-10-CM has introduced the ability to code the laterality of several musculoskeletal deformities, as well as to differentiate between partial and complete dislocation of the hip. What other details can you identify that may be considered for future additional specificity in reporting?

CHAPTER 20 REVIEW

Chapter Summary

Learning Outcome	Key Concepts/Examples
20.1 Interpret coding guidelines for congenital malformations, deformations, and chromosomal abnormalities to determine appropriate codes for these conditions. **(pages 311–312)**	• Codes from Chapter 17 may be used throughout the life of the patient. • For the birth admission, the appropriate code from category Z38, Liveborn infants, according to place of birth and type of delivery, should be sequenced as the principal diagnosis, followed by any congenital anomaly codes, Q00–Q89.
20.2 Apply coding guidelines for congenital malformations of the nervous system, eye, ear, face, and neck. **(pages 312–316)**	• Coding of spina bifida requires documentation regarding spinal level and presence or absence of hydrocephalus. • Although coding of congenital malformations of the eye, ear, face, and neck is very straightforward, coders should be aware of "excludes" notes.
20.3 Use knowledge of disease processes to assign appropriate codes for congenital malformations of the circulatory and respiratory systems. **(pages 317–319)**	• Congenital malformations of the circulatory system have straightforward coding guidelines, but several require knowledge of the disease processes to identify the appropriate code category. • Assignment of codes from the subsection of codes for congenital malformations of the respiratory system is very straightforward, without any special instructions and very few "excludes" notes.
20.4 Identify circumstances in which combination codes are required for coding cleft lip, cleft palate, and congenital malformations of the digestive system. **(pages 319–320)**	• Coding guidelines for cleft palate and cleft lip have changed significantly from ICD-9-CM to ICD-10-CM, eliminating the option to report as complete or incomplete and adding the ability to report laterality. • If there is documentation of any associated malformation of the nose with cleft palate or cleft lip, code Q30.2, fissured, notched, and cleft nose, should be assigned as a secondary code. • Many of the categories for reporting congenital malformations of the digestive system provide significantly greater specificity in reporting than was available in ICD-9-CM.
20.5 Classify congenital malformations of genital organs and urinary system according to ICD-10-CM coding guidelines. **(pages 321–322)**	• Be alert for codes requiring documentation of laterality with the genital organs and urinary system. • ICD-10-CM classifies hypospadias as a congenital malformation of the genital organs, but it classifies epispadias as a congenital malformation of the urinary system.
20.6 Analyze increased specificity in reporting codes for congenital malformations and deformations of the musculoskeletal system, other congenital malformations, and chromosomal abnormalities. **(pages 323–325)**	• Codes for hip dislocations in ICD-10-CM specify partial dislocation versus complete dislocation versus instability of the hip, which were not coded in ICD-9-CM. • Coders need to be aware of instructional notes to report associated documented manifestations.

Applying Your Skills

Assign codes for the following diagnoses, using both ICD-9-CM and ICD-10-CM.

Condition	ICD-9-CM Codes	ICD-10-CM Codes
1. *[LO 20.3]* Arteriovenous malformation of digestive system vessel		
2. *[LO 20.4]* Cleft uvula		
3. *[LO 20.6]* Fetal alcohol syndrome		
4. *[LO 20.5]* Left renal agenesis		
5. *[LO 20.3]* Congenital mitral insufficiency		
6. *[LO 20.2]* Congenital entropion		
7. *[LO 20.2]* Lumbar spina bifida with hydrocephalus		
8. *[LO 20.4]* Esophageal web		
9. *[LO 20.6]* Longitudinal reduction defect of the left tibia		
10. *[LO 20.6]* Congenital diaphragmatic hernia		
11. *[LO 20.5]* Congenital hypoplasia of uterus		
12. *[LO 20.6]* Congenital flat foot		
13. *[LO 20.4]* Congenital stenosis of ileum		
14. *[LO 20.5]* Scrotal transposition		
15. *[LO 20.2]* Arnold-Chiari syndrome, type III, frontal		
16. *[LO 20.6]* Congenital partial dislocation of the right hip		
17. *[LO 20.4]* Tongue tie		
18. *[LO 20.3]* Atresia of pulmonary artery		
19. *[LO 20.6]* Congenital kyphosis of the thoracic region		
20. *[LO 20.3]* Arteriovenous malformation of vessel of leg		

Checking Your Understanding

Select the letter that best answers the question or completes the sentence.

1. *[LO 20.2]* The physician documents that a patient has sacral spina bifida with hydrocephalus. What is the appropriate code assignment?

   a. Q05.3 and Q03.8
   b. Q05.3
   c. Q03.8
   d. Q05.9, Q03.9

2. *[LO 20.3]* What code(s) should be assigned for a congenital anomaly that involves ventricular septal defect, pulmonary stenosis or atresia, dextroposition of aorta, and hypertrophy of the right ventricle?

   a. Q21.0, Q20.3, Q25.6, Q24.8
   b. Q21.2, Q20.3, Q25.6, Q24.8
   c. Q21.3
   d. Q21.0, Q20.3, Q22.1, Q24.8

3. *[LO 20.6]* What is the correct code assignment for congenital diaphragmatic hernia?

   a. K44.9   b. Q40.1
   c. Q79.0, K44.9   d. Q79.0

4. *[LO 20.6]* Which of the following chromosomal abnormalities is a female phenotype?

   a. Klinefelter syndrome karyotype 47, XXY
   b. karyotype 47, XYY
   c. karyotype 47, XXX
   d. mosaicism 45, XY

5. *[LO 20.1]* Identify the most appropriate code assignment for the newborn record of an infant that was a twin, delivered by cesarean section, born missing the left forearm and hand.

   a. Q71.22
   b. Q71.22, Z38.31
   c. Z38.31, Q71.22
   d. Z38.31

6. *[LO 20.5]* Which of the following genital organ congenital anomalies provides codes to differentiate between bilateral and unilateral conditions?

   a. bicornuate uterus
   b. ectopic testis
   c. accessory ovary
   d. embryonic cyst of the fallopian tube

7. *[LO 20.4]* Which of the following aspects of documentation is no longer necessary to impact the coding of cleft lip in ICD-10-CM?

   a. laterality
   b. median cleft lip
   c. presence of cleft palate
   d. complete vs. incomplete

8. *[LO 20.1]* A patient was born with a congenital malformation, which was surgically corrected. What is the correct method of reporting for future encounters?

   a. Assign the code for the malformation.
   b. Assign a code for history of congenital malformation.
   c. Assign a code for history of congenital malformation, plus the code for the malformation to specify the condition.
   d. There is no need to assign any codes for the condition, since it no longer exists.

9. *[LO 20.1]* Which of the following scenarios would be appropriate for assignment of a code from Chapter 17?

   a. A 10-year-old child with a history of surgical correction of ventricular septal defect as an infant is seen in the office for an annual cardiology checkup.

b. A 48-year-old pregnant woman has an amniocentesis, which indicates
   that her fetus has Down syndrome.
   c. A 39-year-old pregnant woman with a bicornuate uterus is admitted for
   delivery.
   d. A 45-year-old pregnant woman is seen for amniocentesis to screen for
   chromosomal abnormalities.

10. *[LO 20.5]* Which of the following conditions is classified as a congenital malformation of the urinary system?

   a. hypospadias
   b. congenital chordee
   c. aplasia of penis
   d. epispadias

Online Activity

[LO 20.1] Search online for information about malformations, deformations, or
chromosomal abnormalities that may not be identified until later in life. Why
do you think it is important to identify and code these congenital conditions
together with disorders that manifest in a newborn? Explain your findings in a
brief report.

Real-World Application

[LO 20.3] Assign ICD-10-CM diagnosis codes for the following discharge
summary.

Discharge Diagnosis:
   1. Pulmonary atresia.
   2. Atrioventricular septal defect.
   3. Nonmosaicism Down syndrome.
   4. Moderate mental retardation

Hospital Course: The patient is a 6-year-old male with nonmosaicism Down syndrome,
moderate mental retardation, atrioventricular septal defect, and pulmonary atresia. He was
admitted following an echocardiogram, which reflected a significant branch of pulmonary artery
stenosis with a well-functioning Contegra valve. Lung perfusion scan demonstrated 48% flow to
the left lung and 55% flow to the right lung. The patient underwent cardiac catheterization with
angiogram of the main pulmonary artery, which demonstrated stable stent configuration of the
proximal branch pulmonary arteries. Balloon pulmonary arterioplasty of the branch of
pulmonary arteries was performed.

Discharge Plan: Pediatric cardiology follow up in two weeks; then routine care through
pediatrician. Discharge home with no medication changes. Limit activity for 48 hours. Diet as
tolerated.

---

21 SKIN AND SUBCUTANEOUS TISSUE

Learning Outcomes *After studying this chapter, students should be able to*

21.1 Describe coding guidelines for assignment of codes to report infections of the skin and subcutaneous tissue.

21.2 Discuss how to code conditions classified as bullous disorders, dermatitis, and eczema.

21.3 Identify codes for papulosquamous disorders, urticaria, erythema, and radiation-related disorders of the skin and subcutaneous tissue.

21.4 Select appropriate code classifications for disorders of skin appendages.

21.5 Apply codes for procedure-related complications and other disorders of the skin and subcutaneous tissue.

Key Terms

alopecia
apocrine
bullous
carbuncle
cellulitis
cicatricial
dermatitis
dyshidrosis
eccrine
eczema
erythematous
furuncle
hidradenitis
impetigo
keloid
keratosis
lymphangitis
pemphigus
pilonidal
prurigo
pruritus
psoriasis
pyoderma
rosacea
vitiligo

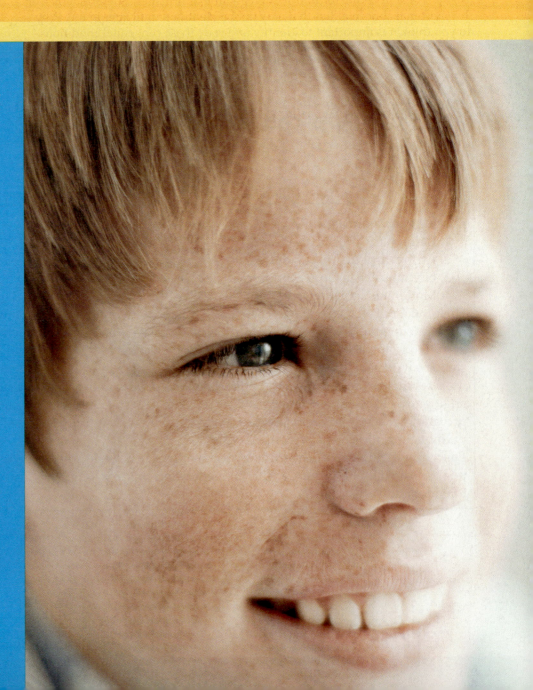

Introduction

The skin is the largest organ of the body. Also known as the integumentary system, the skin provides a protective barrier against infection and maintains thermoregulatory control by way of its innervations with the nervous and musculoskeletal systems. When the skin is wounded, a person is more susceptible to infections that can progress to impair vital organ function and bring about deregulation in metabolic processes overall. A careful understanding of skin diseases will aid you in the selection of their diagnosis codes. ICD-9-CM classifies these conditions in Chapter 12, "Diseases of the Skin and Subcutaneous Tissue." This chapter includes code categories 680–709. ICD-10-CM also classifies these conditions in Chapter 12, "Diseases of the Skin and Subcutaneous Tissue," which includes code categories L00–L99.

Spotlight on A&P

The skin is protective and has an abundant blood supply consisting of both red and white blood cells which protect against infection and aid in the healing process. The nervous system integrates with the skin by way of sense receptors that allow you to feel pain, light and deep touch, and temperature changes.

21.1 Infections of the Skin and Subcutaneous Tissue

When the skin is broken down due to injury or invasive surgery, it is more susceptible to infection. The skin acts as the first line of defense against microorganisms. If bacteria, viruses, fungi, and parasites invade the skin's protective barrier, progressive infection can ensue within the bloodstream, thereby affecting the vital functions of the internal organs that maintain life. There are many different skin conditions, and they have known and unknown causes. Coders should follow the etiology/manifestation convention as outlined in the guidelines for sequencing decisions when coding these diseases. Infectious conditions of the skin and subcutaneous tissue were reported with codes 680–686 in ICD-9-CM; they are reported with codes L00–L08 in ICD-10-CM.

L00–L08 Infections of the Skin and Subcutaneous Tissue

Codes in this subsection of ICD-10-CM correspond with those in categories 680–686 in ICD-9-CM. Conditions coded in this subsection include

impetigo Infection of the skin, producing thick, yellow crusts.

furuncle Infected hair follicle; the infection spreads into the tissues around the follicle.

carbuncle Infection of many hair follicles in a small area, often on the back of the neck.

cellulitis Infection of skin or subcutaneous connective tissue, commonly caused by bacteria.

lymphangitis Inflammation of one or more lymphatic vessels.

pilonidal Of or involving the growth of hairs embedded under the skin.

pyoderma Any pus-producing infection of the skin, such as impetigo.

erythematous Red or ruddy, as skin.

staphylococcal scalded skin syndrome, **impetigo,** cutaneous abscess, **furuncle, carbuncle, cellulitis,** acute **lymphangitis, pilonidal** cyst and sinus, **pyoderma,** erythrasma, pyoderma vegetans, omphalitis not of newborn, and other specified local infections of the skin and subcutaneous tissue.

When assigning codes from this subsection, an additional code from the B95–B97 range should be assigned to report the infectious agent, if documented. Coding of L00, staphylococcal scalded skin syndrome, requires an additional code to report the percentage of skin exfoliation with a code from category L49-, exfoliation due to **erythematous** conditions according to extent of body surface involved.

> **CODING TIP ▶**
>
> A code from category L49-, exfoliation due to erythematous conditions according to extent of body surface involved, is required as an additional code when reporting L00, staphylococcal scalded skin syndrome.

Impetigo codes are further specified as non-bullous, Bockhart's, bullous, and other. Codes in categories L02 for cutaneous abscess, furuncle, and carbuncle; category L03 for cellulitis and acute lymphangitis; and category L04 for acute lymphadenitis are further specified by site.

Think About It 21.1   also available in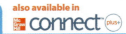

Assign ICD-10-CM codes for the following situations, applying any appropriate sequencing guidelines.

1. Ritter's disease with 40-49 percent erythematous exfoliation, caused by group A *Streptococcus* _____

2. Deep folliculitis of the neck due to *Staphylococcus aureus* _____

3. Acute lymphangitis of the right axilla caused by other *Staphylococcus* _____

4. Acute lymphadenitis of the lymph nodes of the neck caused by cytomegalovirus _____

5. Purulent dermatitis _____

Beyond the Code: ICD-9-CM only required the specification of percent of body impacted when coding for burns. Why is it important to do the same for a staph infection of the skin in L00?

21.2 Bullous Disorders, Dermatitis, and Eczema

pemphigus Any of a group of skin diseases marked by successive, recurring blisters on the skin and mucous membranes.

Bullous skin disorders are characterized by the presence of blisters and erosions on the skin and mucous membranes. They can be acquired, induced, or brought on by **pemphigus,** which is an autoimmune disease. **Dermatitis** involves bumps, rash, itching, redness, swelling, oozing, and scarring of the skin caused by an allergic reaction. **Eczema** is a chronic skin disorder with scaly rashes and itching, which may also be brought on by an allergic reaction. Skin conditions may be associated with respiratory conditions, such as allergies, asthma, or hay fever. Bullous disorders, dermatitis, and eczema conditions were reported with categories 690–694 and 697–698 in ICD-9-CM. They are reported with codes L10–L30 in ICD-10-CM.

dermatitis Inflammation of the skin.

eczema Chronic inflammatory skin disease, often with a serous discharge.

L10–L14 Bullous Disorders

Codes in this subsection of ICD-10-CM correspond with those in category 694 of ICD-9-CM. Conditions coded in this subsection include pemphigus, acquired **keratosis** follicularis, transient acantholytic dermatosis, pemphigoid, dermatitis herpetiformis, subcorneal pustular dermatitis, and **bullous** disorders in diseases classified elsewhere. This subsection provides greater specificity for conditions than previously available in ICD-9-CM. Category L10 provides codes to further specify pemphigus as pemphigus vulgaris, pemphigus vegetans, pemphigus foliaceous, Brazilian pemphigus, pemphigus erythematosus, and drug-induced pemphigus. Category L12 allows for greater specification of pemphigoid, including bullous, **cicatricial,** chronic bullous disease of childhood, and acquired epidermolysis bullosa.

keratosis Excessive growth of the horny layers of the skin.

bullous Of or involving large blisters filled with fluid.

cicatricial Scar.

L15–L19

Note that there are no categories L15–L19.

L20–L30 Dermatitis and Eczema

Codes in this subsection of ICD-10-CM correspond with those in categories 690–693 and 698 in ICD-9-CM. Conditions coded in this subsection include atopic dermatitis, seborrheic dermatitis, diaper dermatitis, allergic contact dermatitis, irritant contact dermatitis, exfoliative dermatitis, dermatitis due to substances taken internally, lichen simplex chronicus, **prurigo, pruritus,** nummular dermatitis, **dyshidrosis,** cutaneous autosensitization, infective dermatitis, erythema intertrigo, and pityriasis alba.

prurigo Skin condition with itching papules.

pruritus Itching.

dyshidrosis Condition in which small blisters form on the hands and feet.

The terms *dermatitis* and eczema are used synonymously in this subsection of ICD-10-CM. Allergic dermatitis codes in category L23 allow coders to report specific classifications of causative agents. These include metals, adhesives, cosmetics, topical medications, dyes, chemical products, food coming in contact with skin, non-food plants, pet dander, and other items. Note that the causative agents reported in category L23 are just those coming in contact with the skin, not those that are ingested, as ingested allergens are reported in category L27.

CODING TIP ▸

The terms *dermatitis* and *eczema* are used synonymously in ICD-10-CM.

Spotlight on A&P

Irritant contact dermatitis differs from allergic dermatitis in that it lacks the pathologic reaction to an allergen. Instead, it is a local reaction to contact with a substance.

Category L24 provides the ability to specify irritants, which include detergents, oils, greases, solvents, cosmetics, topical medications, chemicals, food

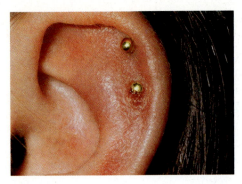
Figure 21.1 Dermatitis of Ear Due to Nickel Sensitivity

coming in contact with skin, non-food plants, metals, and other agents. Figure 21.1 demonstrates dermatitis caused by sensitivity to nickel. Similar to the rule for category L23, this category is only for reporting contact dermatitis for irritants coming in contact with the skin, not those that are ingested.

Dermatitis caused by substances taken internally is reported in category L27. Note that this category includes an instructional note to first assign a code from the range T36–T65 to report the drug or substance responsible. Substances that are specified by codes in this category include drugs and medicaments and other items. Coders need to keep in mind that this category is used only to report dermatitis reactions, not systemic reactions.

L31–L39

Note that there are no categories L31–L39.

Think About It 21.2 also available in **connect** plus+

Assign ICD-10-CM codes for the following situations, applying any appropriate sequencing guidelines.

1. Irritant contact dermatitis due to accidental exposure to detergents _____

2. Generalized skin eruption due to drugs and medicaments taken internally, adverse effects of drug; initial encounter _____

3. Dermatitis due to accidental ingestion of shellfish _____

4. Allergic contact dermatitis due to cat dander _____

5. Allergic contact dermatitis due to cosmetics _____

Beyond the Code: Although the terms *dermatitis* and *eczema* are used synonymously in this subsection of ICD-10-CM, they are different conditions. Locate information about both conditions. Discuss whether you think it makes sense to treat them the same for coding purposes or to report them separately. Justify your answer.

21.3 Papulosquamous Disorders, Urticaria, Erythema, and Radiation-Related Disorders of the Skin and Subcutaneous Tissue

Papulosquamous disorders, such as psoriasis, lichen, and tinea, are characterized by papules and scales on the skin. They can be caused by diaper dermatitis, candidiasis (yeast), fungus, sunburn, and reactions to drugs.

Urticaria is another skin eruption that can occur due to adverse effects of medication, such as penicillin (PCN), sulfa drugs, and nonsteroidal anti-inflammatory drugs (NSAIDs). Allergic reactions to food and ultraviolet (UV) light exposure can also cause urticaria of the skin. Any disease, such as lupus (autoimmune), herpes (viral), or bacterial infection, may cause a form of red rash called erythema. Tissue may also be damaged when it is exposed to radiation during the diagnosing and treating of diseases such as cancer. Papulosquamous disorders, urticaria, erythema, and radiation-related disorders of the skin and subcutaneous tissue are reported with categories L40–L59 in ICD-10-CM. They were reported with portions of category 692, along with categories 695–697 and 708, in ICD-9-CM.

L40–L45 Papulosquamous Disorders

Codes in this subsection of ICD-10-CM correspond with those in categories 696 and 697 in ICD-9-CM. Conditions coded in this subsection include **psoriasis,** parapsoriasis, pityriasis rosea, lichen planus, pityriasis rubra pilaris, lichen nitidus, lichen striatus, lichen ruber moniliformis, infantile papular acrodermatitis, and papulosquamous disorders in diseases classified elsewhere.

psoriasis Skin condition characterized by reddish, silver-scaled patches. (See Figure 21.2.)

Psoriasis is further specified in category L40 with classifications that include psoriasis vulgaris, generalized pustular psoriasis, acrodermatitis continua, pustulosis palmaris et plantaris, guttate psoriasis, arthropathic psoriasis, distal interphalangeal psoriatic arthropathy, psoriatic arthritis mutilans, psoriatic spondylitis, and psoriatic juvenile arthropathy.

Spotlight on A&P

Many diseases can be related to one another. They can be the underlying cause or the manifestation of a primary disease, or they can co-exist with another condition. Psoriasis is one such disease. It is characterized by thick, scaly patches on the skin. It is an autoimmune disease thought to be associated with arthritis and onychomycosis of the nails. Autoimmune diseases come about when the body is no longer able to recognize self from nonself.

Specific classifications of parapsoriasis found in category L41 include pityriasis lichenoides et varioliformis acuta, pityriasis lichenoides chronica, lymphomatoid papulosis, small plaque parapsoriasis, large plaque parapsoriasis, and retiform parapsoriasis. Lichen planus may be reported in category L43 with codes specifying hypertrophic lichen planus, bullous lichen planus, lichenoid drug reaction, and subacute lichen planus.

Code assignment for this subsection is straightforward. The only direction for additional codes is the requirement for code L43.2, lichenoid drug reaction to be assigned as a secondary code, following a code from the range of T36–T50 to report the drug responsible for the reaction.

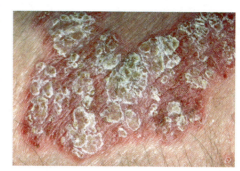

figure 21.2 Psoriasis

L46–L48

Note that there are no categories L46–L48.

L49–L54 Urticaria and Erythema

Codes in this subsection of ICD-10-CM correspond with those in categories 695 and 708 in ICD-9-CM. Conditions coded in this subsection include exfoliation due to erythematous conditions according to extent of body surface involved, urticaria, erythema multiforme, erythema nodosum, toxic erythema, erythema annulare centrifugum, erythema marginatum, and erythema in diseases classified elsewhere. Codes in category L49, exfoliation due to erythematous conditions according to extent of body surface involved, are to be assigned as secondary codes, following the condition causing the exfoliation. These codes are used to report the percentage of the body surface area impacted by the causative condition. Urticaria may be reported by specific type, using codes in category L50, which includes classifications for allergic urticaria, idiopathic urticaria, urticaria due to cold and heat, dermatographic urticaria, vibratory urticaria, cholinergic urticaria, and contact urticaria.

Erythema multiforme code assignment must follow a variety of guidelines provided with category L51. If the condition is caused by a medication, the code from category L51 should be assigned secondary to a code from the T36–T50 range, to first report the causative medication. If the condition being reported by a code from category L51 has associated manifestations, a secondary code is necessary to report any manifestations of the condition. Coding the conditions reported in category L51 also requires a secondary code from category L49 to report the percentage of skin exfoliation involved. Specific conditions reported in category L51 include nonbullous erythema multiforme, Stevens-Johnson syndrome, toxic epidermal necrolysis, and SJS-TEN overlap syndrome.

L55–L59 Radiation-Related Disorders of the Skin and Subcutaneous Tissue

Codes in this subsection of ICD-10-CM correspond with codes 692.70–692.79 and 692.82 in ICD-9-CM. Conditions coded in this subsection include sunburn, other acute skin changes due to ultraviolet radiation, skin changes due to chronic exposure to nonionizing radiation, radiodermatitis, and erythema ab igne. Acute skin changes due to ultraviolet radiation, reported in category L56, include phototoxic response to medication, photoallergic response to medication, photocontact dermatitis, solar urticaria, polymorphous light eruption, and disseminated superficial actinic porokeratosis. Skin changes due to chronic exposure to nonionizing radiation, reported in category L57, include actinic keratosis, actinic reticuloid, cutis rhomboidalis nuchae, poikiloderma of Civatte, cutis laxa senilis, actinic granuloma, farmer's skin, sailor's skin, and solar dermatitis. An additional code should be assigned with codes from categories L56, L57, and L58 to report the source of the ultraviolet radiation.

CODING TIP ▶

Categories L56, L57, and L58 require an additional code to report the source of the ultraviolet radiation.

Assign ICD-10-CM codes for the following situations, applying any appropriate sequencing guidelines.

1. Second-degree sunburn _____

2. Solar keratosis due to chronic exposure to nonionizing radiation of the tanning bed; subsequent encounter _____

3. Acute radiodermatitis due to exposure to radiofrequency; initial encounter _____

4. Drug photoallergic response due to an adverse effect of systemic antibiotic; initial encounter _____

5. Erythema ab igne _____

Beyond the Code: What is the significance of differentiating conditions caused by ultraviolet radiation from conditions caused by nonionizing radiation?

21.4 Disorders of Skin Appendages

Skin appendages include structures such as nails, hair, hair follicles, and sudoriferous eccrine and apocrine sweat glands, as well as sebaceous glands (oil glands). These structures are identified in Figure 21.3. **Eccrine** sweat glands are found all over the body, whereas **apocrine** sweat glands are found only in the armpits and the areolar, genital, and anal areas. There are a wide variety of disorders of the skin appendages, including **alopecia** (hair loss), acne, **rosacea** (red, inflamed cheeks, nose, and forehead), follicular cysts, **keloid scars,** pseudofolliculitis barbae (bumps from razor burn), and **hidradenitis** suppurative, which is a condition of swollen lesions of the axilla and groin and is thought to be a form of acne. Nail disorders such as horizontal Beau lines are the result of metabolic disturbance, disease, trauma, or chemotherapy or radiation therapy. Rhinophyma, a disorder of the nose, is characterized by a large, bulbous, ruddy appearance of the nose caused by a hypertrophic condition of the sebaceous glands. This wide variety of disorders of skin appendages is reported using codes in categories L60–L75 in ICD-10-CM. It was reported with categories 704–706 in ICD-9-CM.

L60–L75 Disorders of Skin Appendages

Codes in this subsection of ICD-10-CM correspond with those in categories 704–706 in ICD-9-CM. Conditions coded in this subsection include nail disorders, **alopecia** areata, androgenic alopecia, acne, **rosacea,** perioral dermatitis, rhinophyma, follicular cysts of skin and subcutaneous tissue, acne **keloid,** pseudofolliculitis barbae, **hidradenitis** suppurativa, **eccrine** sweat disorders, and **apocrine** sweat disorders.

alopecia Partial or complete loss of hair, naturally or from medication.

rosacea Persistent erythematous rash of the central face.

keloid Raised, irregular, lumpy, shiny scar due to excess collagen fiber production during healing of a wound.

hidradenitis Infection or inflammation of the sweat glands.

eccrine Major sweat glands, which occur in the skin all over the body. (See Figures 21.5 and 21.6.)

apocrine Related to apocrine sweat glands, which occur in the skin of the armpits, breasts, and genitoanal region.

CODING TIP

Coders should remember to use the *x* as a placeholder when appropriate.

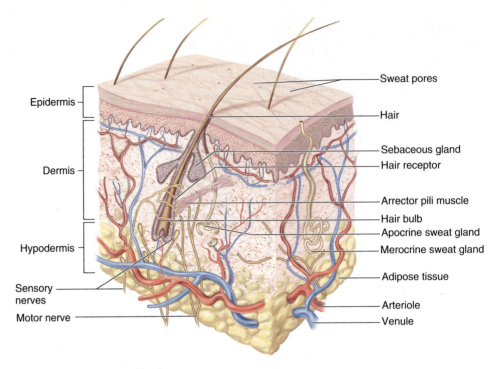

figure 21.3 Dermis and Its Organs

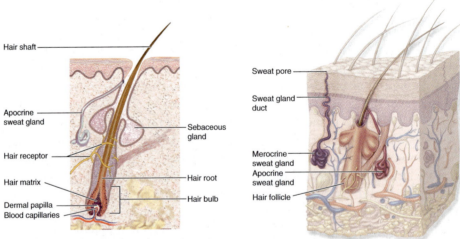

figure 21.4 Hair Follicle and Sebaceous Gland

figure 21.5 Sweat Glands

Nail disorders reported in category L60 include ingrown nails, onycholysis, onychogryphosis, nail dystrophy, Beau lines, and yellow nail syndrome. Structures of the nails are identified in Figure 21.6. Note that code L62 is only to be assigned as a secondary code, with the underlying condition reported first.

ICD-10-CM codes allow the reporting of hair loss, excessive hair, and abnormalities of hair color and hair shaft. Hair loss coding in ICD-10-CM provides significantly greater specificity than previously available in ICD-9-CM. Category L63 provides specific codes for alopecia totalis, alopecia universalis, and ophiasis. Androgenic alopecia, more commonly referred to as "male pattern baldness," is classified as drug-induced, other, or unspecified in category L64. Non-scarring hair loss, including telogen effluvium, anagen effluvium, and alopecia mucinosa, is reported in category L65. Scarring, or cicatricial, alopecia is reported in category L66, which includes specific codes for pseudopelade, lichen planopilaris, folliculitis decalvans, perifolliculitis capitis abscedens, and folliculitis ulerythematosa reticulata.

Hypertrichosis, or excessive hair, disorders are reported in category L68, which includes codes that specify hirsutism, acquired hypertrichosis lanuginosa, localized hypertrichosis, and polytrichia. Trichorrhexis nodosa, variations in hair color, fragilitas crinium, and other abnormalities of the hair shaft or hair color are reported in category L67.

Category L70 provides the ability to report a variety of types of acne (see Figure 21.7), which include acne vulgaris, acne conglobata, acne varioliformis, acne tropica, infantile acne, and acné excoriée des jeunes filles.

Follicular cysts of the skin and subcutaneous tissue, such as epidermal cysts, trichoderma cysts, pilar cysts, sebaceous cysts, and steatocystoma multiplex, are reported in category L72. Sweat disorders of the eccrine gland are reported in category L74 and include the conditions miliaria rubra, miliaria crystallina, miliary profunda, anhidrosis, and focal hyperhidrosis. Apocrine sweat disorders are reported in category L75 and include bromhidrosis, chromhidrosis, and apocrine miliaria.

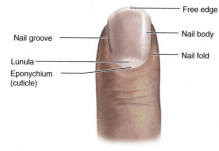

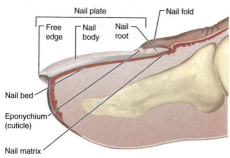

figure 21.6 Anatomy of the Fingernail

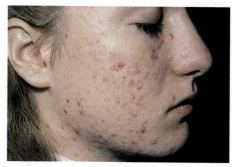

figure 21.7 Acne

Assign ICD-10-CM codes for the following situations, applying any appropriate sequencing guidelines.

1. Acne vulgaris   _____

2. Onycholysis   _____

3. Drug-induced androgenic alopecia; accidental poisoning with beta-adrenoreceptor agonist; subsequent episode   _____

4. Pachydermoperiostosis clubbed nail   _____

5. Bromhidrosis   _____

Beyond the Code: What kind of documentation issues might you anticipate with the increased specificity for coding alopecia? What steps might help you overcome these issues?

21.5 Procedure-Related Complications and Other Disorders of the Skin and Subcutaneous Tissue

Whenever a patient undergoes an invasive surgical procedure, there is risk of damage to the skin and tissue. A variety of skin disorders occur due to many types of disease processes, including accidental punctures, lacerations, hemorrhage, hematoma, and surgical complications. Advances in technology and new techniques are continuously being developed, as seen in minimally invasive techniques that spare surrounding tissue, such as stereotactic radiosurgery, fine needle aspiration, laparoscopic surgery, da Vinci procedures, and sentinel lymph node biopsies for breast cancer. Despite these less invasive techniques, there is always risk for complication. Procedure-related complications and other disorders of the skin and subcutaneous tissue are identified through categories L76–L99 in ICD-10-CM. Some of these disorders were reported with codes in categories 700–709 in ICD-9-CM, whereas others do not directly correspond to ICD-9-CM codes.

L76 Intra-operative and Postprocedural Complications of Skin and Subcutaneous Tissue

Codes in this subsection of ICD-10-CM do not directly correspond with any specific codes in ICD-9-CM. Conditions coded in this subsection are all reported in category L76 and include intra-operative hemorrhage and hematoma, accidental puncture and laceration, postprocedural hemorrhage and hematoma, and other postprocedural complications of skin and subcutaneous tissue. The conditions coded in this category are further specified by whether the procedure was dermatologic or not.

L77–L79

Note that there are no categories L77–L79.

L80–L99 Other Disorders of the Skin and Subcutaneous Tissue

Codes in this subsection of ICD-10-CM correspond with those in categories 700–709 in ICD-9-CM. Conditions coded in this subsection include **vitiligo,** disorders of pigmentation, seborrheic keratosis, acanthosis nigricans, corns, callosities, epidermal thickening, keratoderma in diseases classified elsewhere, transepidermal elimination disorders, pyoderma gangrenosum, pressure ulcers, atrophic disorders of the skin, hypertrophic disorders of the skin, hypertrophic scar, keloid, granulomatous disorders of the skin and subcutaneous tissue, lupus erythematosus, discoid lupus erythematosus, subacute cutaneous lupus erythematosus, localized connective tissue disorders, vasculitis of the skin, livedoid vasculitis, erythema elevatum diutinum, non-pressure chronic ulcers, pyogenic granuloma, factitial dermatitis, febrile neutrophilic dermatosis, eosinophilic cellulitis, mucinosis of the skin, and disorders of the skin and subcutaneous tissue in diseases classified elsewhere.

vitiligo Nonpigmented white patches on otherwise normal skin.

Spotlight on A&P

Livedoid vasculitis is a disease that affects young to middle-aged women. It is associated with many different diseases. Some of those diseases are hypertension, varicosities, circulatory disorders, and blood coagulation disorders. The signs of this disease are ulcers and blood clots in the lower legs.

Pigmentation disorders, which are reported in category L81, include postinflammatory hyperpigmentation, chloasma, freckles, café au lait spots, lentigo, leukoderma, and pigmented purpuric dermatosis. When assigning codes for seborrheic keratosis in category L82, the coder needs to be alert to whether or not the documentation indicates that the condition is inflamed.

Epidermal thickening conditions classified in category L85 include acquired ichthyosis, acquired keratosis palmaris et plantaris, keratosis punctata, xerosis cutis, and cutaneous horn. Note that code L86, keratoderma in diseases classified elsewhere is to be assigned as a secondary code, following the code for the underlying disease. Category L87 classifies transepidermal elimination disorders, which include keratosis follicularis et parafollicularis in cutem penetrans, reactive perforating collagenosis, and elastosis perforans serpiginosa.

Pressure ulcers, or decubitus ulcers (Figure 21.8), are classified to a significantly greater level of specificity in ICD-10-CM than they were in ICD-9-CM. This category is an excellent example of the expandability of ICD-10-CM. The format of ICD-9-CM only allowed expansion to include a maximum of 100 codes per category, due to the five-digit length and only numeric characters. Category L89 contains a total of 150 codes, yet it has

CODING TIP ▶

When coding seborrheic keratosis in category L82, the coder should watch for documentation regarding the presence or absence of inflammation.

CHAPTER **21** REVIEW

Chapter Summary

Learning Outcome	Key Concepts/Examples
21.1 Describe coding guidelines for assignment of codes to report infections of the skin and subcutaneous tissue. **(pages 332–333)**	• When coding infections of the skin and subcutaneous tissue, an additional code from the B95–B97 range should be assigned to report the infectious agent, if documented. • Coding of L00, staphylococcal scalded skin syndrome requires an additional code to report the percentage of skin exfoliation with a code from category L49-, exfoliation due to erythematous conditions according to extent of body surface involved. • Codes for cutaneous abscess, furuncle, carbuncle, cellulitis, acute lymphangitis, and acute lymphadenitis are further specified by site.
21.2 Discuss how to code conditions classified as bullous disorders, dermatitis, and eczema. **(pages 333–335)**	• The terms *dermatitis* and *eczema* are used synonymously in this subsection of ICD-10-CM. • Categories L23, L24, and L27 provide the ability to report specific agents responsible for dermatitis reactions.
21.3 Identify codes for papulosquamous disorders, urticaria, erythema, and radiation-related disorders of the skin and subcutaneous tissue. **(pages 335–337)**	• Code assignment for papulosquamous disorders is straightforward, containing only a single direction for additional code assignment and related sequencing instruction. • Codes in category L49, exfoliation due to erythematous conditions according to extent of body surface involved, are to be assigned as secondary codes, following the condition causing the exfoliation. • An additional code should be assigned with codes from categories L56, L57, and L58 to report the source of ultraviolet radiation.
21.4 Select appropriate code classifications for disorders of skin appendages. **(pages 338–340)**	• Hair loss coding in ICD-10-CM provides significantly greater specificity than previously available in ICD-9-CM.
21.5 Apply codes for procedure-related complications and other disorders of the skin and subcutaneous tissue. **(pages 340–343)**	• This subsection includes a variety of instructional notes, of which coders should be aware. • The comprehensive nature of category L89 for reporting of pressure ulcers demonstrates the expandability of the ICD-10-CM coding system.

Applying Your Skills

Assign codes for each of the following conditions using ICD-9-CM and ICD-10-CM.

Condition	ICD-9-CM Codes	ICD-10-CM Codes
1. *[LO 21.2]* Pemphigus erythematosus		
2. *[LO 21.3]* Contact urticaria		
3. *[LO 21.1]* Cellulitis of finger on the left hand		
4. *[LO 21.2]* Diffuse neurodermatitis		
5. *[LO 21.4]* Male pattern baldness		
6. *[LO 21.3]* Stevens-Johnson syndrome involving 35% of the body surface		
7. *[LO 21.4]* Acne vulgaris		
8. *[LO 21.1]* Pilonidal sinus without abscess		
9. *[LO 21.5]* Stage 2 pressure ulcer of the left lower back		
10. *[LO 21.1]* Bullous impetigo		
11. *[LO 21.2]* Infective dermatitis		
12. *[LO 21.4]* Primary focal hyperhidrosis of the soles of the feet		
13. *[LO 21.2]* Cradle cap		
14. *[LO 21.5]* Freckles		
15. *[LO 21.1]* Furuncle of chest wall		
16. *[LO 21.5]* Discoid lupus erythematosus		
17. *[LO 21.3]* First-degree sunburn		
18. *[LO 21.4]* Yellow nail syndrome		
19. *[LO 21.1]* Cutaneous abscess of the left hand		
20. *[LO 21.1]* Paronychia of right great toe		

Checking Your Understanding

Select the letter that best answers the question or completes the sentence.

1. *[LO 21.1]* _____ categories in the skin and subcutaneous tissue provide greater specificity in ICD-10-CM than was previously available in ICD-9-CM.

    a. All   **b.** Most   **c.** Two   **d.** No

2. *[LO 21.2]* What is the most appropriate code to assign for a patient who developed allergic dermatitis after eating peanuts?

    a. L24.6   **b.** L23.6
    c. L27.2   **d.** None of these

3. *[LO 21.1]* Paronychia is a type of

    a. eczema.   **b.** cellulitis.   **c.** impetigo.   **d.** pyoderma.

4. *[LO 21.5]* Which of the following conditions is not reported with a code in category L89?

    a. decubitus ulcer   **b.** bed sore

    c. diabetic ulcer   **d.** pressure ulcer

5. *[LO 21.4]* Which of the following categories classifies disorders of the hair shaft?

    a. L67   **b.** L74   **c.** L70   **d.** L85

6. *[LO 21.4]* Category L75 classifies disorders of the

    a. sebaceous gland.   **b.** apocrine sweat gland.

    c. merocrine sweat gland.   **d.** hair follicle.

7. *[LO 21.4]* Sebaceous gland disorders are classified in which of the following categories?

    a. L67   **b.** L74   **c.** L70   **d.** L85

8. *[LO 21.5]* Conditions of which structure are reported in category L85?

    a. dermis   **b.** epidermis

    c. subcutaneous fat   **d.** hair follicle

9. *LO 21.4]* Category L74 classifies conditions of which of the following?

    a. hair follicle   **b.** sebaceous gland

    c. apocrine sweat gland   **d.** merocrine sweat gland

10. *[LO 21.4]* Hair follicle conditions are classified in category

    a. L67.   **b.** L70.   **c.** L66.   **d.** L74.

Online Activity

[LO 21.4] Search online for information about the Rule of Nines. Using this information, explain why there is a difference between adults and children.

Real-World Application

[LO 21.3, LO 21.4] Assign ICD-10-CM diagnosis codes for the following dermatology office note.

Subjective: This is a 52-year-old white male, who comes in today as a referral from Dr. Stevens for evaluation of concerns related to scalp lesions and hair loss.

Past Family, Medical, and Social History: No known drug allergies. No significant medical history. No previous hospitalizations. No significant family history. The patient is a nonsmoker. Works outdoors as a landscaper.

Current Medications: None.

Physical Examination: The patient has several 2–4 mm diameter rough, red areas with white and yellowish scaling on the top of the scalp. Receding hairline noted with thinning hair.

Impression: Actinic keratosis and male pattern baldness.

Plan:

1. Apply diclofenac gel daily to reddened, scaly area.
2. Propecia 1 mg daily.
3. Keep scalp covered by wearing a hat outdoors.
4. Recheck in 1 month.

---

22 MUSCULOSKELETAL AND CONNECTIVE TISSUE

Learning Outcomes *After studying this chapter, students should be able to*

22.1 Interpret coding guidelines for diseases of the musculoskeletal and connective tissue in order to determine appropriateness of code assignment and sequencing for conditions in the chapter.

22.2 Identify codes for arthropathies, polyarthropathies, osteoarthritis, and other joint disorders.

22.3 Classify dentofacial anomalies, jaw disorders, and systemic connective tissue disorders.

22.4 Apply coding guidelines to dorsopathies and spondylopathies.

22.5 Use coding guidelines to classify disorders of muscles, synovium, tendons, and other soft tissue.

22.6 Identify codes for osteopathies, chondropathies, disorders of bone density and structure, and other disorders of the musculoskeletal system and connective tissue.

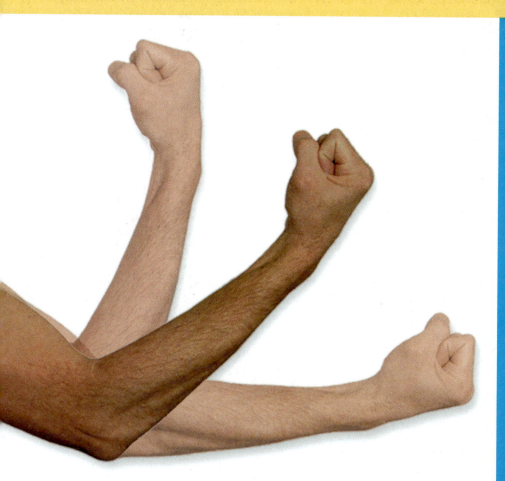

Key Terms

arthrodesis
arthropathy
dorsopathy
effusion
enthesopathy
gout
impingement syndrome
kyphosis
malunion
myelopathy
nonunion
ossification
osteoarthritis
osteomyelitis
pathological fracture
radiculopathy
rheumatoid arthritis
spondylolisthesis
spondylolysis
subluxation
systemic lupus erythematosus (SLE)
valgus deformity
varus deformity

Introduction

The musculoskeletal system consists of bones, joints, ligaments, muscles, and tendons. The skeleton and muscles provide support and protection to the internal organs of the body in addition to physical movement. Conditions affecting the musculoskeletal system can cause significant pain and immobility. Physical immobility, pain, and associated psychological stressors can further compromise a patient's health and level of functioning.

Disorders of the musculoskeletal system and connective tissue include arthropathies, arthritis, dorsopathies, spondylopathies, disorders of muscles, disorders of the synovium and tendon, soft tissue disorders, disorders of bone density and structure, chondropathies, and procedural complications of the musculoskeletal system. They can be caused by genetics, inflammatory processes, an abnormal immune system, environmental factors, or new or old trauma from injury; some disorders have no known cause. When classifying conditions in this chapter, coders must be aware of documentation of laterality, acuity, and the exact location of the condition being reported. ICD-9-CM classifies these conditions in Chapter 13, "Diseases of Musculoskeletal and Connective Tissue," which includes code categories 710–739. ICD-10-CM classifies these conditions in Chapter 13, "Diseases of the Musculoskeletal System and Connective Tissue," which includes code categories M00–M99.

22.1 Coding Guidelines for Diseases of Musculoskeletal and Connective Tissue

The musculoskeletal system is integrated with other body systems. Muscle tissue consists of not only skeletal muscle but also smooth muscle of organs and cardiac muscle. Muscle movement generates heat to help regulate the body's temperature. Bones are responsible for blood cell formation, which is critical to all organ function. Because there are causes, comorbidities, secondary manifestations, and complications of musculoskeletal disorders, the coding guidelines provide direction to sequence the many different considerations to be made when coding for these disorders. An overview of the anatomic skeletal structures is provided in Figure 22.1.

Although a variety of coding guidelines are pertinent to specific subsections of this chapter, more general guidelines also apply. The general musculoskeletal system coding guidelines address laterality and acuity of conditions. When assigning codes for musculoskeletal conditions, coders must also assign external cause codes for applicable causes of the conditions.

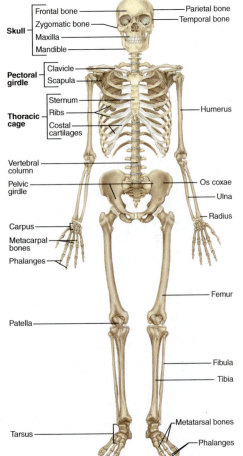

figure 22.1 Adult Skeleton

Laterality is specified for most of the codes in Chapter 13, along with a designation of the site as the specific bone, joint, or muscle. Sometimes multiple bones, joints, or muscles are involved. This is addressed in coding guideline *I.13.a. Site and Laterality.* In these cases, the code for "multiple sites" should be assigned. However, not all categories have codes for "multiple sites," so the coder should assign multiple codes to identify each of the sites involved. One example of a condition that can be classified as having multiple sites is osteoarthritis. If documentation is for post-traumatic osteoarthritis of multiple joints, the appropriate code assignment is M15.3, secondary multiple arthritis.

Previous injury or trauma is the cause of many musculoskeletal conditions, whereas others are recurrent. Coding guideline *I.13.b. Acute Traumatic versus Chronic or Recurrent Musculoskeletal Conditions* instructs the coder that it is appropriate to assign bone, joint, or muscle conditions that are chronic, recurrent, or due to healed injuries with codes in Chapter 13. However, if the condition is due to a current acute injury, the condition is classified to Chapter 19. Documentation that does not clearly identify the condition as acute or chronic should lead to a physician query for clarification.

Think About It 22.1

also available in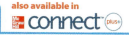

Assign ICD-10-CM codes for the following situations, applying any appropriate sequencing guidelines.

1. Erosive osteoarthritis of multiple sites _____

2. Primary osteoarthritis of the left knee _____

3. Post-traumatic osteoarthritis of the right hip _____

4. Loose body in the right elbow _____

5. Ankylosis of the left wrist _____

Beyond the Code: Why is it important to assign applicable external cause codes and designate the difference between traumatic and nontraumatic conditions of the musculoskeletal system?

22.2 Arthropathies, Polyarthropathies, Osteoarthritis, and Other Joint Disorders

Disorders of the joints include **arthropathies,** polyarthropathies, **osteoarthritis,** and other conditions, such as gout. Arthropathies include inflammation and have systemic effects on other organs. They may be due to an infection,

arthropathy Disease of a joint.

osteoarthritis Chronic inflammatory disease of the joints with pain and loss of function.

rheumatoid arthritis Disease of joints, with arthritis as a major manifestation.

a parasite, or a reaction to some other disease affecting the body. **Rheumatoid arthritis** is an inflammatory polyarthropathy that affects the lungs, heart, and other organs and tissues.

Osteoarthritis is a common condition in patients seen for complications related to obesity, since there is increased strain and load on weight-bearing joints. Pain and immobility render the obese patient with osteoarthritis incapable of exercise to lose the weight. This may lead to further health care risks and complications and a corresponding increase in health care cost associated with utilization of resources in the delivery of health care when treating these patients. For example, gout can lead to deformity and disability when there is associated renal dysfunction as evidenced by increased urea in the blood.

Arthritis involves an inflammatory process of the joint tissues, which can lead to joint derangements, deformities, and immobility. Osteoarthritis and rheumatoid arthritis are the most common types of arthritis. Arthritic conditions are not limited to joint tissues, as some may have systemic effects. Rheumatoid arthritis and gout are examples of arthritic conditions that may affect other organs. Viral, parasitic, and bacterial infections can invade synovial fluid and musculoskeletal tissues, which can lead to a number of chronic and progressive diseases. Arthropathy conditions classified to codes in the M00–M25 range are those disorders that predominantly affect the peripheral joints.

Spotlight on A&P

While the anatomic knowledge requirements for this section are generally focused on the various joints involved, coders may find it helpful to become familiar with the many pathological terms used to describe infectious conditions of the joint, such as pyogenic arthritis, reactive arthropathy, and rheumatoid polyneuropathy.

M00–M02 Infectious Arthropathies

Codes in this subsection of ICD-10-CM correspond with those in category 711 in ICD-9-CM. Conditions coded in this subsection include pyogenic arthritis, direct infections of joints in infectious and parasitic diseases classified elsewhere, and postinfective and reactive arthropathies.

Codes in this subsection classify arthropathies that are due to microbiological agents. Distinction is made between direct and indirect infection of the joint. A direct infection involves invasion of the organism into the synovial tissue with microbial antigens present in the joint. Indirect infection is classified into two types, reactive and postinfective. In a reactive indirect infection, microbial infection of the body is established but neither organisms nor antigens can be identified in the joint. In a postinfective indirect infection, a microbial antigen is present but there is inconsistent recovery of an organism and no evidence of local multiplication. Table 22.1 classifies arthropathies caused by microbiological agents.

Pyogenic arthritis codes are further classified to the 4th-character specification by organism, including staphylococcal, pneumococcal, streptococcal, and other specified bacteria. The 5th character provides specification of the joint involved, and the 6th character provides the ability to report

Table 22.1 Classification of Arthropathies Due to Microbiological Agents

Type of Agent	Description
Direct	• The microorganism has invaded the synovial tissue. • Microbial antigens are present in the joint.
Indirect	Reactive • Microbial infection of the body is established. • Neither organisms nor antigens can be identified in the joint. Postinfective • Microbial antigen is present. • There is inconstant recovery of an organism. • There is no evidence of local multiplication.

laterality for paired joints. Note that there are instructions to assign a secondary code to identify the causative bacterial agent for many of the codes in this range.

Codes in category M01, direct infections of joint in infectious and parasitic diseases classified elsewhere, are to be listed as secondary codes only. These codes should be preceded by codes for the underlying disease. Codes in this category are arranged by the site of the joint, with laterality specification where appropriate.

Postinfective and reactive arthropathies, coded in category M02, should be preceded by codes for the underlying disease. This category specifies the causative conditions at the 4th-character level, including arthropathy following intestinal bypass, postdysenteric arthropathy, postimmunization arthropathy, Reiter's disease, and other reactive arthropathies. The 5th character provides specification of the joint involved, and the 6th character provides the ability to report laterality for paired joints.

M03–M04

Note that there are no categories M03 and M04.

M05–M14 Inflammatory Polyarthropathies

Codes in this subsection of ICD-10-CM correspond with those in categories 274, 713, 714, 716, and 719 in ICD-9-CM. Conditions coded in this subsection include rheumatoid arthritis with rheumatoid factor, rheumatoid arthritis without rheumatoid factor, enteropathic arthropathies, juvenile arthritis, chronic **gout,** gout, other crystal arthropathies, hydroxyapatite

gout Painful arthritis of the big toe and other joints caused by buildup of uric acid.

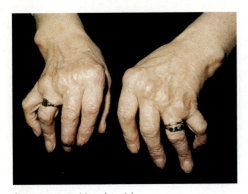

figure 22.2 Hands with Rheumatoid Arthritis

deposition disease, familial chondrocalcinosis, other arthropathies, chronic postrheumatic arthropathy, Kashin-Beck disease, villonodular synovitis, palindromic rheumatism, intermittent hydrarthrosis, traumatic arthropathy, arthritis, polyarthritis, monoarthritis, Charcot's joint, and arthropathies in other diseases classified elsewhere. Note that most codes in this subsection provide the ability to specify the joint involved through a 5th character, as well as the ability to report laterality for paired joints through a 6th-character specification.

Rheumatoid arthritis (see Figure 22.2) with rheumatoid factor is further classified by the involvement of other systems in category M05, which includes Felty syndrome, rheumatoid lung disease with rheumatoid arthritis, rheumatoid vasculitis with rheumatoid arthritis, rheumatoid heart disease with rheumatoid arthritis, rheumatoid myopathy with rheumatoid arthritis, rheumatoid polyneuropathy with rheumatoid arthritis, rheumatoid arthritis with involvement of other organs and systems, rheumatoid arthritis without involvement of other organs and systems, and other rheumatoid arthritis with rheumatoid factor. The 5th character provides specification of the joint involved, and the 6th character provides the ability to report laterality for paired joints.

Other types of rheumatoid arthritis are classified in category M06, which includes rheumatoid arthritis without rheumatoid factor, adult-onset Still disease, rheumatoid bursitis, rheumatoid nodule, and inflammatory polyarthropathy. Codes in this range also include 5th-character specification of the joint involved, and the 6th character provides the ability to report laterality for paired joints.

Enteropathic arthropathies are reported in category M07, with 5th-character specification of joint involvement and 6th-character specification of laterality. This category also has instructions to assign an additional code to report documented associated enteropathy, such as Crohn's disease or ulcerative colitis.

> **CODING TIP ▶**
>
> When reporting enteropathic arthropathies in category M07, a secondary code should be assigned for documented associated enteropathy, such as Crohn's disease or ulcerative colitis.

Juvenile arthritis is reported in category M08; it also requires a secondary code for any documented underlying conditions, such as Crohn's disease or ulcerative colitis. Juvenile arthritis is further specified in this section as juvenile ankylosing spondylitis, juvenile rheumatoid arthritis with systemic onset, polyarthritis, and pauciarticular. The codes in this range also include 5th-character specification of the joint involved, and the 6th character provides the ability to report laterality for paired joints.

Category M1a, chronic gout, is further specified through codes for idiopathic chronic gout, lead-induced chronic gout, drug-induced chronic gout, chronic gout due to renal impairment, and secondary chronic gout. When assigning codes from this category, an additional code should be used to identify associated conditions, such as autonomic neuropathy, urinary stones, cardiomyopathy, external ear disorders, glomerular disorders, and disorders of the iris or ciliary body. As included in previous categories in this subsection, there is also a 5th-character specification for joint involvement and a 6th character for laterality. In addition, category M1a requires the assignment of a 7th character to report the presence or absence of tophus.

> **CODING TIP ▸**
>
> Category M1a requires the assignment of a 7th character to report the presence or absence of tophus.

Gout is reported in category M10, which includes idiopathic gout, lead-induced gout, drug-induced gout, gout due to renal impairment, and other secondary gout. Additional code assignment instructions are similar to those for chronic gout, in category M1a. Fifth-character specification for joint involvement and a 6th character for laterality also apply to this category.

Codes in the range of M14.80–M14.89 are manifestation codes and are for use only as secondary codes. The underlying disease for these arthropathic conditions should be assigned prior to codes in this range.

M09

Note that there is no category M09.

M15–M19 Osteoarthritis

Codes in this subsection of ICD-10-CM correspond with those in category 715 in ICD-9-CM. Conditions coded in this subsection include polyosteoarthritis, osteoarthritis of the hip, osteoarthritis of the knee, osteoarthritis of the first carpometacarpal joint, and other and unspecified osteoarthritis.

Polyosteoarthritis is specified in category M15, which includes codes for primary generalized arthritis, Heberden's nodes, Bouchard's nodes, secondary multiple arthritis, and erosive arthritis. Osteoarthritis of the hip reported in category M16, osteoarthritis of the knee in category M17, and osteoarthritis of the first carpometacarpal joint in category M18 are all further specified as bilateral, unilateral (with the ability to specify laterality), due to hip dysplasia, and post-traumatic. Other arthritis conditions, primary, secondary, and post-traumatic, are reported with category M19, which provides the ability to report the site and laterality of the conditions.

M20–M25 Other Joint Disorders

Codes in this subsection of ICD-10-CM correspond with those in categories 717 and 734–736 in ICD-9-CM. Conditions coded in this subsection include acquired deformities of the fingers and toes, other acquired deformities of the limbs, disorder of the patella, internal derangement of the knee, other specific joint derangements, and other joint disorders that are not elsewhere classified.

Deformities of fingers and toes in M20 are specified as far as laterality of hand or foot, but not specific to the finger or toe involved. Conditions reported in this category include mallet finger, boutonnière deformity,

valgus deformity Permanent abnormal outward twist or bend of bone.

varus deformity Permanent abnormal inward twist or bend of bone.

subluxation Incomplete dislocation in which some contact between the joint surfaces remains.

effusion Collection of fluid that has escaped from blood vessels into a cavity or tissues.

swan-neck deformity, hallux valgus (more commonly known as bunions), hallus rigidus, hallus varus, and hammer toe. Category M21 provides codes for other acquired limb deformities, including **valgus deformity, varus deformity,** flexion deformity, flatfoot, clawhand, clubhand, clawfoot, clubfoot, and unequal limb length. The patella disorders coded in category M22 include recurrent dislocation, recurrent **subluxation,** patellofemoral disorders, derangements of the patella, and chondromalacia.

Internal derangement of the knee, including cystic meniscus, old injury of meniscus, loose body in the knee, chronic instability, and spontaneous and disruption of knee ligaments, are coded with category M23. When assigning codes for internal derangement of the knee, additional variables are addressed, so documentation regarding the part of the meniscus or specific ligament involved may be necessary, in addition to the need for laterality documentation. Other specific joint derangements are coded in category M24, which provides the ability to report loose body in joint, cartilage disorders, ligament disorders, pathological dislocation, recurrent joint dislocation, joint contracture, ankylosis of joint, and protrusio acetabuli. Other joint disorders, not elsewhere classified, reported in category M25 include hemarthrosis, fistula of joint, flail joint, instability of joint, **effusion** of joint, pain in joint, stiffness of joint, and osteophyte.

Think About It 22.2

also available in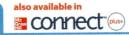

Assign ICD-10-CM codes for the following situations, applying any appropriate sequencing guidelines.

1. Primary osteoarthritis of both knees _____

2. Hammer toe, left foot _____

3. Reactive arthropathy of the left shoulder following acute infective endocarditis _____

4. Right hip stiffness _____

5. Gouty bursitis of the right hip _____

Beyond the Code: What documentation needs might you anticipate when coding arthropathies, polyarthropathies, osteoarthritis, and other joint disorders?

22.3 Dentofacial Anomalies, Jaw Disorders, and Systemic Connective Tissue Disorders

Dentofacial anomalies and other disorders of the jaw have been reclassified to Chapter 13, "Diseases of the Musculoskeletal System and Connective Tissue," in ICD-10-CM; they were classified with digestive system disorders in ICD-9-CM. Although these disorders do impact the digestive system, they are structural in that they are deformities and disorders of the musculoskeletal structures. Structural malformations of the nose, mouth, or jaw interfere with one's ability to eat and swallow.

Connective tissue is collagen- and protein-rich material that holds together and supports other body structures. Since connective tissue is present all over the body, disorders of connective tissue have great potential for systemic disease, such as systemic lupus erythematosus (SLE). Autoimmune diseases are also defined as those in which the body is unable to recognize self from non-self. Antibodies increase in response to what the body perceives as foreign invasion and begins to attack otherwise healthy tissue. This is referred to as autoimmunity. Autoimmune diseases, such as lupus and rheumatoid arthritis, are caused by a malfunctioning immune response that has local and systemic effects throughout the body. This malfunction may be inherited through genetic mutations or may be secondary to injury, trauma, adverse environmental exposure, cancer, or infection. Dentofacial anomalies, disorders of the jaw, and systemic connective tissue disorders are classified in categories M26–M36 in ICD-10-CM. In ICD-9-CM, they were coded from categories 446, 520–529, and 710.

M26–M27 Dentofacial Anomalies (Including Malocclusion) and Other Disorders of Jaw

Codes in this subsection of ICD-10-CM correspond with those in categories 524–526 in ICD-9-CM. It is noteworthy that this is a significant reclassification from ICD-9-CM to ICD-10-CM, as these conditions were classified as diseases of the digestive system.

> **CODING TIP** ▸
>
> Dentofacial anomalies and other disorders of the jaw were classified as diseases of the digestive system in ICD-9-CM. Exercise caution when coding these conditions.

Conditions coded from category M26, dentofacial anomalies, include major anomalies of jaw size, anomalies of jaw-cranial base relationship, anomalies of dental arch relationship, anomalies of tooth position of fully erupted tooth or teeth, malocclusion, dentofacial functional abnormalities, temporomandibular joint disorders, and dental alveolar anomalies. Category M27, other diseases of jaws, provides codes to report developmental disorders of jaws, giant cell granuloma, inflammatory conditions of jaws, osteitis of jaws, **osteomyelitis** of jaw, osteoradionecrosis of jaw, periostitis of jaw, sequestrum of jaw bone, alveolitis of jaws, dry socket, cyst of jaw, perforation of root canal space due to endodontic treatment, endodontic overfill or underfill, and endosseous dental implant failure.

osteomyelitis Infection of bone tissue.

M30–M36 Systemic Connective Tissue Disorders

Codes in this subsection of ICD-10-CM correspond with those in 446 and 710 in ICD-9-CM. Conditions coded in this subsection include polyarteritis nodosa and related conditions, other necrotizing vasculopathies, **systemic lupus erythematosus (SLE),** systemic sclerosis, other systemic involvement of connective tissue, and systemic disorders of the connective tissue in diseases classified elsewhere.

systemic lupus erythematosus (SLE) Autoimmune disease of the connective tissue characterized by systemic inflammation, fever, skin lesions, joint pain, arthritis, and anemia; often affects the kidneys, spleen, and other organs.

Conditions reported in categories M30 and M31 of ICD-10-CM as systemic connective tissue disorders were classified in category 446 of ICD-9-CM as diseases of the circulatory system. Category M30 includes polyarteritis nodosa, polyarteritis with lung involvement, juvenile polyarteritis, and mucocutaneous lymph node syndrome. Conditions classified to category M31 include hypersensitivity angiitis, thrombotic microangiopathy, lethal midline granuloma, Wegener's granulomatosis, aortic arch syndrome, giant cell arteritis with polymyalgia rheumatica, microscopic polyangiitis, and other specified necrotizing vasculopathies.

CODING TIP ▶

Conditions reported in categories M30 and M31 of ICD-10-CM as systemic connective tissue disorders were classified in category 446 of ICD-9-CM as diseases of the circulatory system.

SLE coding expanded from only one code in ICD-9-CM to an entire category, with 10 codes available to report variants of the condition. Code M32.0, drug-induced systemic lupus erythematosus, is accompanied by a note that this code should follow the code for the medication. Other codes in this category report SLE with organ or system involvement, including endocarditis, pericarditis, lung involvement, glomerular disease, and tubulointerstitial nephropathy. Another condition in this subsection with expanded reporting in ICD-10-CM is dermatopolymyositis, which now includes codes in category M33 to specify juvenile dermatopolymyositis and polymyositis with myopathy and respiratory or other organ involvement. This is similar to reporting systemic sclerosis in category M34, which had only a single code in ICD-9-CM but now has codes for specific reporting of progressive systemic sclerosis, CREST syndrome, systemic sclerosis induced by drugs and chemicals, and other forms of systemic sclerosis with lung involvement, myopathy, or polyneuropathy.

Other systemic involvement of connective tissue is reported through categories M35 and M36, which classify sicca syndrome, mixed connective tissue disease, Behçet's disease, polymyalgia rheumatica, diffuse fasciitis, multifocal fibrosclerosis, relapsing panniculitis, hypermobility syndrome, and systemic disorders of connective tissue diseases classified elsewhere. Codes from category M36 are for use only as secondary codes, following codes for the underlying conditions. These underlying conditions include neoplastic disease, hemophilia, other blood disorders, hypersensitivity reactions, and other diseases.

M37–M39

Note that there are no categories M37–M39.

Think About It 22.3

also available in **McGraw Hill connect** (plus+)

Assign ICD-10-CM codes for the following situations, applying any appropriate sequencing guidelines.

1. Arthropathy due to factor IX deficiency _____

2. Deep overbite _____

3. Polymyalgia rheumatica _____

4. Systemic lupus erythematosus causing pleural effusion _____

5. Thrombotic thrombocytopenic purpura _____

Beyond the Code: What implications may exist relative to the coding and retrieval of data for the conditions reclassified to this chapter after previously being classified as diseases of the digestive system and circulatory system?

22.4 Dorsopathies and Spondylopathies

Dorsopathy literally means "disease of the back." It is a broad term that encompasses many disorders, such as **kyphosis,** scoliosis, lordosis, and other disorders that can be deforming and disabling. Pain and chronic fatigue are common symptoms. Kyphosis, scoliosis, and lordosis may be caused by congenital spinal defects, genetic diseases, vascular disorders that impede bone growth, tumors, trauma, infection, tuberculosis, endocrine disorders (such as Cushing's disease), prolonged steroid therapy, or aging. *Spondylopathy*, a similarly broad term, means "disease of the vertebrae." Spondylopathies may involve infection, inflammation, stiffness, stress fractures, and collapsed vertebrae. Dorsopathies and spondylopathies are reported by codes in categories M40–M54 in ICD-10-CM. They were coded from category 720 in ICD-9-CM.

dorsopathy Disease of the back or spine.

kyphosis Spinal curvature appearing as a hunchback, roundback, or slouched posture.

22.5 Disorders of Muscles, Synovium, Tendons, and Other Soft Tissue

Muscles are a type of connective tissue that controls body movements. Muscles are connected to bones by tendons, which are fibrous connective tissue. Figure 22.3 illustrates a cross-section of skeletal muscle. Synovium is a thin layer of smooth tissue, which lines joints and produces synovial fluid to facilitate joint movement. Disorders of muscles and tendons commonly involve inflammation, calcification, or rupture. Synovium and other soft tissue disorders frequently manifest as inflammation and infectious processes. Codes in categories M60–M79 are used to classify disorders of muscles, synovium, tendons, and soft tissue. Also, several codes in this subsection identify symptoms, such as pain in various limbs. The conditions discussed in this section were reported from categories 726–729 in ICD-9-CM. They are reported with codes in categories M60–M79 in ICD-10-CM.

> **CODING TIP** ▸
>
> Most disorders of muscles, synovium, tendons, and other soft tissue are specified by type at the 4th-character classification, and the 5th- and 6th-character specification identifies the exact location and laterality, if applicable.

M60–M63 Disorders of Muscles

ossification Process of bone formation.

Codes in this subsection of ICD-10-CM correspond with those in category 728 in ICD-9-CM. Conditions coded in this subsection include myositis, calcification and **ossification** of muscle, other disorders of muscle, and disorders of muscle in diseases classified elsewhere.

Myositis is further specified in category M60 to include infective myositis, interstitial myositis, and foreign body granuloma of soft tissue. An additional code should be assigned to identify the infectious agent, if documented for infective myositis. The type of foreign body should be reported with an additional code from category Z18- for codes in subcategory M60.2.

Category M61, calcification and ossification of muscle, classifies conditions including myositis ossificans traumatica, myositis ossificans progressiva, myositis ossificans associated with burns, other calcification of muscle, and other ossification of muscle. Other disorders of muscle, which are classified in category M62, include nontraumatic separation of muscle, nontraumatic rupture of muscle, nontraumatic ischemic infarction of muscle, immobility syndrome, contracture of muscle, muscle wasting and atrophy, generalized muscle weakness, rhabdomyolysis, and muscle spasm.

Codes in category M63 are for use only as secondary codes, following a code for the underlying disease. Underlying diseases related to conditions in this category include but are not limited to leprosy, neoplasms, schistosomiasis, and trichinellosis. Muscle disorders are classified according to location and laterality in category M63. Note that there is no category M64.

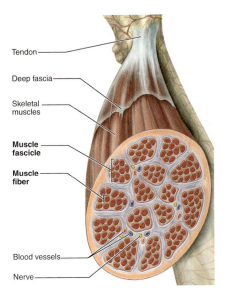

Tendon

Deep fascia

Skeletal muscles

Muscle fascicle

Muscle fiber

Blood vessels

Nerve

figure 22.3 Structure of Skeletal Muscle

M65–M67 Disorders of Synovium and Tendon

Codes in this subsection of ICD-10-CM correspond with those in category 727 in ICD-9-CM. Conditions coded in this subsection include synovitis, spontaneous rupture of synovium and tendon, and other disorders of synovium and tendon. When assigning codes from subcategory M65.0, an additional code should be assigned from B95–B96 to report the infectious agent.

M68–M69

Note that there are no categories M68 and M69.

M70–M79 Other Soft Tissue Disorders

Codes in this subsection of ICD-10-CM correspond with those in categories 726–729 in ICD-9-CM. Conditions coded in this subsection include bursopathies, fibroblastic disorders, palmar fascial fibromatosis, knuckle pads, plantar fasciitis, nodular fasciitis, necrotizing fasciitis, shoulder lesions, **enthesopathies** of the lower limb, and soft tissue disorders related to use, overuse, and pressure. An instructional note appears at the start of category M70, instructing coders to assign a secondary code to report activity documented as being the cause of the disorder.

Soft tissue disorders related to use, overuse, and pressure, reported in category M70, are further specified as crepitant synovitis, bursitis, olecranon bursitis, prepatellar bursitis, and trochanteric bursitis. Category M71 classifies other bursopathies, such as bursa abscess, infective bursitis, Baker cyst of the popliteal space, calcium deposits in the bursa, and other bursitis. When reporting codes from M71.1-, an additional code should be assigned to identify the infectious organism from B95–B96.

Shoulder lesions classified to category M75 include adhesive capsulitis, rotator cuff syndrome, bicipital tendinitis, calcific tendinitis, **impingement syndrome,** and bursitis. In category M76, enthesopathies of the lower limb, except for the foot, are classified, including gluteal tendinitis, psoas tendinitis, iliac crest spur, iliotibial band syndrome, tibial collateral bursitis, patellar tendinitis, Achilles tendinitis, peroneal tendinitis, anterior tibial syndrome, and posterior tibial tendinitis. Other enthesopathies are classified in category M77, which specifies the conditions medial epicondylitis, lateral epicondylitis, periarthritis, calcaneal spur, and metatarsalgia.

Category M79 classifies other disorders, many of which are considered to be symptoms. Conditions in this category include rheumatism, myalgia, neuralgia, neuritis, panniculitis, fat pad hypertrophy, residual foreign body in soft tissue, pain in limb, fibromyalgia, and nontraumatic compartment syndrome. Coders should be aware of the excludes1 note associated with code M79.5, residual foreign body in soft tissue, as close attention should be focused on documentation of the location of the foreign body to ensure that the appropriate code is assigned. Coding of limb pain is significantly expanded in ICD-10-CM, providing the ability to identify the specific body part through 31 codes with laterality, in comparison to ICD-9-CM, which had only a single code to report pain in any limb without specificity to site.

Spotlight on A&P

When a normal force is applied to tissues that are determined to have less than normal strength, a spontaneous rupture may occur. Note that this is classified differently than a traumatic rupture.

enthesopathy Disorder of the attachments to a bone, such as muscular tissue or tendons.

impingement syndrome Disorder of the tendons, most commonly of the rotator cuff muscles, which become irritated and inflamed as they pass through the subacromial space, resulting in pain, weakness, and loss of movement.

Chapter Summary

Learning Outcome	Key Concepts/Examples
22.1 Interpret coding guidelines for diseases of the musculoskeletal and connective tissue in order to determine appropriateness of code assignment and sequencing for conditions in the chapter. **(pages 348–349)**	• It is necessary to assign additional applicable codes for external cause conditions when assigning codes for musculoskeletal conditions. • Most diseases of the musculoskeletal and connective tissue have codes that designate laterality. • Coders should be aware of whether a bone, joint, or muscle condition is an acute traumatic injury or a chronic or recurring condition.
22.2 Identify codes for arthropathies, polyarthropathies, osteoarthritis, and other joint disorders. **(pages 349–354)**	• Most codes in this subsection provide the ability to specify the joint involved through a 5th character and to report laterality for paired joints through a 6th-character specification. • When reporting enteropathic arthropathies in category M07, a secondary code should be assigned for documented associated enteropathy, such as Crohn's disease or ulcerative colitis. • Category M1a requires assignment of a 7th character to report the presence or absence of tophus.
22.3 Classify dentofacial anomalies, jaw disorders, and systemic connective tissue disorders. **(pages 354–357)**	• Dentofacial anomalies (including malocclusion) and other disorders of the jaw, classified in categories M26 and M27, were classified as diseases of the digestive system in ICD-9-CM. • Conditions reported in categories M30 and M31 of ICD-10-CM as systemic connective tissue disorders were classified in category 446 of ICD-9-CM as diseases of the circulatory system. • Codes from category M36, systemic disorders of connective tissue diseases classified elsewhere, are for use only as secondary codes, following codes for the underlying conditions.
22.4 Apply coding guidelines to dorsopathies and spondylopathies. **(pages 357–359)**	• Dorsopathies and spondylopathies are specified by type at the 4th-character classification, while the 5th- and 6th-character specification identifies the region of the spine impacted. • A 7th-character classification is required for subcategories M48.4 and M48.5 to identify the encounter for fracture treatment. • Several conditions in category M54 may be considered to be symptoms, so it is important that coders are aware of any related billing and reimbursement requirements and limitations.

22.5 Use coding guidelines to classify disorders of muscles, synovium, tendons, and other soft tissue. **(pages 360–362)**	•	Most disorders of muscles, synovium, tendons, and other soft tissue are specified by type at the 4th-character classification, whereas the 5th- and 6th-character specification identifies the exact location and laterality, if applicable.
	•	ICD-10-CM provides the ability to report 31 site-specific codes for pain in a limb, compared to the solitary code that existed in ICD-9-CM, which did not provide any specificity of site.
22.6 Identify codes for osteopathies, chondropathies, disorders of bone density and structure, and other disorders of the musculoskeletal system and connective tissue. **(pages 363–367)**	•	For certain conditions, the bone may be affected at the upper or lower end (e.g., avascular necrosis of bone, M87, Osteoporosis, M80, M81). Although the portion of the bone affected may be at the joint, the site designation is the bone, not the joint.
	•	Do not assign a code from category M99 if the condition can be classified elsewhere.

Applying Your Skills

Assign codes for each condition, using both ICD-9-CM and ICD-10-CM codes.

Condition	ICD-9-CM Codes	ICD-10-CM Codes
1. *[LO 22.3]* Wegener's granulomatosis without renal involvement	_____	_____
2. *[LO 22.6]* Postlaminectomy syndrome of the lumbar region	_____	_____
3. *[LO 22.5]* Abscess of tendon sheath of right thigh	_____	_____
4. *[LO 22.2]* Rheumatoid lung disease with rheumatoid arthritis of the left hip	_____	_____
5. *[LO 22.4]* Torticollis	_____	_____
6. *[LO 22.6]* Paget's disease of bone in the left forearm	_____	_____
7. *[LO 22.3]* Endocarditis in systemic lupus erythematosus	_____	_____
8. *[LO 22.6]* Acute slipped upper femoral epiphysis of the left hip with chondrolysis	_____	_____
9. *[LO 22.2]* Gouty bursitis of the right foot	_____	_____
10. *[LO 22.4]* Left-sided sciatica	_____	_____
11. *[LO 22.3]* Polymyalgia rheumatica	_____	_____
12. *[LO 22.2]* Detached anterior horn of lateral meniscus of the left knee	_____	_____
13. *[LO 22.5]* Pain in left upper arm	_____	_____
14. *[LO 22.6]* Cauliflower ear, right ear	_____	_____
15. *[LO 22.3]* Polyarteritis nodosa	_____	_____

23

INJURY, POISONING, AND CERTAIN OTHER CONSEQUENCES OF EXTERNAL CAUSES

Learning Outcomes *After studying this chapter, students should be able to*

23.1 Interpret coding guidelines for injuries, poisonings, and certain other consequences of external causes.

23.2 Classify injuries according to type, site, and presence or absence of complications.

23.3 Explain the rationale for guidelines for coding injuries of multiple regions, unspecified regions, and foreign bodies entering through a natural orifice.

23.4 Apply knowledge of coding guidelines for burns, corrosions, and frostbite.

23.5 Identify terms associated with poisoning and toxic effects.

23.6 Discuss documentation needs related to other effects of external causes, trauma, and complications of care.

Key Terms

abrasion
accidental
anaphylactic shock
asphyxiation
assault
barotrauma
blister
closed fracture
contusion
corrosion
dislocation
frostbite
intentional
neglect
open fracture
poisoning
Rule of Nines
sprain
submersion
superficial injury
underdosing

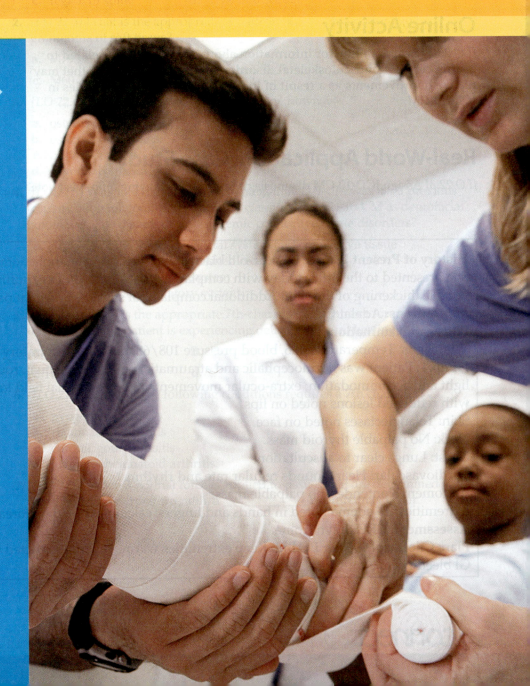

Introduction

Injury is a wound or damage to the structure and function of the body. It can be caused by some internal insult secondary to disease or by an external force. Injury can result from drowning, falls, traffic accidents, overcrowding, poor sanitation, or a hazardous work environment, among many other possible causes. Injuries include bruises, wounds, burns, sprains, concussions, and shock. They can be either accidental or intentional. Intentional infliction of harm is seen in child abuse and violence against others. Poisonings can occur due to misuse or adverse effects of prescribed medication, accidental exposure to chemical toxins, food poisoning, or other poisonings.

Injuries and poisonings are not only life-threatening, but can also lead to long-term physical and psychological debilitation. As health care services are delivered to meet an increased demand for the treatment of these conditions, cost of health care rises. Reporting of these conditions can drive preventive policy and safety measures. This chapter covers a wide range of codes in ICD-10-CM, which includes categories S00–T98. These codes are consistent with categories 800–999 in ICD-9-CM.

23.1 Coding Guidelines for Injuries, Poisonings, and Certain Other Consequences of External Causes

ICD-9-CM classifies injuries, poisonings, and other consequences of external causes in Chapter 17, "Injury and Poisoning." This chapter includes code categories 800–999. ICD-10-CM classifies these conditions in Chapter 19, "Injury, Poisoning, and Certain Other Consequences of External Causes," which includes code categories S00–T98. The S section of the chapter contains codes for classifying different types of injuries as they relate to single body regions, whereas the T section of the chapter contains codes to report injuries for unspecified body regions, poisoning, and certain other consequences of external causes.

There are two important instructional notes at the beginning of this chapter. The first instructs the coder to assign an additional code to identify the retention of a foreign body, if applicable, using a code from category Z18. The other instructional note directs the coder to assign secondary codes from Chapter 20, "External Causes of Morbidity," for the purpose of reporting cause of injury. The exception for this instruction is codes in the T section, which already state the external cause.

Coding guideline *I.C.19.a. Code Extensions* specifies that, in Chapter 19, a 7th-character extension is required for applicable codes for most categories. Aside from the fracture codes, most of the codes requiring a 7th character have three extension options:

- A, initial encounter—assigned if the patient is receiving care for the initial acute injury
- D, subsequent encounter—used for encounters following the initial treatment for acute injury when the patient is healing or recovering
- S, sequela—assigned for complications or other conditions that occur and are documented to be directly resulting from the injury

> **CODING TIP ▶**
>
> When assigning codes from Chapter 19 of ICD-10-CM, a secondary code from Chapter 20 should be assigned to report the cause of injury unless the code already states the external cause.

Active treatment examples include, but are not limited to, a visit to the emergency department, urgent care clinic, physician office, or surgical treatment as the first encounter with healthcare services for an acute injury. Subsequent care may involve the changing of a cast, removal of a fixation device, dressing change, or other follow-up after the initial treatment of the injury. It is not appropriate to assign a Z code for aftercare of an injury, as the acute injury code appended with the 7th-character extension of D should be assigned instead.

An example of a sequela is a scar from a burn or laceration. When reporting sequelae of an injury, the injury code should also be assigned with the code for the sequela, appending the S extension to the injury code, rather than the sequela, since it is identifying the injury that is responsible for the sequela. Sequencing of codes for sequelae should have the type of sequela listed first, with the injury code sequenced as a secondary code. Coding guideline *I.C.19.b. Coding of Injuries* directs the coder to assign a separate code for each injury when multiple injuries are being reported, unless an appropriate combination code is available. It is important for the coder to remember that, although a code may be available for multiple injuries, they are for use only if more specific documentation is not available to specify sites of injuries. Codes S00–T14.9 are for traumatic injury, and coders should refrain from assigning them for non-traumatic wounds, such as healing surgical wounds and complicated surgical wounds.

When sequencing injuries, the most serious one that is the focus of treatment should be sequenced first, followed by those with less severity. If a more severe injury coexists with a **superficial injury** (**abrasion** or **contusion**) of the same site, no code should be assigned for the superficial injury. When damage to peripheral nerves or blood vessels occurs with a primary injury, codes are assigned for both conditions, sequencing the primary injury code first, followed by secondary codes for the injuries of nerves, the spinal cord, and blood vessels. However, if the nerve or blood vessel injury is documented as the primary injury, it is appropriate to sequence the condition first.

> **superficial injury** Injury of less severity that does not penetrate to bones or organs.
>
> **abrasion** Area of skin or mucous membrane that has been scraped off.
>
> **contusion** Bruising of a tissue, including the brain.

> **CODING TIP** ▸
>
> When coding injuries, assign separate codes for each injury unless a combination code is provided, in which case the combination code is assigned.

Coding guideline *I.C.19.c. Coding of Traumatic Fractures* directs the coder to follow the same principles of coding multiple injury sites when reporting fractures. If multiple fracture sites are specified in the documentation, each site should be coded separately. If fracture documentation does not indicate if the fracture is open or closed, the default is to code it as a closed fracture. Similarly, if documentation does not indicate if a fracture is displaced or not, the default code is for a displaced fracture.

There are 7th-character extensions for fractures that are more specific than those for other injuries, as follows:

> **closed fracture** Fracture in which the bone is broken but the skin over it is left intact.
>
> **open fracture** Fracture in which the skin over the fracture is broken.

- A—initial encounter for **closed fracture**
- B—initial encounter for **open fracture** type I or II

- C—initial encounter for open fracture type IIIA, IIIB, or IIIC
- D—subsequent encounter for closed fracture with routine healing
- E—subsequent encounter for open fracture type I or II with routine healing
- F—subsequent encounter for open fracture type IIIA, IIIB, or IIIC with routine healing
- G—subsequent encounter for closed fracture with delayed healing
- H—subsequent encounter for open fracture type I or II with delayed healing
- J—subsequent encounter for open fracture type IIIA, IIIB, or IIIC with delayed healing
- K—subsequent encounter for closed fracture with nonunion
- M—subsequent encounter for open fracture type I or II with nonunion
- N—subsequent encounter for open fracture type IIIA, IIIB, or IIIC with nonunion
- P—subsequent encounter for closed fracture with malunion
- Q—subsequent encounter for open fracture type I or II with malunion
- R—subsequent encounter for open fracture type IIIA, IIIB, or IIIC with malunion
- S—sequela

The 7th characters A, B, and C are appended to codes reporting encounters for the initial encounter for fracture treatment. Note that the 7th characters for subsequent encounters for fractures not only indicate if the fracture is open or closed with the type of fracture but also indicate if the subsequent care is for a routinely healing fracture versus one with delayed healing, nonunion, or malunion. Seventh characters for subsequent encounters should be appended to the acute injury codes when reporting encounters for injury aftercare, rather than a Z code for aftercare.

When reporting multiple fractures, they should be sequenced according to severity. This may require a physician query to obtain documentation that specifies the order of severity. If a patient has known osteoporosis and suffers a fracture, a code from category M80, Osteoporosis with current pathological fracture, should be assigned instead of a code for a traumatic fracture. This applies even if a minor fall or trauma that would not break a normal, healthy bone was a contributing factor.

> **CODING TIP ▶**
>
> A fracture not indicated as open or closed should be coded as closed. A fracture not indicated as displaced or not displaced should be coded as displaced.

Think About It 23.1

also available in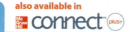

Why do you think that aftercare Z codes should not be used for aftercare for injuries?

23.2 Injuries

Injury can happen to any site in the body. Some examples of injury are sports injuries, violent gunshot wounds, and accidents resulting from the use of various types of mechanical equipment or transportation. Injuries can also result from poor judgment, lack of awareness, negligent actions, or failure to act with caution. Injuries can also result from poor judgement, lack of awareness or knowledge, negligent acts and/or ommissions. Injuries may require prolonged and costly hospital stays and an application for disability assistance via a government supported insurance program when the patient also suffers loss of earned income or does not have private short-term or long-term disability insurance coverage. Caregiving is often needed, and individuals may not be able to afford this due to a lack of access to insurance coverage, discretionary funds, or other assets that can be divested to pay for personal home care services. Health care complications can occur secondary to injury, requiring repeat utilization of services. Fragmentation in service delivery and lack of transportation in some instances can make it especially difficult for some patients to get the care they need. Patient's health status may decline or become complicated by comorbid conditions. Reporting the prevalence of these conditions may drive preventive policies and safety regulations with the goal of reducing costs associated with injury and its complications. Patients may experience increased quality of life, when the delivery of health care services is efficient and effective.

ICD-10-CM classifies injuries differently than ICD-9-CM. In ICD-9-CM, conditions were classified according to type of injury. ICD-10-CM classifies them according to the site of injury on the body. The conditions discussed in this section are reported with ICD-10-CM category codes S00–S99, which correspond with categories 800–929 in ICD-9-CM. A comparison of the ICD-10-CM and ICD-9-CM classifications is presented in Table 23.1, which demonstrates how ICD-10-CM now classifies the injuries primarily according to anatomic location, as opposed to the primary classification according to type of injury in ICD-9-CM.

Spotlight on A&P

Injury may result in extensive internal organ damage or superficial external wounds that interfere with vital, life-sustaining functions.

S00–S09 Injuries to the Head

Codes in this subsection of ICD-10-CM correspond with those in categories 800–804, 830, 850–854, 870–873, 905–908, 910, 918, 920, 921, and 925 in ICD-9-CM. Conditions coded in this subsection include injuries of the ear, eye, face, gum, jaw, oral cavity, palate, periocular area, scalp, temporomandibular joint area, tongue, and tooth. The types of injuries classified include superficial injuries, open wounds, fractures, dislocations, sprains, nerve injuries, crushing injuries, avulsions, traumatic amputations, and other specified injuries.

Table 23.1 Comparison of ICD-10-CM and ICD-9-CM Classification of Injuries

ICD-10-CM Categories	Corresponding ICD-9-CM Categories
S00–S09 Injuries to the head	800–804, 830, 850–854, 870–873, 905–908, 910, 918, 920, 921, and 925
S10–S19 Injuries to the neck	805, 806, 874, 900, 905–908, 910, 920, and 925
S20–S29 Injuries to the thorax	805–807, 860–862, 875, 901, 905–908, 911, 922, and 926
S30–S39 Injuries to the abdomen, lower back, lumbar spine, pelvis, and external genitals	805, 806, 808, 846, 847, 863–868, 876–879, 902, 905–908, 911, 922, and 926
S40–S49 Injuries to the shoulder and upper arm	810–812, 831, 840, 880, 903, 905–908, 912, 923, and 927
S50–S59 Injuries to the elbow and forearm	813, 832, 841, 881, 887, 903, 905–908, 913, 923, and 927
S60–S69 Injuries to the wrist, hand, and fingers	814–817, 833, 834, 842, 881–883, 885–887, 905–908, 913–915, 923, and 927
S70–S79 Injuries to the hip and thigh	820, 821, 835, 843, 890, 904, 905–908, 916, 924, and 928
S80–S89 Injuries to the knee and lower leg	822, 823, 836, 844, 891, 897, 904–908, 916, 924, and 928
S90–S99 Injuries to the ankle and foot	824–826, 837, 838, 845, 892, 893, 895,896, 905–908, 916, 917, 924, and 928

Superficial injuries of each of the areas in this subsection are further classified in category S00 to specify the type of injury, including abrasion, **blister,** contusion, external constriction, superficial foreign body (such as a splinter), and insect bite. The type of superficial injury is specified at the 4th character, and the location is specified at the 5th- and 6th-character levels. Category S00 also requires the assignment of a 7th character to report the encounter. Table 23.2 specifies these 7th characters.

Category S01 classifies open wounds of the head for the areas previously listed. The 4th character identifies the specific location, whereas the 5th

blister Thin, bubblelike sac on the surface of the skin, usually filled with watery liquid, or serum.

Table 23.2 Encounters Specified by 7th Characters for Categories S00, S01, and S03–S06

Seventh Character	Meaning
A	Initial encounter
D	Subsequent encounter
S	Sequela

Table 23.3 Encounters Specified by 7th Characters for Category S02

Seventh Character	Meaning
A	Initial encounter for closed fracture
B	Initial encounter for open fracture
D	Subsequent encounter for fracture with routine healing
G	Subsequent encounter for fracture with delayed healing
K	Subsequent encounter for fracture with nonunion
S	Sequela

digit provides additional detail about the open wound, including laceration without foreign body, laceration with foreign body, puncture wound without foreign body, puncture wound with foreign body, and open bite. The 6th character designates laterality, where applicable. This category also requires the assignment of a 7th character of A, D, or S to report the encounter.

Category S02 classifies fractures of the vault of the skull, base of the skull, nasal bones, orbital floor, malar bones, maxillary bones, zygoma bones, tooth, and mandible. Note that there is a difference between a broken tooth and a cracked tooth for coding purposes. A broken tooth is that which is fractured traumatically, whereas a cracked tooth is non-traumatic and reported with code K03.81. Fractures of the mandible are further specified as condylar process, subcondylar process, coronoid process, ramus, angle, symphysis, and alveolus. Table 23.3 specifies the 7th characters used to report encounters when coding from category S02. Figure 23.1

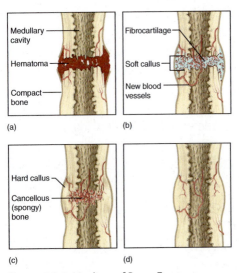

(a)

(b)

(c)

(d)

figure 23.1 Healing of Bone Fracture

illustrates the process of fracture healing, which is necessary to comprehend when assigning 7th characters.

Dislocations and **sprains** are reported in category S03, according to site. The 7th characters A, D, and S are required with category S03 to identify if it is the initial encounter, a subsequent encounter, or a sequela.

Category S04 classifies injuries of cranial nerves. Note that laterality for the side of the body being affected should be identified as either left or right. A code for any documented intracranial injury should be reported and listed prior to codes in this category. If an injury of the optic nerve and pathways is reported, an additional code should be reported to identify any documentation of an associated visual field defect or blindness with code H53.4- or H54.

Categories S05–S09 require a 7th character of A, D, or S to identify if it is the initial encounter, a subsequent encounter, or a sequela. When reporting an intracranial injury, any documentation of an associated open wound of the head or a skull fracture should be reported with an additional code. Crushing injuries of the head, reported in category S07, should have an additional code assigned to identify any associated intracranial injuries or skull fractures. Injury of a muscle or tendon of the hand should have an additional code assigned to report an associated open wound.

sprain Joint or muscle injury caused by overexertion or overextension.

> **CODING TIP ▸**
>
> When identifying laterality for injuries of the cranial nerve, the side of the body being affected is the basis of code assignment.

S10–S19 Injuries to the Neck

Codes in this subsection of ICD-10-CM correspond with those in categories 805, 806, 874, 900, 905–908, 910, 920, and 925 in ICD-9-CM. Conditions coded in this subsection include category classifications similar to those for injuries to the head, then are further specified to the structures in the neck. The categories are superficial injuries; open wound; fracture; injury of nerves; injury of blood vessels; injury of muscle, fascia, and tendon; crushing injury; and other and unspecified injuries. Categories S10 and S11 require a 7th character of A, D, or S to identify if it is the initial encounter, a subsequent encounter, or a sequela. Seventh digits of A, B, D, G, K, or S are to be assigned with category S12.

S20–S29 Injuries to the Thorax

Codes in this subsection of ICD-10-CM correspond with those in categories 805–807, 860–862, 875, 901, 905–908, 911, 922, and 926 in ICD-9-CM. Conditions coded in this subsection follow similar, although not identical, category classifications as previous subsections. However, they are further specified to include structures of the thorax. The categories are superficial injuries, open wound, fracture, injury of nerves, injury of blood vessels, injury of the heart, crushing injury, and other and unspecified injuries.

S30–S39 Injuries to the Abdomen, Lower Back, Lumbar Spine, Pelvis, and External Genitals

Codes in this subsection of ICD-10-CM correspond with those in categories 805, 806, 808, 846, 847, 863–868, 876–879, 902, 905–908, 911, 922, and 926 in ICD-9-CM. Conditions coded in this subsection follow similar, although not identical, category classifications as previous subsections, then are further specified to the structures in the abdomen, lower back, lumbar spine,

dislocation Separation of bones from normal position at a joint.

pelvis, and external genitals. The categories are superficial injuries, open wound, fracture, **dislocation** and sprain, injury of nerves, injury of blood vessels, injury of intra-abdominal organs, injury of urinary and pelvic organs, crushing injury, and other and unspecified injuries.

S40–S49 Injuries to the Shoulder and Upper Arm

Codes in this subsection of ICD-10-CM correspond with those in categories 810–812, 831, 840, 880, 903, 905–908, 912, 923, and 927 in ICD-9-CM. Conditions coded in this subsection follow similar, although not identical, category classifications as previous subsections, then are further specified to the shoulder and upper arm. The categories are superficial injuries; open wound; fracture (see Figure 23.2 for types of fractures); dislocation and sprain; injury of nerves; injury of blood vessels; injury of the muscle, fascia, and tendon; crushing injury; traumatic amputation; and other and unspecified injuries.

S50–S59 Injuries to the Elbow and Forearm

Codes in this subsection of ICD-10-CM correspond with those in categories 813, 832, 841, 881, 887, 903, 905–908, 913, 923, and 927 in ICD-9-CM.

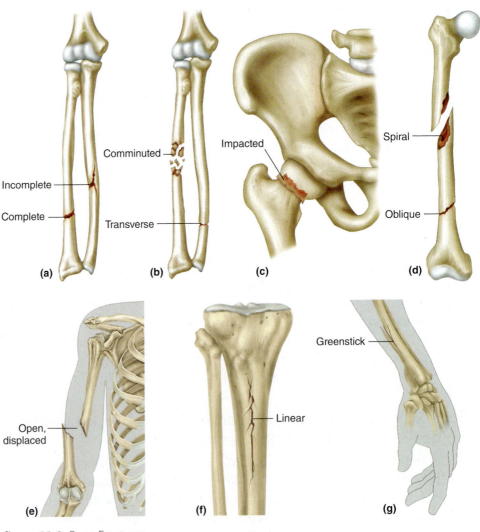

figure 23.2 Bone Fractures

Conditions coded in this subsection follow similar, although not identical, category classifications as previous subsections, then are further specified to the elbow and forearm. The categories are superficial injuries; open wound; fracture; dislocation and sprain; injury of nerves; injury of blood vessels; injury of the muscle, fascia, and tendon; crushing injury; traumatic amputation; and other and unspecified injuries.

S60–S69 Injuries to the Wrist, Hand, and Fingers

Codes in this subsection of ICD-10-CM correspond with those in categories 814–817, 833, 834, 842, 881–883, 885–887, 905–908, 913–915, 923, and 927 in ICD-9-CM. Conditions coded in this subsection follow similar, although not identical, category classifications as previous subsections, then are further specified to the wrist, hand, and fingers. The categories are superficial injuries; open wound; fracture; dislocation and sprain; injury of nerves; injury of blood vessels; injury of the muscle, fascia, and tendon; crushing injury; traumatic amputation; and other and unspecified injuries.

S70–S79 Injuries to the Hip and Thigh

Codes in this subsection of ICD-10-CM correspond with those in categories 820, 821, 835, 843, 890, 904, 905–908, 916, 924, and 928 in ICD-9-CM. Conditions coded in this subsection follow similar, although not identical, category classifications as previous subsections, then are further specified to the hip and thigh. The categories are superficial injuries; open wound; fracture; dislocation and sprain; injury of nerves; injury of blood vessels; injury of the muscle, fascia, and tendon; crushing injury; traumatic amputation; and other and unspecified injuries.

S80–S89 Injuries to the Knee and Lower Leg

Codes in this subsection of ICD-10-CM correspond with those in categories 822, 823, 836, 844, 891, 897, 904–908, 916, 924, and 928 in ICD-9-CM. Conditions coded in this subsection follow similar, although not identical, category classifications as previous subsections, then are further specified to the knee and lower leg. The categories are superficial injuries; open wound; fracture; dislocation and sprain; injury of nerves; injury of blood vessels; injury of the muscle, fascia, and tendon; crushing injury; traumatic amputation; and other and unspecified injuries. Several of these knee injuries are illustrated in Figure 23.3.

S90–S99 Injuries to the Ankle and Foot

Codes in this subsection of ICD-10-CM correspond with those in categories 824–826, 837, 838, 845, 892, 893, 895, 896, 905–908, 916, 917, 924, and 928 in ICD-9-CM. Conditions coded in this subsection follow similar, although not identical, category

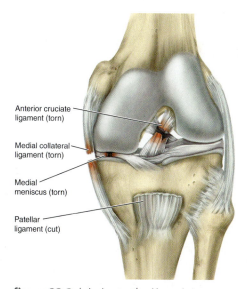

figure 23.3 Injuries to the Knee Joint

Anterior cruciate ligament (torn)

Medial collateral ligament (torn)

Medial meniscus (torn)

Patellar ligament (cut)

classifications as previous subsections, then are further specified to the ankle and foot. The categories are superficial injuries; open wound; fracture; dislocation and sprain; injury of nerves; injury of blood vessels; injury of the muscle, fascia, and tendon; crushing injury; traumatic amputation; and other and unspecified injuries.

Assign ICD-10-CM codes for the following situations, applying any appropriate sequencing guidelines.

1. Minor laceration of the internal, extra-cranial portion of the right carotid artery of the neck from a foreign body of other part of the neck; initial encounter with associated open wound

   _____

2. Open wound of the trachea with infection as a result of a puncture wound with foreign body; associated incomplete spinal cord injury of the central cord at C8 with transient paralysis; subsequent encounter

   _____

3. Subsequent encounter for malunion of posterior displaced fracture of sternal end of left clavicle

   _____

4. Initial encounter to treat hair tourniquet syndrome of left small toe

   _____

5. Initial encounter for type IIIB displaced fracture of coronoid process of right ulna _____

   Beyond the Code: What do you think is the rationale for identifying laterality for injuries of the cranial nerve by the side of the body being affected?

23.3 Injuries of Multiple Regions, Unspecified Regions, and Foreign Bodies Entering through Natural Orifice

Depending on the nature and extent of the injury, multiple regions may be affected by superficial injuries, open wounds, open or closed fracture, dislocation, sprains, blood vessel damage, injury to internal organs, and crushing trauma. In some instances, there can also be injury to unspecified regions, and three codes are available for reporting them. A foreign body, or material that does not normally belong in an orifice of the body or organ system, can lead to injury and death. There are a variety of ways this may occur. Children can get food items or small objects stuck in their mouth, nose, or throat. Anyone who drinks alcohol can aspirate on his or her own vomit, which can lead to lung disease or death. Adults have been known to choke or asphyxiate on food that is not properly chewed. Foreign objects can lead to tears and lacerations in any anatomic tissue, which can lead to an inability to use that part of the body again. Foreign objects in the mouth, nose, or throat can interfere with digestive processes. Foreign objects in the anus or rectum can cause colon damage, which can result in a surgical colostomy. Genital injuries can impair the ability to eliminate toxins from the body and result in kidney disease.

Ultimately, any foreign object can cause an obstruction in a vital function within the body. Injuries in this section are classified in ICD-10-CM categories T00–T19, which are equivalent to ICD-9-CM categories 930–939 for foreign bodies and a variety of codes in ICD-9-CM Chapter 17 for injuries involving multiple body regions.

Spotlight on A&P

Anyone with an injury or a disease can end up with a foreign object lodged in an orifice of the body. Some stroke patients have difficulty swallowing due to paralysis and weakness. Understanding the physiology of an underlying condition can shed light on the injury.

T00–T06

Categories T00–T06 have been deactivated. Conditions previously classified to these categories are now classified to individual injury codes.

T07 Injuries involving Multiple Body Regions

Codes in this subsection of ICD-10-CM correspond with those in a variety of categories, scattered throughout Chapter 17 of ICD-9-CM. Code T07, unspecified multiple injuries is the only code in this subsection. It is only allowed for use if there is no available documentation to identify the specific injuries and is not for use in the inpatient setting. Note that categories T00–T06 and T08–T13 have been deactivated.

T14 Injury of Unspecified Body Region

Codes in this subsection of ICD-10-CM correspond with those in a variety of categories, scattered throughout Chapter 17 in ICD-9-CM. There are only three codes in this subsection: T14.8, other injury of unspecified body region; T14.90, unspecified injury; and T14.91, suicide attempt. Code T14.8 is used to report unspecified contusions, crush injuries, fractures, skin injuries, and vascular injuries. Code T14.90 is only for use when there is no documentation to identify specific injuries, and it should not be assigned in an inpatient setting.

CODING TIP ▸

Codes T07, unspecified multiple injuries, and T14.90, unspecified injury, are only for use when there is no documentation to identify specific injuries, and they should not be assigned in an inpatient setting.

from category T86 are reported only if the function of the transplanted organ is impacted. When reporting transplant complications, a code from category T86 must be accompanied by a secondary code to report the documented complication.

If a patient has received a kidney transplant, there may still be some chronic kidney disease (CKD) present, as function may not be fully restored by the transplanted organ. The presence of CKD following a transplant is not considered a complication unless there is documentation of rejection or failure of the transplant. If the coder is unable to determine if the condition is related to failure or rejection of the transplanted kidney, a physician query should be performed for clarification.

Some T codes that report complications also include the external cause in the code. This may include both the nature of the complication and the type of procedure responsible for the complication. If this is the case, it is not necessary to report an additional external cause code, as that would be redundant. If a code from a specific body system chapter exists to report an intra-operative or postprocedural complication, the body system–specific code should be sequenced first, followed by any applicable codes to identify the specific complication.

Documentation must exist to confirm the relationship between mechanical ventilation and pneumonia in order to report code J95.851, ventilator associated pneumonia. When reporting ventilator associated pneumonia (VAP), an additional code should be assigned to identify the causal organism. If a patient is admitted with one type of pneumonia and documentation exists that the patient developed VAP following admission, the type of pneumonia that was diagnosed at admission is listed first, with code J95.851 assigned as a secondary code.

Think About It 23.6

also available in **connect** plus+

Assign ICD-10-CM codes for the following situations, applying any appropriate sequencing guidelines.

1. Hypothermia; initial encounter   _____

2. Caisson disease; subsequent encounter   _____

3. Initial encounter for treatment of dislocated internal right knee prosthesis   _____

4. Subsequent encounter to treat condition from confirmed physical abuse of an adult   _____

5. Late effects of psychological abuse of a child   _____

Beyond the Code: What documentation challenges might you anticipate related to codes T80–T88? What methods might you use to overcome them?

Chapter Summary

Learning Outcome	Key Concepts/Examples
23.1 Interpret coding guidelines for injuries, poisonings, and certain other consequences of external causes. **(pages 373–375)**	• When assigning codes from Chapter 19 of ICD-9-CM, a secondary code from Chapter 20 should be assigned to report the cause of injury, unless the code already states the external cause. • When coding injuries, assign separate codes for each injury unless a combination code is provided, in which case the combination code is assigned.
23.2 Classify injuries according to type, site, and presence or absence of complications. **(pages 376–382)**	• Injuries were classified according to type of injury in ICD-9-CM, whereas ICD-10-CM classifies them according to the site of injury on the body. • Injuries in this section are classified specific to site and then further specified as superficial injuries; open wound; fracture; injury of nerves; injury of blood vessels; injury of muscle, fascia, and tendon; crushing injury; and other and unspecified injuries. • Seventh characters are to be assigned to identify the encounter as initial encounter, subsequent encounter, or sequela.
23.3 Explain the rationale for guidelines for coding injuries of multiple regions, unspecified regions, and foreign bodies entering through a natural orifice. **(pages 382–384)**	• Codes T07, unspecified multiple injuries, and T14.90, unspecified injury, are for use only when there is no documentation to identify specific injuries and should not be assigned in an inpatient setting.
23.4 Apply knowledge of coding guidelines for burns, corrosions, and frostbite. **(pages 384–387)**	• Burns and corrosions are classified in categories by general site, with a 4th character to specify the degree, a 5th character to specify the site, a 6th character to specify applicable laterality, and a 7th character to specify the encounter. • When assigning codes from categories T20–T25, an additional code from category T31 or T32 should be assigned to report the extent of body surface involved.
23.5 Identify terms associated with poisoning and toxic effects. **(pages 390–394)**	• When reporting poisonings, adverse effects, and underdosing, the first code listed is a code from categories T36–T65, followed by codes for all documented manifestations of the adverse effect, poisoning, or toxic effect. It is not necessary to assign an additional external cause code for poisonings, toxic effects, adverse effects, and underdosing codes. • Codes for underdosing should never be assigned as principal or first-listed codes. If a patient has a relapse or an exacerbation of the medical condition for which the drug is prescribed because of the reduction in dose, the medical condition itself should be coded.

- Asphyxiation, reported with codes in category T71, is classified according to method of asphyxiation, with further specification of whether it was accidental, intentional self-harm, assault, or undetermined.

- Confirmed cases of abuse, reported in category T74, should have an additional code assigned from Y07.- to identify the perpetrator, if known.

Applying Your Skills

Assign codes for each condition, using both ICD-9-CM and ICD-10-CM codes.

Condition	ICD-9-CM Codes	ICD-10-CM Codes
1. *[LO 23.2]* Fracture of the nasal bones; initial encounter with no loss of consciousness	_____	_____
2. *[LO 23.2]* Traumatic subarachnoid hemorrhage following injury with open intracranial wound; with brief loss of consciousness 30 minutes or less; initial encounter	_____	_____
3. *[LO 23.2]* Nonvenomous insect bite of the throat without infection; initial encounter	_____	_____
4. *[LO 23.2]* Non-displaced fracture of the 4th cervical vertebra; initial encounter for open fracture; with central cord syndrome	_____	_____
5. *[LO 23.3]* Foreign body in the stomach; initial encounter	_____	_____
6. *[LO 23.4]* First-degree burn of cheek; initial encounter	_____	_____
7. *[LO 23.5]* Nosebleed as an adverse effect of Coumadin taken according to prescription; initial encounter	_____	_____
8. *[LO 23.5]* Subsequent encounter to follow patient for palpitations caused by accidental overdose of Synthroid	_____	_____
9. *[LO 23.5]* Initial encounter for hypotension caused by intentional overdose of losartan for the purpose of self-harm	_____	_____
10. [LO 23.5] Accidental ingestion of toxic berries, causing nausea and vomiting; initial encounter	_____	_____
11. *[LO 23.6]* Anaphylactic shock due to peanuts; initial encounter	_____	_____
12. *[LO 23.6]* Exhaustion due to excessive exertion; initial encounter	_____	_____
13. *[LO 23.5]* Initial encounter for coughing and throat pain following inhalation of chlorine fumes from bleach	_____	_____
14. *[LO 23.6]* Sinus barotrauma; initial encounter	_____	_____
15. *[LO 23.5]* Initial encounter—patient in coma, no motor response, no verbal response, eyes not opening to any stimuli for first three days of hospital admission; determined to be toxic effect of arsenic pesticide; undetermined if accident or purposely inflicted	_____	_____
16. *[LO 23.6]* Confirmed sexual abuse of child; subsequent encounter	_____	_____
17. *[LO 23.6]* Displacement of indwelling urethral catheter; initial encounter	_____	_____
18. *[LO 23.6]* Subsequent visit for treatment of mechanical complication of cardiac device; breakdown of surgically created arteriovenous shunt	_____	_____

19. *[LO 23.6]* Asphyxiation due to a plastic bag; intentional self-harm; initial encounter

_____ _____

20. *[LO 23.1]* Accidental overdose of caffeine, causing intractable headache; initial encounter

_____ _____

Checking Your Understanding

Select the letter that best answers the question or completes the sentence.

1. *[LO 23.4]* Which of the following conditions is classified as a corrosion?

    a. chemical burn   **b.** electrical burn

    c. radiation burn   **d.** thermal burn

2. *[LO 23.5]* How does the classification of poisonings differ between ICD-9-CM and ICD-10-CM?

    a. ICD-9-CM did not classify poisonings and adverse effects.

    b. ICD-9-CM included manifestations in combination codes for poisonings.

    c. ICD-9-CM classified poisonings by type, rather than by substance involved.

    d. ICD-9-CM classified poisonings by substance, rather than by type of poisoning.

3. *[LO 23.2]* Which type of injury should have an additional code assigned to report documentation of an associated open wound of the hand?

    a. superficial injury of the hand

    b. injury of muscle or tendon of the hand

    c. open fracture of the hand

    d. closed fracture of the hand

4. *[LO 23.1]* Which 7th character should be assigned for a scar as a result of a burn?

    a. A   **b.** D

    c. S   **d.** It is never appropriate to assign an injury code for a scar.

5. *[LO 23.1]* What is the appropriate action if a fracture is not indicated as open or closed?

    a. Assign the code for unspecified fracture.

    b. Assign the code for closed fracture.

    c. Assign the code for displaced fracture.

    d. Assign the code for open fracture.

6. *[LO 23.3]* An inpatient was recently discharged and transferred to another facility for specialized trauma care. The discharge diagnosis documented by the physician is "multiple traumatic injuries." There is very limited documentation anywhere in the record. What action should you take?

    a. Assign code T07.

    b. Assign code T14.90.

    c. Contact the facility where the patient was transferred to find out the details of the patient's injuries.

    d. Query the physician for specification of the injuries.

7. *[LO 23.2]* A patient with a history of a closed femur fracture is seen by the orthopedic surgeon for treatment of nonunion of the fracture. What is the appropriate 7th digit to be assigned for the visit?

    a. A   **b.** G

    c. K   **d.** S

McGraw Hill **connect** ᵖˡᵘˢ⁺ **Enhance your learning by completing these exercises and more at mcgrawhillconnect.com**

CHAPTER 23 INJURY, POISONING **401**

8. *[LO 23.1]* How is the most serious injury determined?

   a. chief complaint stated by the patient
   b. code with the highest number in the section
   c. physician documentation
   d. coder opinion

9. *[LO 23.6]* A two-month-old baby is treated in the emergency department for asphyxiation. The mother, who had been home alone with the baby, reported that she went to check on the baby and found the baby tangled in bedding in the crib. Which code should be assigned?

   a. T71.131
   c. T71.133

   b. T71.132
   d. T71.134

10. *[LO 23.6]* Which of the following conditions should not be coded in category T67, effects of heat and light?

   a. heat exhaustion
   c. sunburn

   b. sunstroke
   d. heat edema

Online Activity

[LO 23.1] Search online for information about reimbursement issues related to coding of injuries. Summarize your findings in a brief report.

Real-World Application: Case Study

[LO 23.5] Assign ICD-10-CM codes to the following discharge summary.

Date of Admission: 6/17/XX
Date of Discharge: 6/18/XX
Admitting Diagnosis: 1. Atrioventricular block, complete
Procedure(s): Continuous cardiac monitoring. Echocardiogram on 6/18/XX
History of Present Illness: A 26-year-old female with a history of SVT presented to the emergency room with the complaint of an uncomfortable heartbeat in her throat. Cardiac monitoring in the emergency room revealed no T waves. She was admitted with complete atrioventricular block after an accidental overdose of Cordarone. The patient has no history of health problem other than mild hypothyroidism.
Physical Examination: The patient's vital signs were normal. Temperature: 98.6; Respiratory rate: 16; Pulse: 76; Blood Pressure: 118/76. Lungs are clear. Few ectopic beats are heard on auscultation. Pulses are present in the extremities. PERRLA. Skin is normal with no discoloration. The patient is alert and oriented.
Hospital Course: The patient was admitted to a telemetry unit for continuous cardiac monitoring and detoxification. No medication was administered. The patient was provided with supplemental oxygen as needed. An echocardiogram revealed no cardiac damage. The patient successfully detoxed and was discharged home.
Discharge Instructions: No prescriptions were given. The patient is to follow up with her cardiologist within 2 weeks.
Discharge Diagnosis: Complete atrioventricular block following overdose of Cordarone.

---

24 EXTERNAL CAUSES OF INJURY, POISONING, AND MORBIDITY

Learning Outcomes *After reading this chapter, students should be able to*

24.1 Interpret coding guidelines for external causes of morbidity.

24.2 Classify external causes of injury for transport accidents.

24.3 Select appropriate codes for injuries due to falls and exposure.

24.4 Identify factors related to causes of injuries due to self-harm, assault, or undetermined intent.

24.5 Analyze documentation to report legal, military, and medical causes and supplementary factors.

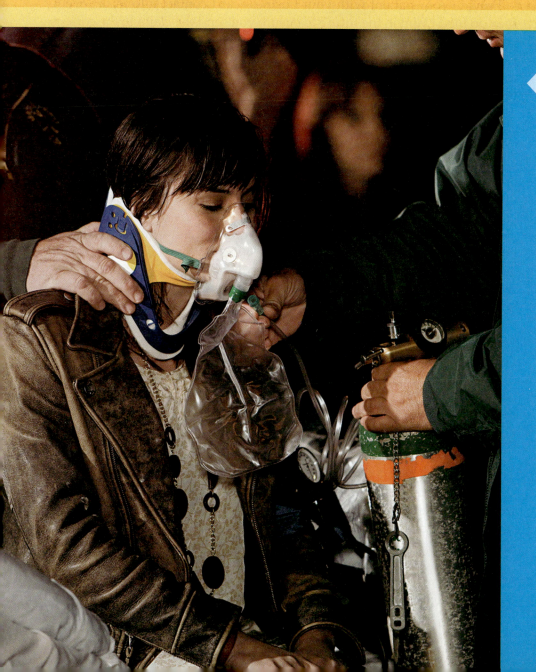

Key Terms

assault
cataclysmic event
collision
external cause
misadventure
morbidity
non-collision transport accident
non-traffic accident
nosocomial
pedestrian
place of occurrence
terrorism
transport accident

Introduction

Based upon the nature of a patient's injuries or illness and manner by which they were sustained, the patient may have filed a claim with his or her automobile insurance company, homeowner's, or other premises liability insurance company, or worker's compensation office. Reasons for wounds or injuries should be accurately identified to ensure that medical claims are sent to the appropriate payer. This can be done by asking the patient the following series of questions:

1. How did the injury occur?
2. Where were you when the injury occurred?
3. Were there any contributing factors to the injury?
4. Has a liability claim been filed?

   If the patient has filed a claim, ask

5. What insurance provider received the liability claim?

Provide your patient with your business card contact info in the event they do file a claim in the future to ensure you send the claim to the correct payer for adjudication. In the event your patient has hired an attorney to represent them, you may need to place the attorney and any other insurance parties on notice that the patient has outstanding medical claims in need of adjudication and settlement.

6. What is the claim number?

The patient may have filed a claim with his or her automobile insurance company, homeowner's or other premises liability insurance, or worker's compensation.

Coding of poisonings and adverse effects of medications also require circumstances to be reported. The insurance company and claim number should be obtained in order to send the medical claim to the appropriate payer. External causes of morbidity in this section are classified as injury due to transport accidents, falls and exposure, self-harm, assault, undetermined intent, and legal, military, and medical causes. ICD-9-CM classifies these causes with code categories from Chapter 19, "Supplemental Classification of External Causes of Injury and Poisoning," which includes codes E800–E999. ICD-10-CM classifies these factors in Chapter 20, "External Causes of Morbidity," which includes code categories V00–Y99.

24.1 Coding Guidelines for External Causes of Morbidity

There are a variety of coding guidelines that apply to all of Chapter 20 of ICD-10-CM. They provide the coder with explanations and purposes of the standardized use of codes for external causes of morbidity, along with direction regarding sequencing, number of codes to be assigned, and special circumstances, such as unknown intent, undetermined intent, and late effects or sequelae of injuries.

Coding guideline *I.C.20* presents an explanation of the standardized use of external causes of **morbidity** codes, along with a purpose for their use. **External cause** codes are secondary codes for use in any healthcare setting

morbidity Incidence of disease.

external cause Cause of injury not stemming from the patient's own status or condition.

for the purpose of providing data for injury research and evaluation of strategies for injury prevention. The codes identify the cause, intent, and location where the injury occurred, along with the patient's status and the activity that was being performed.

The Index to External Causes follows the alphabetic index to diseases. Although they generally apply to injuries, any code in the ranges of A00.0–T88.9 or Z00–Z99, which are used to report a health condition that is due to an external cause, may be followed by an external cause code. For example, a patient may experience an acute myocardial infarction when performing a strenuous physical activity.

Coding guideline *I.C.20.a. General External Cause Coding Guidelines* further specifies that external cause codes are for use only as secondary diagnoses and should never be reported as principal or first-listed diagnoses. If the external cause and intent are included in a code from another chapter, it is not appropriate to report an external cause code from Chapter 20. When assigning external cause codes, the appropriate 7th character should be assigned to identify if the visit is the initial encounter, a subsequent encounter, or a sequela.

Coders may assign as many codes as necessary to provide a comprehensive description of the injury, and the full range of external cause codes should be used in order to identify the intent, place, activity, and status of the patient. There may be instances where only one external cause code can be reported. In these cases, the code most closely related to the principal diagnosis should be assigned. This is further supported by coding guideline *I.C.20.e. If the Reporting Format Limits the Number of External Cause Codes.*

Some combination codes describe sequential events that result in injuries. Although the injury may be caused by either or both of the events, the combination code should correspond to the sequence of events as they are documented.

> **CODING TIP** ▶
>
> Although they are most applicable to injuries, external cause codes are also valid for use with such things as infections or diseases due to an external source and other health conditions, such as a heart attack that occurs during strenuous physical activity.

Coding guideline *I.C.20.d. Place of Occurrence, Activity, and Status Codes Used with other External Cause Code* specifies that codes to report **place of occurrence,** activity, and external cause status codes are to be sequenced secondarily, following the main external cause code(s). The guideline also specifies that it is only appropriate to report one place of occurrence code, one activity code, and one external cause status code to an encounter, no matter how many other external cause codes are assigned.

Coding guideline *I.C.20.f. Multiple External Cause Coding Guidelines* provides instructions for sequencing external cause codes when more than one is assigned:

1. External codes to report child and adult abuse take sequencing priority over all other external cause codes.

2. The next priority for external cause codes are those reporting **terrorism** events.

3. This is followed by external cause codes for **cataclysmic events.**

place of occurrence Geographical location of a patient when an injury occurred.

terrorism Unlawful use of force or violence against persons or property to intimidate or coerce a government, the civilian population, or any segment thereof in furtherance of a political or social objective.

cataclysmic event Events causing widespread injury and upheaval, such as a natural disaster or an act of war.

transport accident Accident involving a device designed primarily for, or used at the time primarily for, conveying persons or goods from one place to another.

assault Threat of bodily harm to another.

4. External cause codes for **transport accidents** are next in the list of priorities.

5. The first-listed external cause code is that which corresponds most closely to the cause of the most serious diagnosis due to an **assault,** an accident, or self-harm, following the order of hierarchy listed.

Coding guideline *I.C.20.h. Unknown or Undetermined Intent Guideline* specifies that the default for the intent of an injury cause, if not known or documented, is accidental. Transport accidents are assumed to be accidental unless otherwise specified by documentation. Undetermined intent is reported only if the documentation specifies that no determination of intent can be made.

External cause codes not only are used at the time of the original injury but also are used to report additional detail for patients experiencing late effects of injuries. When reporting external cause codes for late effects, the code should have the 7th character of S for *sequela*. Coding guideline *I.C.20.i. Late Effects of External Cause Guidelines* also provides direction about the importance of being aware of the difference between subsequent visits for follow-up care for an injury and a late effect. It is not appropriate to report a late effect external cause code with an injury that is still being treated as an acute condition.

Think About It 24.1

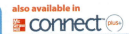
also available in connect plus+

Some healthcare settings have limitations on the number of codes that may be reported on a claim. What action may be taken to supplement the coding and billing process to ensure that the payer has complete information about the circumstances of an injury?

24.2 External Causes of Injury for Transport Accidents

Codes for external causes of injury for transport accidents reflect the victim's mode of transport with further classifications to identify the type of accident. Transportation accidents can involve pedestrians, cycle riders, animal riders, automobile operators, and other occupants injured while operating any type of vehicle on land, on water, or in the air. Injuries sustained may be the result of personal negligence or mechanical failure. There are 12 subsections of codes classifying transport accidents.

The first two characters identify the vehicle occupied by the injured person. A transport accident is any accident involving machine or equipment designed for transporting persons or goods from one place to another. In order to report transport accident codes, the machine, equipment, or vehicle must have been moving, running, or in use for transport purposes at the time the accident occured. Table 24.1 defines the transport terms used in ICD-10-CM.

When reporting transport accidents, additional codes should be reported if there is documentation of an injury by the vehicle airbag or use of a cellular telephone or other electronic equipment at the time of the transport accident. The type of street or road should also be identified. The conditions in this section s are reported with ICD-10-CM codes V00–V99. By comparison, ICD-9-CM uses category codes E800–E848.

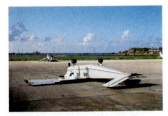
Accidents involving aircraft are among those reported with specific cause codes in ICD-10-CM.

Table 24.1 Definitions of Transport Terms

Term	Definition
Aircraft	Any device for transporting passengers or goods in the air. This includes hot-air balloons, gliders, helicopters, and airplanes.
Bus (coach)	A motor vehicle designed or adapted primarily for carrying more than 10 passengers and requiring a special driver's license.
Car (automobile)	A four-wheeled motor vehicle designed primarily for carrying up to 7 persons. A trailer being towed by a car is considered part of the car.
Driver	An occupant of a transport vehicle who is operating or intending to operate it.
Heavy transport vehicle	A motor vehicle designed primarily for carrying property, meeting local criteria for classification as a heavy goods vehicle in terms of weight, and requiring a special driver's license.
Military vehicle	Any motorized vehicle, operating on a public roadway, owned by the military and being operated by a member of the military.
Motorcycle	A two-wheeled motor vehicle with one or two riding saddles and sometimes with a third wheel for the support of a sidecar. The sidecar is considered part of the motorcycle.
Motorcycle rider	Any person riding a motorcycle or in a sidecar or trailer attached to the motorcycle.
Non-traffic accident	Any vehicle accident that occurs entirely in any place other than a public highway.
Passenger	Any occupant of a transport vehicle other than the driver, except a person traveling on the outside of the vehicle.
Pedal cycle	Any land transport vehicle operated solely by non-motorized pedals, including a bicycle or tricycle.
Pedal cyclist	Any person riding a pedal cycle or in a sidecar or trailer attached to a pedal cycle.
Pedestrian	Any person involved in an accident who was not at the time of the accident riding in or on a motor vehicle, railway train, streetcar or animal-drawn or other vehicle, or a pedal cycle or animal. This includes a person changing a tire or working on a parked car. It also includes the use of a pedestrian conveyance, such as a baby carriage, ice-skates, roller skates, a skateboard, a non-motorized or motorized wheelchair, a motorized mobility scooter, and a non-motorized scooter.

(continued)

V07–V08

Note that there are no categories V07 and V08.

V10–V19 Pedal Cycle Rider Injured in Transport Accident

Codes in this subsection of ICD-10-CM correspond with those in categories E800–E829 in ICD-9-CM. Seventh characters A, D, or S are required to identify if the visit is for the initial encounter, a subsequent encounter, or a sequela of the accident.

Codes in this subsection are used to report pedal cycle rider injuries involving collision with pedestrian or animal, other pedal cycle, two- or three-wheeled motor vehicle, heavy transport vehicle or bus, railway train or railway vehicle, other non-motor vehicle, fixed or stationary object, car, pickup truck, or van. Pedal cycle riders injured in non-collision transport accidents and other and unspecified transport accidents are also classified in this subsection.

V20–V29 Motorcycle Rider Injured in Transport Accident

Codes in this subsection of ICD-10-CM correspond with those in categories E810–E829 in ICD-9-CM. This subsection classifies injuries to motorcycle riders injured in collisions with pedestrian or animal, pedal cycle, two- or three-wheeled motor vehicle, heavy transport vehicle or bus, railway train or railway vehicle, other non-motor vehicle, fixed or stationary object, and car, pickup truck, or van. Categories V28 and V29 in this subsection classify injuries to motorcycle riders in **non-collision transport accidents** and in other and unspecified transport accidents.

non-collision transport accident Vehicular accident not involving collision, such as falling or being thrown from a motorcycle.

V30–V39 Occupant of Three-Wheeled Motor Vehicle Injured in Transport Accident

Codes in this subsection of ICD-10-CM correspond with those in categories E810–E825 in ICD-9-CM. This subsection classifies injuries to the occupant of a three-wheeled motor vehicle in collision with a pedestrian or animal, pedal cycle, two- or three-wheeled motor vehicle, heavy transport vehicle or bus, railway train or railway vehicle, other non-motor vehicle, fixed or stationary object, and car, pickup truck, or van. Also included in this subsection are codes to report injuries to the occupant of a three-wheeled motor vehicle in a non-collision transport accident or other and unspecified transport accidents.

V40–V49 Car Occupant Injured in Transport Accident

Codes in this subsection of ICD-10-CM correspond with those in E810–E825 in ICD-9-CM. This subsection classifies injuries to car occupants in collision with a pedestrian or animal, pedal cycle, two- or three-wheeled motor vehicle, heavy transport vehicle or bus, railway train or railway vehicle, other non-motor vehicle, fixed or stationary object, and car, pickup truck, or van. Also included in this subsection are codes to report injuries to the occupant of a car in a non-collision transport accident or other and unspecified transport accidents.

V50–V59 Occupant of Pickup Truck or Van Injured in Transport Accident

Codes in this subsection of ICD-10-CM correspond with those in categories E810–E825 in ICD-9-CM. This subsection classifies injuries to the occupant of a pickup truck or van in collision with a pedestrian or animal, pedal cycle, two- or three-wheeled motor vehicle, heavy transport vehicle or bus, railway train or railway vehicle, other non-motor vehicle, fixed or stationary object, and car, pickup truck, or van. Also included in this subsection are codes to report injuries to the occupant of a pickup truck or van in a non-collision transport accident or other and unspecified transport accidents.

V60–V69 Occupant of Heavy Transport Vehicle Injured in Transport Accident

Codes in this subsection of ICD-10-CM correspond with those in categories E810–E825 in ICD-9-CM. This subsection classifies injuries to the occupant of a heavy transport vehicle in collision with a pedestrian or animal, pedal cycle, two- or three-wheeled motor vehicle, heavy transport vehicle or bus, railway train or railway vehicle, other non-motor vehicle, fixed or stationary object, and car, pickup truck, or van. Also included in this subsection are codes to report injuries to the occupant of a heavy transport vehicle in a non-collision transport accident or other and unspecified transport accidents.

V70–V79 Bus Occupant Injured in Transport Accident

Codes in this subsection of ICD-10-CM correspond with those in categories E810–E825 in ICD-9-CM. This subsection classifies bus occupant injuries caused by collision with a pedestrian or animal, pedal cycle, two- or three-wheeled motor vehicle, heavy transport vehicle or bus, railway train or railway vehicle, other non-motor vehicle, fixed or stationary object, and car, pickup truck, or van. Also included in this subsection are codes to report injuries to bus occupants in a non-collision transport accident or other and unspecified transport accidents.

V80–V89 Other Land Transport Accidents

Codes in this subsection of ICD-10-CM correspond with those in categories E810–E829 and E846 in ICD-9-CM. This subsection classifies injuries involving land transport modes, including animal-riders and occupants of animal-drawn vehicles, railway trains, railway vehicles, powered streetcars, special vehicles used mainly on industrial premises, vehicles mainly used in agriculture, special construction vehicles, special all-terrain or other motor vehicles, or unknown mode of transport. Many of the codes in this subsection specify injuries caused by collisions similar to those discussed in the previous subsections; however, due to the unique nature of several modes of land transport in categories V80-V89, there are also codes to identify accidents caused by means specific to corresponding transport methods.

Accidents causing injuries to animal riders may also involve falls or being thrown from the animal. Causes of injuries to occupants of railway trains, railway vehicles, or powered streetcars may be identified as due to derailment. Codes for the causes of accidents involving the occupants of railway trains, railway vehicles, powered streetcars, special vehicles used mainly on industrial premises, vehicles mainly used in agriculture, special construction vehicles, or special all-terrain vehicles include accidents while boarding or alighting. Special all-terrain or other motor vehicles, reported in category V86, may be identified with codes to specific vehicles, such as ambulances, fire engines, snowmobiles, dune buggies, or military vehicles.

V90–V94 Water Transport Accidents

Codes in this subsection of ICD-10-CM correspond with those in categories E830–E838 in ICD-9-CM. Codes further specify the type of watercraft, including merchant ship, passenger ship, fishing boat, other powered watercraft, sailboat, canoe or kayak, inflatable craft, other unpowered watercraft, and unspecified watercraft. Category V90 classifies drowning and submersion due to watercraft accidents, including those due to the watercraft overturning or sinking or from an individual falling or jumping from burning or crushed watercraft. Other injuries due to accident to watercraft are classified in category V91, which includes codes for burn due to watercraft on fire, crushed between watercraft and other watercraft or other object due to collision, fall due to collision between watercraft and other watercraft or other object, hit or struck by falling object due to accident to watercraft, and other injury due to other accident to watercraft.

Category V92 classifies drowning and submersion due to accident on board watercraft without accident to watercraft, which includes codes for injuries due to a fall off watercraft, being thrown overboard by motion of watercraft, and being washed overboard from watercraft. Other injuries due to accident on board watercraft without accident to watercraft are classified in category V93, which provides codes for burn due to localized fire on board watercraft, other burn on board watercraft, heat exposure on board watercraft, fall on board watercraft, being struck by falling object on board watercraft, explosion on board watercraft, machinery accident on board watercraft, and other injury due to other accident on board watercraft. Other and unspecified water transport accidents, classified in category V94, include hitting object or bottom of body of water due to fall from watercraft, bather struck by watercraft, rider of non-powered watercraft struck by other watercraft, injury to rider of (inflatable) watercraft being pulled behind other watercraft, injury to barefoot water-skier, and other water transport accident

V95–V97 Air and Space Transport Accidents

Codes in this subsection of ICD-10-CM correspond with those in categories E840–E845 in ICD-9-CM. Category V95 classifies accidents causing injury to occupants of powered aircraft, such as helicopter, ultralight, microlight, powered glider, other private fixed-wing aircraft, commercial fixed-wing aircraft, spacecraft, or other powered aircraft. Accidents involving non-powered aircraft causing injury to occupant, classified to category V96, specify the involvement of balloons, hang gliders, gliders, and other non-powered aircraft. Category V97 includes codes to specify the causes of injury to occupants of other specified air transport accidents, such as injury while boarding or alighting from aircraft, parachutist accident, person on ground injured in air transport accident, and other air transport accidents, not elsewhere classified.

V98–V99 Other and Unspecified Transport Accidents

Codes in this subsection of ICD-10-CM correspond with those in category E848 in ICD-9-CM. Category V98 classifies other specified transport accidents, which include accidents to, on, or involving cable car not on rails, land yacht, ice yacht, ski lift, or other transport accidents. Code V99 is reported to identify an unspecified transport accident and should be coded out to seven characters.

Think About It 24.2

also available in **connect** (plus+)

Assign ICD-10-CM codes for the following situations, applying any appropriate sequencing guidelines.

1. Initial treatment of a passenger in a pick-up truck injured in a collision traffic accident with a car
   _____

2. Follow-up treatment for a passenger in a car injured in a collision traffic accident with a pickup truck
   _____

3. Treatment for a late effect of a motorcycle accident in which the motorcycle overturned when the driver was boarding it
   _____

4. Initial treatment for a fall from a non-motorized scooter
   _____

5. Initial treatment of a baby injured in a stroller when the stroller hit a wall
   _____

Beyond the Code: ICD-10-CM provides a significantly greater level of specificity to some modes of transportation in this section. What stakeholders may benefit from this increased specificity in the reporting of transport accidents, and how might they benefit?

24.3 Injuries Due to Falls and Exposure

Slips, trips, and falls can occur for a variety of reasons. Sometimes they occur because of the health of an individual, such as conditions that may cause dizziness. At other times, the injuries sustained after slips, trips, and falls may occur by accident or due to unfavorable and unsafe environmental conditions, such as faulty mechanical equipment; impaired operators of equipment, tools, and machinery; faulty or dilapidated design or functionally obsolete buildings; sports injuries; rain; ice; and snow. Disease processes such as epilepsy, Parkinson's disease, Alzheimer's dementia, stroke with secondary paralysis, and many others that affect the nervous system's sensory function, motor function, or musculoskeletal system function can lead to improper gait, which results in a slip or fall. Bone disorders can cause fractures and breaks, which result in injury due to falls. Patients with orthostatic hypotension secondary to medications taken for heart disease may fall. The elderly and people with disabilities are at greater risk for falls. Injuries can also be caused by exposure to smoke, fire, other people, plants, animals, mechanical forces, or physical forces, such as extreme air temperature, and pressure.

Many types of falls may be reported with external cause codes, specifying surfaces, items, and levels on which the fall occurred, as well as combination codes to identify other external causes of the injury associated with the fall. A wide variety of external cause codes are provided to identify circumstances, forces, and substances, which have caused an injury. Also in this subsection are codes to report drowning and submersion accidents that are not associated with transport accidents. The conditions are reported with ICD-9-CM code categories E880–E888, E890–E899, E900–E902, E905–E906, E908–E910, E916–E926, and E928. ICD-10-CM reports these conditions with codes from categories W00–W74, W85–W99, X00–X08, X10–X19, X30–X39, and X52–X58.

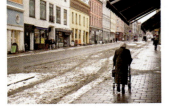

Codes W00–W19 report the type of fall experienced by a patient, such as slipping on an icy sidewalk.

W00–W19 Slipping, Tripping, Stumbling, and Falls

Codes in this subsection of ICD-10-CM correspond with those in categories E880–E888 in ICD-9-CM. This subsection classifies the causes of injuries identified as fall due to ice and snow; fall on same level from slipping, tripping, and stumbling; other fall on same level due to collision with another person; fall while being carried or supported by other persons; fall from non-moving wheelchair, non-motorized scooter, and motorized mobility scooter; fall from bed; fall from chair; fall from other furniture; fall on and from playground equipment; fall on and from stairs and steps; fall on and from ladder; fall on and from scaffolding; fall from, out of, or through building or structure; fall from tree; fall from cliff; fall, jump, or diving into water; and unspecified fall. Table 24.2 outlines the causes of falls reported by categories within W00–W19.

W20–W49 Exposure to Inanimate Mechanical Forces

Codes in this subsection of ICD-10-CM correspond with those in categories E916–E923 in ICD-9-CM. Injury causes classified in this subsection include those caused by being struck by thrown, projected, or falling object; striking against or being struck by sports equipment; being caught, crushed, jammed, or pinched in or between objects; contact with lifting and transmission devices, not elsewhere classified; contact with sharp glass; contact with knife, sword, or dagger; contact with non-powered hand tool; contact with powered lawn mower; contact with other powered hand tools and household machinery; contact with agricultural machinery; contact with other and unspecified machinery; accidental handgun discharge and malfunction; accidental rifle, shotgun, and larger firearm discharge and malfunction; accidental discharge and malfunction from other and unspecified firearms and guns; explosion and rupture of boiler;

Table 24.2 Specified Causes of Falls in Categories W00, W01, W09, W10, W13, W16, W17, and W18

Code Category	Types of Falls Reported
W00 Fall due to ice and snow	• Fall on same level • Fall from stairs and steps • Other fall from one level to another
W01 Fall on same level from slipping, tripping, and stumbling	• With or without subsequent striking against object • With subsequent striking against sharp glass, power tool, or machine; other sharp object; unspecified sharp object; furniture; or other object
W09 Fall on and from playground equipment	• Playground slide • Swing • Jungle gym • Other playground equipment
W10 Fall on and from stairs and steps	• Escalator • Sidewalk curb • Incline • Stairs or steps
W13 Fall from, out of, or through building or structure	• Balcony • Bridge • Roof • Floor • Window • Other building or structure
W16 Fall, jump, or diving into water	• Striking water surface • Striking bottom • Striking side • Causing drowning and submersion or causing other injury

(continued)

Table 24.2 *(continued)*

Code Category	Types of Falls Reported
W17 Other fall from one level to another	• Fall into well • Fall into storm drain or manhole • Fall into hole • Fall into empty swimming pool • Fall from dock • Other fall from one level to another • Fall down embankment (hill) • Fall from (out of) grocery cart • Fall due to grocery cart tipping over • Other fall from one level to another
W18 Other slipping, tripping, and stumbling and falls	• Fall due to bumping against object • Striking against unspecified object with subsequent fall • Striking against sports equipment with subsequent fall • Striking against glass with subsequent fall • Striking against other object with subsequent fall • Fall from or off toilet, further specified as with or without subsequent striking against object • Fall in (into) shower or empty bathtub • Slipping, tripping, and stumbling without falling due to stepping on object • Slipping, tripping, and stumbling without falling due to stepping into hole or opening • Slipping, tripping, and stumbling without falling due to stepping from one level to another

explosion and rupture of gas cylinder; explosion and rupture of pressurized tire, pipe, or hose; explosion and rupture of other specified pressurized devices; discharge of firework; explosion of other materials; exposure to noise; foreign body or object entering through skin; contact with hypodermic needle; and exposure to other inanimate mechanical forces.

Category W20 classifies injuries caused by being struck by thrown, projected, or falling object, including codes to specify falling object in cave-in, object due to collapse of building, and other thrown, projected, or falling objects. When assigning codes from category W20, a code for any associated cataclysm or lightning strike should be sequenced first.

Injuries caused by striking against or being struck by sports equipment are classified to category W21, with codes further specifying the type of sports equipment as football, soccer ball, baseball, golf ball, basketball, volleyball, softball, other hit or thrown ball, baseball bat, tennis racquet, golf club, other bat, racquet, club, hockey stick, ice hockey stick, field hockey stick, hockey puck, ice hockey puck, field hockey puck, shoe cleats, skate blades, other sports footwear, diving board, football helmet, or other sports equipment. If code W21.4 is assigned for striking against a diving board, an additional code from W16.- should be assigned for any subsequent fall into water.

Codes in category W23 for being caught, crushed, jammed, or pinched in or between objects are further specified as between moving objects or stationary objects. When assigning codes in category W25 for contact with sharp glass, any associated transport accident or injury due to flying glass from explosion or firearm discharge should be sequenced first. Category W27, contact with non-powered hand tool includes codes to specify the type of tool as workbench tool, garden tool, scissors, needle, kitchen utensil, paper cutter, or other non-powered hand tool. Note that code W27.3, contact with needle, is not for use to report injury due to hypodermic needle. Types of tools and machinery are also specified through individual codes in category W29, which includes the ability to identify injuries caused by powered kitchen appliance, electric knife, other powered household machinery, powered garden and outdoor hand tools and machinery, and nail gun. Contact with agricultural machinery injuries are specified in category W30 as due to combine harvester, power take-off devices, hay derrick, or grain storage elevator with agricultural machinery. Category W31 provides codes to specify contact with other and unspecified machinery, identified as mining and earth-drilling machinery, metalworking machines, powered woodworking and forming machines, and prime movers.

Categories W32, W33, and W34 provide specific codes for accidental discharge and malfunction of guns according to type, including handgun, larger firearm, shotgun, hunting rifle, machine gun, air gun, and paintball gun. Explosions and ruptures of gas cylinders are specified in category W36 codes to identify explosions of aerosol cans, air tanks, and pressurized gas tanks.

Category W37, explosion and rupture of pressurized tire, pipe, or hose provides the ability to specify the device as a bicycle tire. Explosion of other materials, classified in category W40, has codes to identify the materials as blasting materials or explosive materials. Supersonic waves can be identified as a causal factor in category W42, exposure to noise. Foreign bodies or objects entering through the skin, reported in category W45, includes codes to specify the objects as nails, paper, or the lid of a can. When reporting contact with a hypodermic needle as an external cause in category W46, attention to documentation is necessary to determine if the

application and packing; underdosing and non-administration of necessary drug, medicament, or biological substance; underdosing of necessary drug, medicament, or biological substance; and non-administration of necessary drug, medicament, or biological substance. Reporting of the performance of wrong procedure allows the identification of the circumstances of performance of the wrong procedure on the correct patient, performance of a procedure on a patient not scheduled for surgery, or performance of the correct procedure on the wrong side or wrong body part.

Category Y60 has been deactivated, and coders are directed to see complications within body system chapters. Category Y61 has also been deactivated, with conditions being reported by subcategory T81.5.

Y70–Y82 Medical Devices Associated with Adverse Incidents in Diagnostic and Therapeutic Use

Codes in this subsection of ICD-10-CM correspond with those in categories E870–E871 in ICD-9-CM. The causes of injury in this subsection are related to complications of medical devices as the cause of abnormal reaction of the patient or of later complication, without mention of misadventure at the time of the procedure. This subsection includes the breakdown or malfunction of medical devices after implantation or during ongoing use. Categories in this subsection identify the causative devices as anesthesiology devices, cardiovascular devices, otorhinolaryngological devices, gastroenterology and urology devices, general hospital and personal-use devices, neurological devices, obstetrical and gynecological devices, ophthalmic devices, radiological devices, orthopedic devices, physical medicine devices, or general and plastic surgery devices. Within each category, the 4th character identifies the use of the devices as diagnostic and monitoring; therapeutic (nonsurgical) and rehabilitative; prosthetic and other implants, materials and accessory; surgical instruments or materials; or miscellaneous.

Y83–Y84 Surgical and Other Medical Procedures as the Cause of Abnormal Reaction of the Patient or of Later Complication, without Mention of Misadventure at the Time of the Procedure

Codes in this subsection of ICD-10-CM correspond with those in categories E878–E879 in ICD-9-CM. The causes of injury in this subsection are related to surgical and medical procedures: abnormal reaction of the patient or later complication, not necessarily requiring mention of misadventure at the time of the procedure. Surgical operations as the cause of an abnormal reaction of the patient or of later complication, without mention of misadventure at the time of the procedure, are further specified through individual codes in category Y83 as operations with transplant of whole organ; implant of artificial internal device; anastomosis, bypass, or graft; formation of external stoma; other reconstructive surgery; amputation of limb(s); or removal of other organ. Category Y84 identifies other medical procedures as the cause of an abnormal reaction of the patient or later complication, without mention of misadventure at the time of the procedure, and specifies the procedures through individual codes as cardiac catheterization, kidney dialysis, radiological procedure and radiotherapy, shock therapy, aspiration of fluid, insertion of gastric or duodenal sound, urinary catheterization, or blood sampling. Categories Y85–Y89 have been deactivated and replaced with the 7th character of S for categories V00–Y38.

Y90–Y99 Supplementary Factors Related to Causes of Morbidity Classified Elsewhere

Codes in this subsection of ICD-10-CM correspond with those in categories E000–E030 and E849 in ICD-9-CM. Note that the categories in this subsection may be used to provide supplementary information concerning the causes of morbidity. However, they are not to be used for single-condition coding.

Category Y90 reports evidence of blood alcohol involvement in the cause of injury, as determined by blood alcohol level. This was not previously reported with E codes in ICD-9-CM. Codes in this category specify blood alcohol level. When assigning codes in category Y90, any associated alcohol-related disorders should be assigned first. Table 24.4 presents the blood alcohol level reported by each code in category Y90.

Category Y92, place of occurrence of the external cause, is used to identify the place of occurrence of an external cause. Codes in this category should be used in conjunction with an activity code. The code for place of occurrence should be recorded only at the initial encounter for treatment. This category is significantly expanded from what was previously in ICD-9-CM. There were only 10 codes available in ICD-9-CM to report place of occurrence. Places of occurrence may be identified as a wide variety of residential, educational, public, sporting, recreational, travel-related, healthcare, and other places. Table 24.5 lists some of the types of places that can be reported in ICD-10-CM.

Codes that specify the place as a residence in the Y92.010–Y92.199 range are further classified to identify the specific place in the residence—the kitchen, dining room, bathroom, bedroom, driveway, garage, swimming pool, garden, or yard.

Table 24.4 Classification of Blood Alcohol Level for Involvement as Cause of Injury

Code	Blood Alcohol Level Reported
Y90.0	Less than 20 mg/100 ml
Y90.1	20–39 mg/100 ml
Y90.2	40–59 mg/100 ml
Y90.3	60–79 mg/100 ml
Y90.4	80–99 mg/100 ml
Y90.5	100–119 mg/100 ml
Y90.6	120–199 mg/100 ml
Y90.7	200–239 mg/100 ml
Y90.8	240 mg/100 ml or more
Y90.9	Presence of alcohol in blood, level not specified

Table 24.5 Examples of Locations Reported in ICD-10-CM

Type of Place	Examples
Residential	Single-family house Mobile home Boarding house Institutional residence Nursing home Military base Prison Reform school School Dormitory
Educational	School Daycare center Elementary school Middle school High school College Trade school
Public	Religious institution Courthouse Library Post office City hall Other public administrative building Art gallery Museum Music hall Opera house Theater Other cultural public building Movie house Bank Restaurant Supermarket Shop
Sports and recreation	Basketball court Squash court Tennis court Baseball field Football field Soccer field Ice skating rink Roller skating rink Bike path Public park Amusement park Beach Campsite Zoo

(continued)

Type of Place	Examples
Travel	Airport Bus station Railway station Rest stop Transport vehicle Gas station Dock or shipyard Railroad track Interstate highway Parkway State road Residential street Exit ramp Sidewalk Parking lot
Healthcare	Physician office Urgent care center Hospital Ambulatory surgery center
Other	Building under construction Factory Mine or pit Oil rig Barn Chicken coop Farm field Orchard Desert Forest Military training ground Slaughterhouse

When reporting a hospital as the place of occurrence with Y92.23-, the location may be specified with individual codes for patient room, patient bathroom, corridor, cafeteria, operating room, or other place. Transport vehicles are further specified as car, bus, truck, airplane, boat, train, or subway.

The location of the patient when the injury occurred should be reported using codes from category Y92, place of occurrence of the external cause. Coding guideline *I.C.20.b. Place of Occurrence Guideline* specifies that these codes are only for assignment with the initial encounter for treatment. Therefore, it is not necessary to assign any 7th character to identify the encounter. It is also only appropriate to assign one code from category Y92. If the place of occurrence is not documented, code Y92.9 should not be reported. An activity code from category Y93, activity code, should be reported in conjunction with the place of occurrence to report the activity being performed at the time of the incident.

Category Y93 codes are used to indicate the activity of the person seeking healthcare for an injury or a health condition that resulted from, or was contributed to by, the activity. These codes may be reported with both acute injuries, such as those from Chapter 19, and conditions that are due to the long-term, cumulative effects of an activity, such as those from Chapter 13. In addition, they may be reported with external cause codes if identifying the activity provides additional information on the event. Codes in category Y93 should be used in conjunction with codes for external cause status (Y99) and place of occurrence (Y92). Table 24.6 lists the categories of activities reported by codes Y93.0–Y93.9.

A code from category Y93, activity code, should be assigned to identify the specific activity being performed by the patient at the time of injury. This code is only used on the record for the initial encounter for treatment, and only one code from the category should be reported. Activity codes are not for use with poisonings, adverse effects, misadventures, or late effects. Code Y93.9, unspecified activity, is not assigned if documentation does not identify

Table 24.6 Categories of Activities Reported in ICD-10-CM

Code	Type of Activity
Y93.0	Activities involving walking and running
Y93.1	Activities involving water and watercraft
Y93.2	Activities involving ice and snow
Y93.3	Activities involving climbing, rappelling, and jumping off
Y93.4	Activities involving dancing and other rhythmic movement
Y93.5	Activities involving other sports and athletics played individually
Y93.6	Activities involving other sports and athletics played as a team or group
Y93.7	Activities involving other specified sports and athletics
Y93.a	Activities involving other cardiorespiratory exercise
Y93.b	Activities involving other muscle-strengthening exercises
Y93.c	Activities involving computer technology and electronic devices
Y93.d	Activities involving arts and handcrafts
Y93.e	Activities involving personal hygiene and interior property and clothing maintenance
Y93.f	Activities involving caregiving
Y93.g	Activities involving food preparation, cooking and grilling
Y93.h	Activities involving exterior property and land maintenance, building and construction
Y93.i	Activities involving roller-coasters and other types of external motion
Y93.j	Activities involving playing musical instrument
Y93.k	Activities involving animal care
Y93.8	Activities, other specified
Y93.9	Activity, unspecified

the activity. Coding guideline *I.C.20.c. Activity Code* instructs the coder to assign the 7th character of 2, work-related activity, if the patient is a student injured while performing an activity for income. ICD-10-CM defines a work-related activity as any activity for which payment or income is received.

Category Y95 is used to report a **nosocomial** condition.

In order to be consistent with coding guideline I.C.20.k, external cause status, one code from category Y99, external cause status, should be assigned in addition to the cause for the condition. Be sure to also identify the person involved at the time the event occurred. Examples are seen when reporting events for military activity, civilian activities performed for income, or other activities that are not performed for pay.Codes from category Y99 do not apply to poisonings, adverse effects, misadventures, or late effects. If there is no documentation about the patient's status, it is not appropriate to assign a code from category Y99.

nosocomial Acquired while in the hospital.

Deactivated Categories

Category Y91 has been deactivated, and coders are directed to see category F10. Category Y96 has also been deactivated, with instructions to use code Y99.0. Category Y97 has been deactivated, with direction to see categories Z57 and Z77. Also deactivated is category Y98, with a redirection to categories Z72 and Z73.

Think About It 24.5

also available in **connect** (plus+)

Assign ICD-10-CM codes for the following situations, applying any appropriate sequencing guidelines.

1. Injury occurring in the barracks of a military base while the individual was performing military work _____

2. Adverse incident associated with a prosthetic orthopedic device _____

3. Initial encounter for a civilian condition caused by a confirmed act of terrorism involving biological weapons _____

4. Patient on whom the correct procedure was performed, but on the wrong side of the body _____

5. Initial encounter for treatment of a bystander injured by the use of tear gas in a legal intervention _____

Beyond the Code: What types of stakeholders may use the statistics reported with codes in categories Y35–Y38? How might information from these statistics be used in policy development by these stakeholders?

Chapter Summary

Learning Outcome	Key Concepts/Examples
24.1 Interpret coding guidelines for external causes of morbidity. **(pages 404–406)**	• External cause codes are used to report cause, intent, activity, and place of occurrence for injuries or health conditions. • Although they are most applicable to injuries, external cause codes are also valid for use with such things as infections or diseases due to an external source and other health conditions, such as a heart attack that occurs during strenuous physical activity.
24.2 Classify external causes of injury for transport accidents. **(pages 406–413)**	• Codes for external causes of injury for transport accidents reflect the victim's mode of transport, with further classifications to identify the type of accident. • When reporting transport accidents, additional codes should be reported if there is documentation of an injury by the vehicle airbag or use of a cellular telephone or other electronic equipment at the time of the transport accident. • The type of street or road should also be identified when reporting transport accidents.
24.3 Select appropriate codes for injuries due to falls and exposure. **(pages 413–422)**	• Codes in categories W00–W19 classify causes of injuries identified as falls and allow the coder to report specific circumstances of falls. • Circumstances of injuries caused by animal contact are classified to significantly greater detail in ICD-10-CM regarding the type of animal and may be further specified by codes that report details specific to various animals, including contact with saliva, contact with feces, contact with urine, bitten, struck by, knocked over, stung by, crushed, pecked by, or other contact with animals.
24.4 Identify factors related to causes of injuries due to self-harm, assault, or undetermined intent. **(pages 422–425)**	• Adult and child abuse, neglect, and maltreatment are classified as assault. Any of the assault codes may be used to indicate the external cause of any injury resulting from the confirmed abuse. • Selection of the correct perpetrator code is based on the relationship between the perpetrator and the victim.
24.5 Analyze documentation to report legal, military, and medical causes and supplementary factors. **(pages 425–433)**	• A legal intervention is considered to be any injury sustained as a result of an encounter with any law enforcement official, serving in any capacity at the time of the encounter, whether on-duty or off-duty. • Causes of injury in categories Y62–Y84 are related to surgical and medical procedures: abnormal reaction of the patient or later complication, not necessarily requiring mention of misadventure at the time of the procedure. • Category Y90 reports evidence of blood alcohol involvement in the cause of injury, as determined by blood alcohol level. This was not reported with E codes in ICD-9-CM.

Applying Your Skills

Assign codes for each external cause, using both ICD-9-CM and ICD-10-CM.

External Cause	ICD-9-CM	ICD-10-CM
1. *[LO 24.3]* Initial visit for injury sustained from accidentally being struck by a golf ball	_____	_____
2. *[LO 24.2]* Follow-up visit for injuries sustained by driver of motorcycle in traffic accident collision with car	_____	_____
3. *[LO 24.4]* Abuse of child by stepmother	_____	_____
4. *[LO 24.4]* Abuse of child by biological mother	_____	_____
5. *[LO 24.5]* Late effect of injuries sustained by military personnel involving fragments from munitions during war operations	_____	_____
6. *[LO 24.2]* Initial visit for submersion injuries sustained in overturning kayak accident to occupant of the kayak	_____	_____
7. *[LO 24.4]* Initial visit after being bitten by another person	_____	_____
8. *[LO 24.3]* Follow-up visit for injuries sustained in fall down ice-covered steps	_____	_____
9. *[LO 24.5]* Initial visit for injuries sustained by public safety official as a result of a terrorist mortar bomb	_____	_____
10. *[LO 24.2]* Initial visit for injuries sustained by horse rider being thrown from horse in non-traffic accident	_____	_____
11. *[LO 24.4]* Initial visit for injuries sustained when attacked with a broken beer bottle	_____	_____
12. *[LO 24.3]* Initial visit for injuries sustained from being butted by a goat	_____	_____
13. *[LO 24.2]* Initial visit for injuries sustained in fall while using in-line skates	_____	_____
14. *[LO 24.4]* Initial visit for injuries sustained when teenager attempted suicide by driving car into a tree	_____	_____
15. *[LO 24.5]* Initial visit for police officer with gunshot wound following legal intervention	_____	_____
16. *[LO 24.3]* Initial visit for burn from contact with a hot toaster	_____	_____

17. *[LO 24.5]* Mismatched blood in transfusion   _____   _____

18. *[LO 24.5]* Injury in the bedroom of an apartment   _____   _____

19. *[LO 24.3]* Initial visit for injuries sustained by contact with
a power hedge trimmer   _____   _____

20. *[LO 24.5]* Injury sustained while playing an electronic game
with an interactive device   _____   _____

Checking Your Understanding

Select the letter that best answers the question or completes the sentence.

1. *[LO 24.1]* External cause codes for terrorism events take priority over all
other external cause codes, except for

    a. transport accidents.
    b. child and adult abuse.
    c. cataclysmic events.
    d. self-harm.

2. *[LO 24.4]* Which of the following should be accompanied by a code from
category Y07?

    a. T76.12   **b.** T76.21
    c. T74.31   **d.** T75.89

3. *[LO 24.5]* Which of the following individuals is not specified for category
Y35?

    a. law enforcement official
    b. suspect
    c. bystander
    d. military officer

4. *[LO 24.2]* A patient is injured while "surfing" on the top of a moving automobile. How would this be classified?

    a. passenger
    b. person on the outside of a vehicle
    c. pedestrian
    d. non-traffic accident

5. *[LO 24.1]* What is the maximum number of external cause codes that may be
assigned for an encounter?

    a. one
    b. two
    c. three
    d. There is no maximum; coders should use as many as necessary to fully
explain the cause.

6. *[LO 24.4]* A woman is discovered on the sidewalk behind an apartment
building; she has multiple critical injuries and is in a comatose state. She is
taken to the hospital and admitted to ICU, where she dies the following day.
The balcony door to her apartment is open, the door is not locked, there are
no signs of a struggle, and she did not leave a suicide note. How should the
circumstances be reported?

    a. intentional self-harm
    b. assault
    c. undetermined intent
    d. accident

7. **[LO 24.3]** Which of the following is not reported as a circumstance of injury caused by animal contact?

   a. thrown from a horse
   b. bitten by a dog
   c. pecked by a turkey
   d. struck by an alligator

8. **[LO 24.2]** A semi driver, hauling a bulldozer to a construction site, is injured in an accident while driving on the highway. How is the vehicle classified?

   a. heavy transport vehicle
   b. pickup truck or van
   c. special construction vehicle
   d. special vehicle mainly used on industrial premises

9. When reporting injuries caused by terrorism, what should be listed first?

   a. the injury code
   b. a code from category Y38, terrorism
   c. a code for the place of occurrence (Y92.-)
   d. a code to report the activity

10. **[LO 24.3]** What should be coded before the code for exposure to smoke in an uncontrolled fire in a building?

    a. arson as a cause of the fire
    b. fire caused by lightning
    c. chemical gas exposure
    d. cataclysm

Online Activity

[LO 24.2] Search online for information about how the assignment of codes for external causes of morbidity may impact reimbursement. Summarize your findings in a brief report.

Real-World Application: Case Study

[LO 24.3, LO 24.5] Assign ICD-10-CM codes for the following ER visit.

Emergency Room Note

History of Present Illness: This is a 38-year-old white male, who presented to the emergency department via automobile following a fall while playing softball at a local stadium. The patient complains of shoulder pain.

Past Medical/Surgical History: None.

Medications: None.

Allergies: NKA.

Family History: Negative for heart disease, diabetes, cancer, or stroke.

Social History: The patient is single. He does not smoke or consume drugs. He does use alcohol on occasion.

Review of Systems

Constitutional: The patient denies weight loss/gain, fever, chills.

HEENT: Negative for headaches, blurred vision, or changes in/loss of vision.

CV: No chest pain, palpitations, or edema.

Respiratory: Negative for SOB, wheezing, or cough.

GI: No heartburn, blood in stools, loss of appetite, abdominal pain, or constipation.

GU: No painful/burning urination or flank pain.

Musculoskeletal: Painful left shoulder. Denies other pain.

Neuro: Denies any loss of consciousness.

Integumentary: Denies any lesions or rashes.

Physical Examination

Constitutional: Blood pressure 120/75, pulse 80, respirations 18, temperature 98.6.

Neck: The neck is symmetric, trachea is midline, and no masses are noted. Respiratory: Normal respiratory effort. Normal breath sounds bilaterally with no rhonchi, wheezing, or rubs.

CV: No audible murmur, click, or rub. No audible abdominal bruits. Extremities show no edema or varicosities.

GI: No palpable abdominal tenderness or masses.

Lymphatic: No node enlargement noted in the neck, axillae, or groins.

Musculoskeletal: There is an obvious disruption of the junction of the clavicle and scapula. Normal gait.

Skin: No abrasions noted.

Neurologic: Normal sensation by touch.

Radiology report demonstrated 150% dislocation of right AC joint.

Impression: Right shoulder 150% AC dislocation.

Plan: Sling was applied and prescription for Vicodin given. Patient instructed to follow up with orthopedic surgeon in the morning.

INTRODUCTION TO MEDICAL PROCEDURE CODING

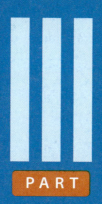

PART

25. Procedure Coding System
Formats and Conventions

26. ICD-9-CM, Volume 3

25 PROCEDURE CODING SYSTEM FORMATS AND CONVENTIONS

Learning Outcomes *After completing this chapter, students should be able to*

25.1 Explain the rationale for HIPAA code set designations for healthcare settings and service types.

25.2 Identify appropriate services and procedures to be reported using the Healthcare Common Procedure Coding System (HCPCS).

25.3 Select the appropriate section of Current Procedure Terminology (CPT) used for reporting surgical procedures, diagnostic testing, medical treatments, and physician services.

25.4 Locate National Drug Codes (NDC) for medications.

25.5 Compare ICD-9-CM, Volume 3, and ICD-10-PCS classification systems.

Key Terms

Advance Beneficiary Notice (ABN)

American Dental Association (ADA)

American Medical Association (AMA)

Code on Dental Procedures and Nomenclature

Current Procedure Terminology (CPT)

Drug Registration and Listing System (DRLS)

electronic data interchange (EDI)

Food and Drug Administration (FDA)

Healthcare Common Procedure Coding System (HCPCS)

Health Insurance Portability & Accountability Act of 1996 (HIPAA)

National Drug Codes (NDC)

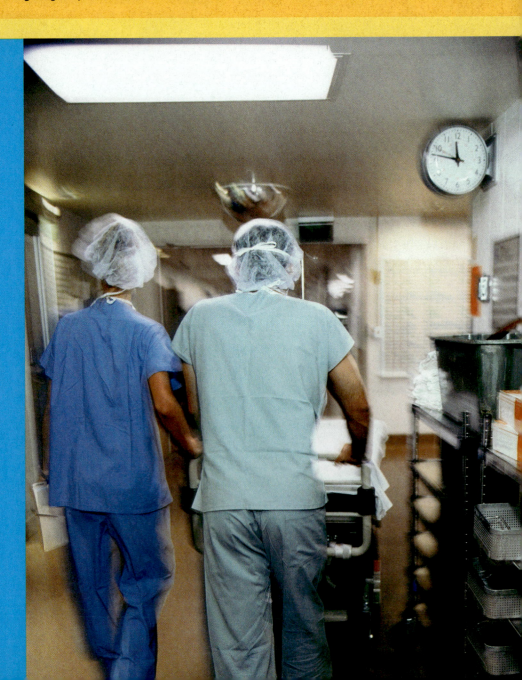

Introduction

A variety of code sets are available for reporting medical and surgical procedures and services. The most commonly thought of procedures and services are surgical in nature. However, other services include the evaluation of patients with the management of treatment by physicians, the administration of medications, dental procedures, and a variety of ancillary services, such as radiology and laboratory services. Reviewing the code sets that report medical and surgical procedures and services helps coders see how the code sets complement each other, enabling them to report the full picture of clinical services for each patient.

Both the ICD-9 and ICD-10 code sets were developed by the World Health Organization (WHO) for the classification of morbidity and mortality information for statistical purposes. Volumes 1 and 2 of ICD-9-CM are used for reporting diagnoses and symptoms. Volume 3 codes are for reporting surgical and nonsurgical procedures in hospital settings. On October 1, 2013, The International Classification of Diseases, tenth revision, Clinical Modification (ICD-10-CM) codes will replace ICD-9-CM, Volumes 1 and 2, and the International Classification of Diseases, tenth revision, Procedure Coding System (ICD-10-PCS) will replace ICD-9-CM, Volume 3.

25.1 HIPAA Code Set Designations

The **Health Insurance Portability & Accountability Act of 1996 (HIPAA)** has mandated the adoption of specified code sets to be used for diagnoses and procedures in all transactions. This was accompanied by another HIPAA mandate, which required the adoption of standards related to transactions for **electronic data interchange (EDI)** of healthcare data. An example of an EDI transaction is the submission of an electronic claim for payment. The EDI standards mandated by HIPAA provide requirements related to content, format, and several other aspects. These standards facilitate the communication of data to ensure the accurate and timely processing of information.

> **CODING TIP ▶**
>
> HIPAA has mandated the adoption of specific code sets, along with standards related to EDI transactions.

Many different code sets are used in a variety of healthcare settings, based on the type of service delivered. Table 25.1 provides a basic overview of which code sets are appropriate for which type of healthcare setting as designated by HIPAA. The Healthcare Common Procedure Coding System (HCPCS); Current Procedure Terminology (CPT); the Code on Dental Procedures and Nomenclature; International Classification of Diseases–9–Clinical Modification, Volume 3 (ICD-9-CM, Vol. 3); International Classification of Diseases–10–Procedure Code System (ICD-10-PCS); and

Health Insurance Portability & Accountability Act of 1996 (HIPAA) US law providing uniform privacy, security, and electronic transaction standards regarding patients' medical records and other health-related information and allowing the continuation of health insurance after termination of employment for a prescribed period.

electronic data interchange (EDI) Transmission of electronic medical insurance claims from providers to payers.

Table 25.1 HIPAA-Designated Procedure and Service Code Sets

Setting/Service Type	Code Set
Ancillary services	Healthcare Common Procedure Coding System (HCPCS)
Physician procedures	Current Procedure Terminology (CPT)
Dental procedures	Code on Dental Procedures and Nomenclature
Inpatient procedures (prior to October 1, 2013)	ICD-9-CM, Volume 3
Inpatient procedures (as of October 1, 2013)	ICD-10-PCS
Pharmaceutical services	National Drug Codes (NDC)

National Drug Codes (NDC) are HIPPA-designated procedure and service code sets reportable by a variety of inpatient and outpatient healthcare facilities. Services include ancillary durable medical equipment and supplies, outpatient physician services, inpatient hospital services, outpatient emergency room services, dental services, assisted living or skilled nursing facilities, and outpatient surgery or other ambulatory care such as that seen in public or rural health clinics.

The code sets serve many purposes. Healthcare providers use them to report the procedures and services they render to treat a variety of diagnoses. Accurate coding based on the medical record documentation is submitted on insurance claim forms for reimbursement from government payers (i.e., Medicare, Medicaid, TRICARE, and CHAMPVA) and private, for-profit commercial third-party payers. Correctly coded medical claims minimize loss through collection and recovery processes. Streamlining payment processes that ultimately cut into a healthcare provider's time and resources to provide better healthcare will bring about increased efficiency and lower-cost utilization to continuously meet the demand for healthcare services. Delivery of health care and its associated costs may be utilized more efficiently when demand for services is realized through the medical reporting of codes.

Codes should be reported according to the official coding guidelines. Proper coordination of benefits, pre-authorizations, and coverage predeterminations will results in fewer claim denials and a reduction in unpaid accounts receivables. The codes are also used to gather statistical data, which can be used by the national, state, and local organizations and agencies that are responsible for providing information and research on disease, monitoring the prevalence of disease, identifying diagnostic trends and progress in treatment modalities, and performing further research in order to make additional advancements in healthcare delivery. The codes are useful for the scientists, clinicians, healthcare administrators, legislators, and public health officials who are responsible for ensuring high-quality healthcare that is evidence-based, with lower-cost utilization, higher efficiency, and better outcomes for patients in need of access to healthcare.

The **American Dental Association (ADA)** was founded in 1859. It is the largest national dental society in the world and acts as a leading source for oral health–related information, public health service, bio-medical ethics, and scientific advancement and professional advocacy, as they pertain to dental care, at national, state, and local levels. The Current Dental Terminology (CDT), or **Code on Dental Procedures and Nomenclature,** was developed by the ADA.

American Dental Association (ADA) Largest national dental society in the world; leading source for oral health–related information, public health service, bio-medical ethics, scientific advancement, and professional advocacy.

Code on Dental Procedures and Nomenclature Standardized way of reporting dental procedures performed in the treatment of dental disease; developed by the ADA.

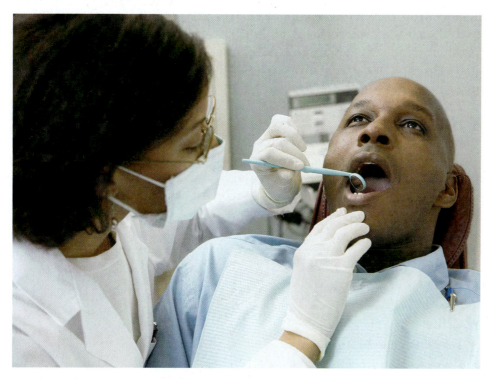

Dental procedures are reported with CDT codes.

The CDT code set provides a standardized way of reporting dental procedures performed in the treatment of dental disease. The CDT code system is updated every two years, with revisions made in every odd-numbered year. As with all reporting on medical insurance claims forms, it is important to code to the highest degree of specificity. In order to fully link the appropriate dental diagnoses with their corresponding procedures, you will find codes for dental procedures in the CDT code book published by the ADA and diagnostic codes in the ICD-9-CM and ICD-10-CM coding manuals. Claims can be submitted either electronically or on paper.

Think About It 25.1

also available in **connect** plus+

Although HIPAA defines EDI guidelines for code submission, other aspects of the electronic billing process are also specified, such as the format of the date. What other elements of a healthcare bill would you also expect to be impacted by HIPAA EDI guidelines?

25.2 Healthcare Common Procedure Coding System

Healthcare Common Procedure Coding System (HCPCS) Coding system, maintained by CMS, that is used in coding procedures, supplies, and nonphysician services not included in CPT.

American Medical Association (AMA) Society that educates the healthcare community; addresses ethical, financial, and political pressures within healthcare; advocates for physicians and their patients; and maintains the CPT code set.

The **Healthcare Common Procedure Coding System (HCPCS)** is established and maintained by the Centers for Medicare and Medicaid Services (CMS). It is used for reporting procedures, supplies, and nonphysician services that are not included in the **American Medical Association (AMA)** CPT codes. The HCPCS code set was established in 1978 to standardize the reporting of medical procedures, supplies, products, and services and has been in use since 1983. The HCPCS coding system was initially introduced to promote uniform reporting of information to Medicare.

There are currently two levels of HCPCS: I and II. Level I HCPCS consists of alphanumeric codes, as found in the American Medical Association's CPT coding manual, which are copyrighted and maintained by the AMA. Level II codes, which are also known as National Codes, are maintained by CMS. Annual updates are published, for use effective on January 1 of each year. Level II HCPCS codes consist of alphanumeric codes that include nonphysician services as follows:

- Ambulance services
- Medical and surgical supplies
- Syringes
- Needles
- Catheters
- Dressing change supplies
- Compression stockings
- Ostomy bags
- Urinary supplies
- Oxygen and ventilation supplies
- Nebulizers
- Total parenteral nutrition
- Nasogastric tube feeding supplies
- Various types of orthotics and prosthetics
- Cardiac pacemakers
- Neurostimulators
- Drugs, chemotherapy, and injections
- Dental procedures
- Canes, crutches, and walkers
- Wheelchairs
- Bedside commodes

Codes also report various screenings for disease, codes for physicians' professional services rendered, documentation, and orders.

The format used for HCPCS codes is five-digit alphanumeric. The first digit is an alphabetic character, followed by four numeric characters.

Table 25.2 HCPCS Level II Sections

Code Category	Services Reported
A	Transportation, Medical & Surgical Supplies, Miscellaneous & Experimental
B	Enteral and Parenteral Therapy
C	Temporary Hospital Outpatient Prospective Payment System
D	Dental Procedures
E	Durable Medical Equipment
G	Temporary Procedures & Professional Services
H	Rehabilitative Services
J	Drugs Administered Other Than Oral Method, Chemotherapy Drugs
K	Temporary Codes for Durable Medical Equipment Regional Carriers
L	Orthotic/Prosthetic Procedures
M	Medical Services
P	Pathology and Laboratory
Q	Temporary Codes
R	Diagnostic Radiology Services
S	Private Payer Codes
T	State Medicaid Agency Codes
V	Vision/Hearing Services

HCPCS codes may not be reimbursed under health insurance coverage and reimbursement policy. HCPCS contains an alphabetic index, revised, new, deleted, and reinstated codes; and an alphabetic table of drugs, which includes drug names, dosage, method of administration, and HCPCS code. The Level II National Codes/HCPCS is a collection of codes that represents procedures, supplies, products, and services that may be provided to Medicare beneficiaries and eligible individuals enrolled in some private health insurance plans.

HCPCS also contains HCPCS modifiers, which are two-digit codes that are numeric, alphanumeric, or two alpha characters in length. These modifiers alter the primary codes to which they are appended to further describe the procedure, supply, or service with more clarity. Modifiers allow for more specific reporting. Table 25.2 presents an overview of how the types of services and devices are classified in HCPCS Level II. Modifiers are grouped by three levels: Level I by the AMA, Level II by HCPCS, and D modifiers by the ADA.

Introduction

Initially, the classification of disease was not created for the purpose of reimbursement but, rather, to track epidemiological data, to identify and monitor the prevalence of disease, and then to reimburse through coded data abstracted from patients' medical records. Physicians use Current Procedural Terminology (CPT) codes in the outpatient setting to document medical and surgical procedures. Inpatient facilities, such as hospitals, use Volume 3 of ICD-9-CM for procedure coding. Inpatient procedure codes are found within the diagnostic coding manual ICD-9-CM, which contains Volumes 1, 2, and 3. Volumes 1 and 2 are for diagnostic coding purposes, and Volume 3 is for inpatient procedure coding purposes. Volume 3 of ICD-9-CM includes inpatient procedures on a variety of body systems.

26.1 Background of ICD-9-CM, Volume 3

The history of ICD-9-CM, Volume 3, differs from that of Volumes 1 and 2. Whereas Volumes 1 and 2 were primarily adopted for the purpose of tracking mortality statistics, the procedure coding component evolved for alternate statistical collection activities. Following the initial implementation of the coding system, additional uses for the data have also appeared.

In 1950, the US Public Health Service and the Veterans Administration began indexing for an international system of classification of diseases (ICD) system. Hospitals and medical centers began using this system. The US National Committee on Vital and Health Statistics keeps hospital data and statistics. In 1956, organizations such as the American Hospital Association (AHA) and the American Association of Medical Record Librarians (AAMRL), which is now known as AHIMA, began looking at ways to make healthcare systems more efficient to meet a growing demand for use of these classification systems. The first edition of the classification system was published in December 1959, then was revised in 1962 with the title *Classification of Operations and Treatments*. Various consultants have reviewed the classification systems and have repeatedly recognized the need for increased specificity and detail for diagnostic indexing, as there is a need for greater detail to be reported through coding hospital morbidity and mortality data. Procedural classifications were not an original part of the International Classification of Diseases. The ICD-9-CM classification for procedures was published separately in 1978 in supplementary documents called fascicles. Each fascicle contains classifications of the modes of therapy, surgery, radiology, laboratory, and other diagnostic procedures. Procedural classifications are necessary in order to analyze the healthcare provided by hospitals.

The roots of ICD-9-CM, Volume 3, can be traced back to the World Health Organization (WHO) document *Fascicle V Surgical Procedures,* modified in 1975. The resulting classification from this modification, the **International Classification of Procedures in Medicine (ICPM),** was published in 1978 by the WHO and adopted for use in 1979. In 1985, the US Department of Health and Human Services (HHS) established the **ICD-9-CM Coordination and Maintenance Committee,** and the committee published the first revision in 1986. The cooperating parties of the ICD-9-CM Coordination and Maintenance

---

International Classification of Procedures in Medicine (ICPM) Classification resulting from the modification of the *Fascicle V Surgical Procedures*, published in 1978 by the WHO and adopted for use in 1979.

Fascicle V Surgical Procedures Document published, by the WHO, that classifies medical and surgical procedures.

ICD-9-CM Coordination and Maintenance Committee Organization founded in 1985 by the US Department of Health and Human Services to revise the International Classification of Procedures in Medicine.

Committee, which includes the AHA, AHIMA, the Centers for Medicare and Medicaid Services (CMS), and the National Center for Health Statistics (NCHS), perform annual reviews and maintenance of ICD-9-CM. The maintenance of Volume 3 is the responsibility of the CMS.

> **CODING TIP ▸**
>
> The following are the cooperating parties of the ICD-9-CM Coordination and Maintenance Committee:
> - American Hospital Association (AHA)
> - American Health Information Management Association (AHIMA)
> - Centers for Medicare and Medicaid Services (CMS)
> - National Center for Health Statistics (NCHS)

Think About It 26.1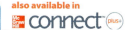

What are the benefits of changing the use of the International Classification of Diseases from reporting mortality to reporting illnesses? Identify the individuals and agencies that may have benefited from this change.

26.2 Settings Using Volume 3 of ICD-9-CM

One of the major differences between ICD-9-CM, Volumes 1 and 2, and ICD-9-CM, Volume 3, is the settings in which they are used. In Volumes 1 and 2, diagnoses are coded in a fairly similar manner across most healthcare settings, with a few exceptions to the general coding guidelines. In October 2013, Volumes 1 and 2 will be replaced by ICD-10-CM. On the other hand, Volume 3 of ICD-9-CM is for use only in the hospital inpatient setting. ICD-9-CM, Volume 3, will be replaced by ICD-10-PCS in October 2013.

Whereas the alphabetic index and tabular list for diagnoses are in separate volumes in ICD-9-CM, the index and tabular list for the procedure codes are both in Volume 3. When purchasing ICD-9-CM code books, it is important to be aware that not all versions of the publication include Volume 3, since it is not used by physician providers.

A variety of unplanned uses for Volume 3 of ICD-9-CM have also been adopted over the years. Although Volume 3 codes are intended for use in the hospital inpatient setting, some facilities have adopted Volume 3 codes for statistical purposes. Some state Medicaid programs have also developed additional uses for Volume 3.

> **CODING TIP ▸**
>
> Volume 3 of ICD-9-CM is intended for use only in the hospital inpatient setting.

Think About It 26.2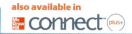

What are some reasons that it would be beneficial for physician providers to have ICD-9-CM code books that do not include Volume 3?

Table 27.5 Meanings for Character 4 according to Section

Section Number	Section Name	Character 4 Meaning
0	Medical and Surgical	Body part
1	Obstetrics	Body part
2	Placement	Body region
3	Administration	Body system/region
4	Measurement and Monitoring	Body system
5	Extracorporeal Assistance and Performance	Body system
6	Extracorporeal Therapies	Body system
7	Osteopathic	Body region
8	Other Procedures	Body region
9	Chiropractic	Body region
B	Imaging	Body part
C	Nuclear Medicine	Body part
D	Radiation Oncology	Treatment site
F	Physical Rehabilitation and Diagnostic Audiology	Body system/region
G	Mental Health	Type qualifier
H	Substance Abuse Treatment	Type qualifier

approach Fifth character of an ICD-10-PCS code in Sections 0–4 and 7-9, identifying the clinical method used to carry out the service or procedure.

device Equipment left in at the end of a procedure, or a substance meant for a specific purpose.

qualifier Seventh character of an ICD-10-PCS code, whose values are unique to individual procedures and treatments.

The 5th character in Sections 0–4 and 7-9 is defined as the **approach.** Whereas Sections 5 and 6 have this character defined as duration, Section B is defined as contrast, Section C is defined as radionuclide, Section D is a modality qualifier, Section E is a type qualifier, and Section F is simply defined as a qualifier. Meanings for the characters have specific definitions for each different section, but they remain constant within each section. Table 27.6 shows the meanings for character 5 according to section.

The 6th character in Sections 0–2 is defined as the **device,** in Section 3 it is defined as substance, in Section 4 it is defined as function/device, in Section 5 it is defined as function, in Sections 6, B, C, G, and H it is defined as qualifier, in Sections 7–9 it is defined as method, in Section D it is defined as isotope, and in Section F it is defined as equipment (as shown in Table 27.7). Meanings for the characters have unique definitions that are specific to each different section, but they remain constant within each section.

The 7th character of each section is defined as a **qualifier.** The qualifier character values are unique to individual procedures and treatments. The Placement, Osteopathic, Chiropractic, Nuclear Medicine, Physical Rehabilitation and Diagnostic Audiology, Mental Health, and Substance Abuse Treatment sections do not use qualifiers; the value of the character for those sections should always be Z.

Table 27.6 Meanings for Character 5 according to Section

Section Number	Section Name	Character 5 Meaning
0	Medical and Surgical	Approach
1	Obstetrics	Approach
2	Placement	Approach
3	Administration	Approach
4	Measurement and Monitoring	Approach
5	Extracorporeal Assistance and Performance	Duration
6	Extracorporeal Therapies	Duration
7	Osteopathic	Approach
8	Other Procedures	Approach
9	Chiropractic	Approach
B	Imaging	Contrast
C	Nuclear Medicine	Radionuclide
D	Radiation Oncology	Modality qualifier
F	Physical Rehabilitation and Diagnostic Audiology	Type qualifier
G	Mental Health	Qualifier
H	Substance Abuse Treatment	Qualifier

Table 27.7 Meanings for Character 6 according to Section

Section Number	Section Name	Character 6 Meaning
0	Medical and Surgical	Device
1	Obstetrics	Device
2	Placement	Device
3	Administration	Substance
4	Measurement and Monitoring	Function/device
5	Extracorporeal Assistance and Performance	Function
6	Extracorporeal Therapies	Qualifier
7	Osteopathic	Method
8	Other Procedures	Method
9	Chiropractic	Method
B	Imaging	Qualifier

(continued)

Chapter Summary

Learning Outcome	Key Concepts/Examples
27.1 Outline the history and development of ICD-10-PCS. (pages 469–470)	• The agency responsible for maintenance of the US procedure code set, the Centers for Medicare and Medicaid Services (CMS), contracted with 3M Health Information Systems to develop a system to replace ICD-9-CM, Volume 3. • Part of the goal in the development of ICD-10-PCS was the incorporation of six major attributes, which are completeness, unique definitions, expandability, multi-axial codes, standardized terminology, and structural integrity.
27.2 Describe the standardized terminology of ICD-10-PCS codes. (pages 471–476)	• The ICD-10-PCS codes consist of seven characters, each with the potential to have up to 34 different values. • Values for each character in an ICD-10-PCS code are alphanumeric and may consist of the numeric digits 0–9 and the letters A–H, J–N, and P–Z. The letters I and O are not used to avoid confusion with the numbers 1 and 0.
27.3 Demonstrate how to build an ICD-10-PCS code. (pages 476–478)	• The process of building an ICD-10-PCS code involves finding the main term in the index, identifying any subterm in the index, locating the first three characters in the tables section, and identifying values for characters 4–7. • Although the process of building an ICD-10-PCS code may appear relatively simple and straightforward, even simple procedures include a significant extent of decision making and knowledge requirements of terminology involved for identification of the correct code.
27.4 Apply the structure of the ICD-10-PCS manual to build codes. (pages 478–480)	• Rather than simply looking up the terms in the alphabetic index, then cross-referencing the tabular list to verify that the code is correct, coders can use ICD-10-PCS to build the most appropriate code possible, taking into account seven different aspects of procedures and services. • The ICD-10-PCS manual includes a procedure index, a tables section, and six appendices. • The need for a detailed level of understanding of anatomy and physiology is demonstrated through the list of anatomic structures associated with body parts in Appendix C.

Learning Outcome	Key Concepts/Examples
27.5 Discuss the documentation and knowledge requirements for the accurate assignment of ICD-10-PCS codes. **(pages 480–481)**	• Coders should have a strong knowledge of anatomy and physiology to be able to identify the locations and functions of all the anatomic structures listed in the body part key in Appendix C of the ICD-10-PCS manual. • Audits help identify any opportunities for improvement in documentation or education related to coding.

Checking Your Understanding

Select the letter that best answers the question or completes the sentence.

1. *[LO 27.2]* How many characters are in an ICD-10-PCS code?

    a. four to six   **b.** five to seven   **c.** six   **d.** seven

2. *[LO 27.1]* What are the six major attributes of ICD-10-PCS?

    a. comprehensiveness, unique definitions, expandability, multi-axial codes, standardized terminology, and structural integrity

    b. completeness, unique definitions, expandability, alphanumeric codes, standardized terminology, and structural integrity

    c. completeness, unique definitions, expandability, multi-axial codes, standardized terminology, and structural integrity

    d. completeness, unique definitions, dependability, multi-axial codes, standardized terminology, and structural expandability

3. *[LO 27.4]* Which of the following is *not* found in the ICD-10-PCS index?

    a. commonly used names of procedures

    b. eponym names of procedures

    c. general types of procedures

    d. root operation names

4. *[LO 27.3]* What is the proper order for building an ICD-10-PCS code?

    a. Find index main term, find index subterm, locate first three characters in tables section, and identify values for characters 4–7.

    b. Find index subterm, find index main term, locate first three characters in tables section, and identify values for characters 4–7.

    c. Locate first three characters in tables section, find index main term, find index subterm, and identify values for characters 4–7.

    d. Identify values for characters 4–7, locate first three characters in tables section, find index main term, and find index subterm.

5. *[LO 27.2]* What is represented by the first digit of an ICD-10-PCS code?

    a. root operation   **b.** body system   **c.** section   **d.** qualifier

6. *[LO 27.5]* Which of the following activities contribute to improvement of documentation related to coding?

   a. audits
   b. performance improvement
   c. quality improvement
   d. all of these

7. *[LO 27. 2]* What is the meaning of character 2 for the Chiropractic section?

   a. body system
   b. root operation
   c. anatomic regions
   d. body region

8. *[LO 27.1]* ICD-10-PCS was developed to replace

   a. CPT.
   b. ICD-9-CM.
   c. ICD-9-CM Volumes 1 and 2.
   d. ICD-9-CM Volume 3.

9. *[LO 27.5]* Which of the following is a benefit of externally administered audits?

   a. awareness of problem areas
   b. a fresh set of eyes looking at the documentation
   c. familiarity with the documents
   d. familiarity with the location of documents in the record

10. *[LO 27.4]* Terms located in the ICD-10-PCS index may provide the coder with all of the following items *except*

    a. the seven-character code.
    b. the first three characters of a code.
    c. the first four characters of a code.
    d. directions to see a different term in the index.

Online Activity

[LO 27.3] Many coders use encoder software on computers to assign codes, rather than using a hard-copy code book. Search online for information about encoders and how they are used to select ICD-10-PCS codes. Summarize your findings in a brief report.

Real-World Application

[LO 27.5] Now that you have been introduced to ICD-9-CM, Volume 3, and ICD-10-PCS, you should have developed an awareness of the differences in the levels of detail needed in medical documentation. The actions of healthcare professionals as they prepare to transition from ICD-9-CM to ICD-10-CM/PCS include the performance of documentation audits and the obtaining of more education. Write an ICD-9-CM to ICD-10-CM/PCS transition plan for use in an acute care hospital. Provide a detailed outline of the activities to be performed, identify which professionals are responsible for each task, and provide a rationale for the importance of each activity.

28

ICD-10-PCS SECTIONS 0–4

Learning Outcomes *After completing this chapter, students should be able to*

28.1 Apply knowledge of root operations, body parts, and other components of procedures in the Medical and Surgical section.

28.2 Discuss the rationale for ICD-10-PCS coding of procedures in the Obstetrics section.

28.3 Identify procedures appropriate for coding in the Placement section.

28.4 Classify procedures in the Administration section according to body system or region.

28.5 Incorporate knowledge of functions and devices into assignment of codes in the Measurement and Monitoring section.

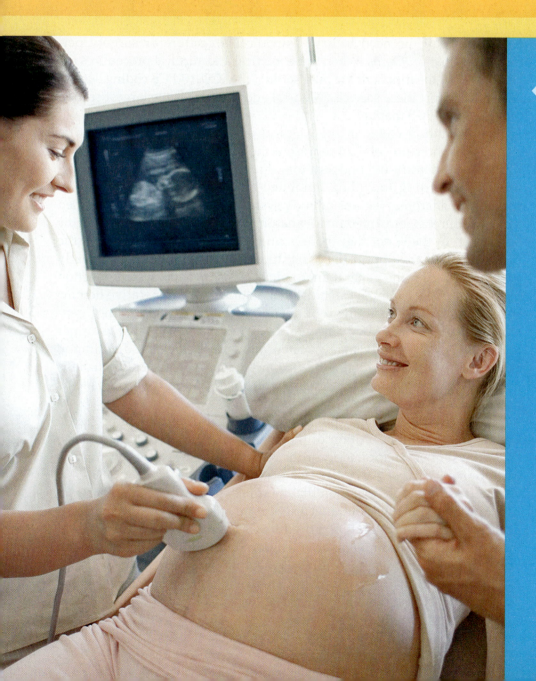

Key Terms
alteration
approach via natural or
     artificial opening
bypass
change
compression
control
detachment
drainage
excision
extirpation
extraction
fragmentation
inspection
introduction
irrigation
map
measurement
monitoring
occlusion
reattachment
replacement
reposition
restriction
transfer
transfusion
transplantation

Introduction

In the ICD-10-PCS coding system, procedures are classified according to sections. The sections identify the general types of procedures. The section value is the first character of the procedure code and may consist of numeric values 0–9 or alphabetic value B, C, D, F, G, or H. The ICD-10-PCS code consists of seven characters, each with the potential for up to 34 different values. The values assigned to each character in an ICD-10-PCS code represent options that are defined as they relate to specific sections. Values for characters 2–7 vary not only by chapter but also sometimes by body system and root operation. The first five sections of ICD-10-PCS—sections 0–4—cover procedures classified as medical and surgical, obstetrics, placement, administration, and measurement and monitoring.

28.1 Medical and Surgical Section

Sometimes patients need to have a medical procedure or surgery performed to treat problems. When these medical and surgical procedures are performed in the inpatient hospital setting, the ICD-10-PCS coding system is used to report these services. Medical and Surgical is the largest section of the ICD-10-PCS manual.

When building codes in the Medical and Surgical section, the first character is the value of 0, to represent the section. Character 2 values in this section identify the body system on which the procedure was performed. According to coding guideline B2.1a., the procedure codes in the general anatomic regions or body systems should be used only when the procedure is performed on an anatomic region, rather than a specific body part. In the event that there is no information documented in the medical record to support the assignment of a code for a specific body part, a code from the general anatomic regions or body systems section may be used. An example can be seen in control of postoperative hemorrhage, which is coded to the root operation Control, found in the "general anatomic regions" body system. Body systems designated as upper and lower contain body parts located above or below the diaphragm, according to coding guideline B2.1b. One example of this coding rule is a vein located above the diaphragm, which is found in the Upper Veins body system.

The 3rd character is the root operation. According to coding guideline B3.1a., the full definition of the root operation as contained in the PCS tables must be applied in order to determine the appropriate root operation.

An *alteration* is an operation that modifies the natural anatomic structure of a body part without affecting the function of the body part. The principal purpose of alteration procedures is to improve the appearance of the body part. An example of an alteration operation is an open bilateral breast augmentation using synthetic substitute. The entire code 0H0V0JZ (see Table 28.1) can be found in the Medical Surgical section under 0H, Skin and Breast, and then the subterm "Alteration."

alteration Operation that modifies the natural anatomic structure of a body part without affecting the function of the body part, principally to improve the appearance of the body part.

Table 28.1 Structure of Code 0H0V0JZ

Section	Body System	Root Operation	Body Part	Approach	Device	Qualifier
Medical and Surgical	Skin and Breast	Alteration	Breast, Bilateral	Open	Synthetic Substitute	No Qualifier
0	H	0	V	0	J	Z

A *bypass* operation alters the route of passage of the contents of a tubular body part. The route may be altered so that it is taken to a place past the body part on the same route, to a similar route and body part, or to a completely different route and different body part. The re-routing includes at least one anastomosis, and a device may or may not be left in at the conclusion of the procedure. An example of a bypass procedure is aortocoronary bypass, which can be found in the ICD-10-PCS coding manual by locating the main procedural name "Bypass" in the alphabetic index or by looking for "Heart and Great Vessels" in the Medical and Surgical section. The main procedure name "Bypass" can then be found and the code built from there up to seven characters; 0 represents the Medical Surgical section, 2 represents "Heart and Great Vessels," and 1 represents the bypass procedure and its definition. The remaining four codes are built from the table to include the affected body part.

The patient may have had one or more sites of blockage in a main coronary artery or the atrium. The 5th character represents how the procedure was performed. In this example, it may have been an open, percutaneous, or percutaneous endoscopic procedure. The 6th character describes the device used. This procedural example can include any one of four characters: 9 represents autologous venous tissue, A represents autologous arterial tissue, J is assigned if a synthetic tissue substitute was used, and Z is coded in the 6th position if no device is used. The 7th character is for a qualifier, which further describes the artery or vein used to perform the bypass. A coronary artery bypass graft (CABG) of two coronary arteries, performed as an open procedure using autologous venous tissue to a coronary artery would be reported with code 0211093 (see Table 28.2).

According to coding guideline *B3.6a.*, bypass procedures are coded by identifying the body part bypassed "from" and the body part bypassed "to." The 4th-character body part specifies the body part bypassed "from," and the 7th-character qualifier specifies the body part bypassed "to." An example can be seen in a bypass from the stomach to the jejunum

bypass Operation that alters the route of passage of the contents of a tubular body part.

Table 28.2 Structure of Code 0211093

Section	Body System	Root Operation	Body Part	Approach	Device	Qualifier
Medical and Surgical	Heart and Great Vessels	Bypass	Coronary Artery, Two Sites	Open	Autologous Venous Tissue	Coronary Artery
0	2	1	1	0	9	3

of the small intestine. The stomach is the body part and the jejunum is the qualifier. According to coding guideline *B3.6b.*, coronary arteries are classified by the number of distinct sites treated, rather than the number of coronary arteries or the anatomic name of a coronary artery (e.g., left anterior descending artery). Rather than identifying the body part bypassed from, the body part identifies the number of coronary artery sites bypassed to, and the qualifier specifies the vessel bypassed from.

An example of this can be seen in an aortocoronary artery bypass of one site on the left anterior descending coronary artery and one site on the obtuse marginal coronary artery. This procedure is classified in the body part axis of classification as two coronary artery sites and the qualifier specifies the aorta as the body part bypassed from. Coding guideline *B3.6c.* states that, if multiple coronary artery sites are bypassed, a separate code is assigned for each coronary artery site that uses a different device and/or qualifier. Aortocoronary artery bypass and internal mammary coronary artery bypass use different sites, so they are coded separately.

Change procedures involve taking out or taking off a device from a body part and putting back an identical or similar device in or on the same body part without cutting or puncturing the skin or a mucous membrane. It is important to note that the approach for all change procedures is external. An example of a change procedure is changing a gastrostomy tube.

To code for a gastrostomy tube change, the coder can go under the main category for medical and surgical procedures and search for 0D Gastrointestinal System, 0D2 Change, and then locate the table where four other codes can be obtained. This example presents two pathways to choose from, as outlined in two rows across for the upper and lower intestine or the omentum, mesentery, or peritoneum and four columns to describe the body part, approach, device, and qualifier. The external approach is the same for each path taken in this example. Path 1 has characters 0, U, and Y for drainage device, feeding device, and other device. Path 2 has characters 0 and Y for drainage device and other device. There is no qualifier for this example on either pathway; therefore, a Z is assigned as the 7th digit. If the health record documentation states that the procedure was for a gastrostomy tube change of the upper intestine with an external drainage device, the correct code for this example is 0D20X0Z (see Table 28.3).

Control procedures are those that stop, or attempt to stop, postprocedural bleeding. When coding control procedures, the site of bleeding is coded as the anatomic region, not to a specific body part. Control of post-tonsillectomy hemorrhage is an example of a control procedure. This procedure is found

change Procedure that involves taking out or taking off a device from a body part and putting back an identical or similar device in or on the same body part without cutting or puncturing the skin or a mucous membrane.

> **CODING TIP ▶**
>
> All change procedures are performed by an external approach.

control Procedure that stops, or attempts to stop, postprocedural bleeding.

Table 28.3 Structure of Code 0D20X0Z

Section	Body System	Root Operation	Body Part	Approach	Device	Qualifier
Medical and Surgical	Gastrointestinal System	Change	Upper Intestinal Tract	External	Drainage Device	No Qualifier
0	D	2	0	X	0	Z

Table 28.4 Structure of Code 0W330ZZ

Section	Body System	Root Operation	Body Part	Approach	Device	Qualifier
Medical and Surgical	Anatomic Regions, General	Control	Oral Cavity and Throat	Open	No Device	No Qualifier
0	W	3	3	0	Z	Z

under the General Anatomic Regions section, coded with a W, and the Oral Cavity and Throat section, coded with a 3. Control procedures can be performed on a wide variety of body parts, as shown in the table for this section. Code character 0 is assigned if the open approach is used. There is no device or qualifier in this case, so the character Z should be assigned for both the 6th and 7th digits. The code for this example is 0W330ZZ (see Table 28.4).

According to coding guideline *B3.7*, the root operation Control is defined as "Stopping, or attempting to stop, postprocedural bleeding." If an attempt to stop postprocedural bleeding is initially unsuccessful, and to stop the bleeding requires performing any of the definitive root operations Bypass, Detachment, Excision, Extraction, Reposition, Replacement, or Resection, that root operation is coded instead of Control. An example can be seen in a resection of the spleen to stop postprocedural bleeding, which is coded to Resection instead of Control.

Creation procedures involve making a new structure that does not physically take the place of a body part. These procedures are unique to sex change operations. An example is the creation of a penis or vagina.

Destruction procedures involve eradicating all or a portion of a body part, using energy, force, or a destructive agent. These procedures do not involve physical removal of the body part. Cauterization of a skin lesion is an example of a destruction procedure. This procedure can be found by looking in the ICD-10-PCS manual under the index or table of contents for medical and surgical procedures of the skin and breast. Once there, the coder will want to find the main category heading Destruction. If the procedural scenario as documented in the health record indicates that multiple skin lesions were eradicated from the left upper arm by an external approach with no device, the correct code assignment is 0H5CXZD (see Table 28.5).

0H5 represents the medical and surgical procedure of destruction of the skin and breast. C represents the left upper arm, X represents the external approach, Z indicates that no device was used during the procedure, and D as a 7th character shows there were multiple lesions destroyed from that site.

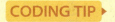

CODING TIP ▶

Creation procedures are unique to sex change operations.

Table 28.5 Structure of Code 0H5CXZD

Section	Body System	Root Operation	Body Part	Approach	Device	Qualifier
Medical and Surgical	Skin and Breast	Destruction	Skin, Left Upper Arm	External	No Device	Multiple
0	H	5	C	X	Z	D

Table 28.6 Structure of Code 0X600ZZ

Section	Body System	Root Operation	Body Part	Approach	Device	Qualifier
Medical and Surgical	Anatomic Regions, Upper Extremities	Detachment	Forequarter, Right	Open	No Device	No Qualifier
0	X	6	0	0	Z	Z

detachment Procedure in which all or a portion of an extremity is cut off.

Detachment procedures are those in which all or a portion of an extremity is cut off. A qualifier should be used with this operation, when applicable, to further specify the level at which the detachment occurred. Above-the-knee amputation is an example of a detachment. If the right forequarter is detached, the code character 0 should be assigned as a 4th digit. With an open approach, the complete code is 0X600ZZ (see Table 28.6). This code can be found under Medical and Surgical: Anatomic Regions, Upper Extremities and then Detachment.

Dilation is the expansion of an orifice or the lumen of a tubular body part. The orifice may be either natural or artificially created. Dilation may be performed by stretching with pressure or by cutting a portion of the orifice or wall of the tubular body part. Esophageal dilation is an example of this operation. In order to assign the correct code for this procedure, a coder needs to know what part of the esophagus was dilated. An endoscopic dilation of the middle part of the esophagus with an intraluminal device is assigned code 0D728DZ (see Table 28.7). The code table can be found under Gastrointestinal System and then Dilation.

Division procedures involve separating or transecting a body part, without removing it and without draining fluids and/or gases from the body part. The operation results in either all or a portion of the body part being separated into at least two portions. An open osteotomy of the left lower femur is assigned code 0Q8C0ZZ (see Table 28.8).

Table 28.7 Structure of Code 0D728DZ

Section	Body System	Root Operation	Body Part	Approach	Device	Qualifier
Medical and Surgical	Gastrointestinal System	Dilation	Esophagus, Middle	Via Natural or Artificial Opening Endoscopic	Intraluminal Device	No Qualifier
0	D	7	2	8	D	Z

Table 28.8 Structure of Code 0Q8C0ZZ

Section	Body System	Root Operation	Body Part	Approach	Device	Qualifier
Medical and Surgical	Lower Bones	Division	Lower Femur, Left	Lumbar Vertebra	No Device	No Qualifier
0	Q	8	C	0	Z	Z

Table 28.9 Structure of Code 0W994ZX

Section	Body System	Root Operation	Body Part	Approach	Device	Qualifier
Medical and Surgical	Anatomic Regions, General	Drainage	Pleural Cavity, Right	Percutaneous	No Device	Diagnostic
0	W	9	9	4	Z	X

Drainage is defined as taking or letting fluids and/or gases out of a body part. Sometimes a drainage procedure is considered a biopsy. In these cases, a qualifier is assigned to identify the procedure as diagnostic. Thoracentesis is an example of a drainage procedure, and the alphabetic index directs the coder to the table for 0W9. If the procedure is performed on the right pleural cavity by way of percutaneous approach with no device and for diagnostic reasons, the correct code assignment is 0W994ZX (see Table 28.9).

Drainage procedures can be performed on many body systems, as reflected in the medical and surgical subcategories 00, 01, 03, 04, 05, 0G, 0M, and so on. The index is helpful to ensure that coders are using the correct table for code assignment.

Excision procedures involve using a sharp instrument for cutting a portion of a body part out or off without replacement of the part. This is another type of procedure that may be used for biopsy and should be identified as diagnostic through the use of a qualifier. Some of the instruments used to perform excisions are scalpel, wire, scissors, and bone saw. A liver biopsy is an example of an excision. An excision can be performed on many body systems, so it is important to code from the correct body system section. A liver biopsy can be found utilizing the alphabetic index or the table under the appropriate body system section. When using the index, the coder is directed to Excision, and then Liver, which is found under table 0FB. If the coder is using the table for a percutaneous liver biopsy of the right lobe of the liver for diagnostic purposes, the correct code assignment is 0FB13ZX (see Table 28.10).

If a diagnostic Excision, Extraction, or Drainage procedure (biopsy) is followed by a more definitive procedure, such as Destruction, Excision, or Resection at the same procedure site, both the biopsy and the more definitive treatment are coded, according to coding guideline *B3.4.* An example

drainage Taking or letting fluids and/or gases out of a body part.

excision Using a sharp instrument for cutting a portion of a body part out or off without replacement of the part.

Table 28.10 Structure of Code 0FB13ZX

Section	Body System	Root Operation	Body Part	Approach	Device	Qualifier
Medical and Surgical	Hepatobiliary System and Pancreas	Excision	Liver, Right Lobe	Percutaneous	No Device	Diagnostic
0	F	B	1	3	Z	X

can be seen in a biopsy of the breast followed by a partial mastectomy at the same procedure site. Both the biopsy and the partial mastectomy procedures are coded.

If the root operation Excision, Repair, or Inspection is performed on overlapping layers of the musculoskeletal system, the body part specifying the deepest layer is coded, in accordance with coding guideline B3.5. An example of coding for overlapping body layers is seen in an Excisional debridement that includes skin, and subcutaneous tissue and muscle, is coded to the muscle body part.

According to coding guideline B3.8, the procedure coding system contains specific body parts for anatomic subdivisions of a body part, such as lobes of the lungs or liver and regions of the intestine. Resection of the specific body part is coded whenever all of the body part is cut out or off, rather than coding Excision of a less specific body part. One such example is a left upper lung lobectomy coded to Resection of Upper Lung Lobe, Left, rather than Excision of Lung, Left.

If an Autograft is obtained from a different body part in order to complete the objective of the procedure, a separate procedure is coded. An example can be seen in a coronary bypass with excision of a saphenous vein graft whereby the excision of the saphenous vein is coded separately. See coding guideline B3.9 for Excision for Graft.

Extirpation procedures take or cut solid matter out of a body part. Solid matter may have a variety of origins, such as an abnormal by-product of a natural biological process or a foreign body. The solid matter may or may not be embedded in the body part or the lumen of a tubular body part. Sometimes a procedure is done to break up the solid matter into smaller pieces prior to the extirpation procedure. An example of extirpation is a thrombectomy. An open thrombectomy on the right pulmonary artery is located under the heading Heart and Great Vessels. The code assigned for this procedure is 02CQ0ZZ (see Table 28.11).

Extraction is a procedure that uses force to pull or strip out or off all or a portion of a body part. This is another type of procedure that may be used for biopsies, which should be identified by assignment of the diagnostic qualifier. Dilation and curettage are an example of an extraction procedure. In ICD-10-PCS terms, the procedure is extraction of the endometrium by way of a natural opening with no device and no qualifier, which is reported with code 0UDB7ZZ (see Table 28.12). This code is found under Female Reproductive and Extraction.

Fragmentation procedures break solid matter in a body part into pieces. This can be accomplished through a physical force, including manual or ultrasonic methods, applied to break up the solid matter. Fragmentation

extirpation Procedure that takes or cuts solid matter out of a body part.

extraction Procedure that uses force to pull or strip out or off all or a portion of a body part.

fragmentation Breaking solid matter in a body part into pieces through a physical force, including manual or ultrasonic methods, applied either directly to the solid matter or indirectly through intervening body parts.

Table 28.11 Structure of Code 02CQ0ZZ

Section	Body System	Root Operation	Body Part	Approach	Device	Qualifier
Medical and Surgical	Heart and Great Vessels	Extirpation	Pulmonary Artery, Right	Open	No Device	No Qualifier
0	2	C	Q	0	Z	Z

Table 28.12 Structure of Code 0UDB7ZZ

Section	Body System	Root Operation	Body Part	Approach	Device	Qualifier
Medical and Surgical	Female Reproductive System	Extraction	Endometrium	Via Natural or Artificial Opening	No Device	No Qualifier
0	U	D	B	7	Z	Z

Table 28.13 Structure of Code 0TF33ZZ

Section	Body System	Root Operation	Body Part	Approach	Device	Qualifier
Medical and Surgical	Urinary System	Fragmentation	Kidney Pelvis, Right	Percutaneous	No Device	No Qualifier
0	T	F	3	3	Z	Z

may be done through direct application to the solid matter, or it may be done indirectly, through intervening body parts. Lithotripsy is an example of a fragmentation procedure. In order to assign the correct code of 0TF33ZZ (see Table 28.13) for a percutaneous lithotripsy of the right renal pelvis, the coder can start searching for this procedure in one of two ways.

If the coder knows what body system the procedure was performed on, he or she can go straight to the table for Fragmentation of the Urinary System to build the code. If the health record documentation is not clear and the coder is not very familiar with the procedure or does not know what body system a lithotripsy pertains to, the coder might be better off starting with the index. The coder should query the provider, if needed, to determine the body part on which the procedure was performed. For example, if the alphabetic index is referenced to look up Lithotripsy, it will guide the coder to see Fragmentation of the Kidney 0TF3.

Fusion is a procedure that involves joining the portions of an articular body part in order to render the articular body part immobile. This may be done by means of a fixation device, a bone graft, or other methods. Spinal fusion is an example of a fusion procedure. This procedure can be located by locating the main procedural term "Fusion" in the alphabetic index to procedures. Once that is located, the anatomic site or spinal location involved should be identified. Then the coder can proceed to the table for further building of the code. The complete code assignment for a posterior percutaneous spinal fusion of the lumbosacral joint using autologous tissue substitute is 0SG3371 (see Table 28.14).

According to coding guideline *B3.10a.*, fusion procedures of the spine, the body part coded for a spinal vertebral joint(s) rendered immobile by a spinal fusion procedure is classified by the level of the spine (e.g., thoracic). There are distinct body part values for a single vertebral joint and for multiple vertebral joints at each spinal level. In one example, body part values may specify lumbar vertebral joint; lumbar vertebral joints, two or more; and lumbosacral vertebral joint. In the event that the procedure was

Table 28.14 Structure of Code 0SG3371

Section	Body System	Root Operation	Body Part	Approach	Device	Qualifier
Medical and Surgical	Lower Joints	Fusion	Lumbosacral Joint	Percutaneous	Autologous Tissue Substitute	Posterior Approach, Posterior Column
0	S	G	3	3	7	1

performed on multiple vertebral joints, a separate procedure is coded for each vertebral joint that uses a different device and/or qualifier, which is outlined in coding guideline *B3.10b*.

Combinations of devices and materials are often used on a vertebral joint to render the joint immobile. When combinations of devices are used on the same vertebral joint, the device value coded for the procedure is as follows:

- If an interbody fusion device is used to render the joint immobile (alone or containing other material, such as bone graft), the procedure is coded with the device value 3, Interbody Internal Fusion Device.

- If internal fixation is used to render the joint immobile and an interbody fusion device is *not* used, the procedure is coded with the device value 4, Internal Fixation Device.

- If bone graft is the *only* device used to render the joint immobile, the procedure is coded with the device value K, Nonautologous Tissue Substitute, or 7, Autologous Tissue Substitute.

- If a mixture of autologous and nonautologous bone graft (with or without biological or synthetic extenders or binders) is used to render the joint immobile, the procedure should be coded with the device value 7, Autologous Tissue Substitute.

An example of this can be seen in a fusion of a vertebral joint using a cage style interbody fusion device containing morselized bone graft, which is coded to the device Interbody Fusion Device. Fusion of a vertebral joint using a bone dowel interbody fusion device made of cadaver bone and packed with a mixture of local morselized bone and demineralized bone matrix is coded to the device Interbody Fusion Device, fusion of a vertebral joint using rigid plates affixed with screws and reinforced with bone cement is coded to the device Internal Fixation Device, and fusion of a vertebral joint using both autologous bone graft and bone bank bone graft is coded to the device Autologous Tissue Substitute. This direction is specified through coding guideline *B3.10c*.

Insertion is a procedure that puts in a non-biological appliance that monitors, assists, performs, or prevents a physiological function. However, the appliance does not physically take the place of a body part. An example of an insertion procedure is insertion of a central venous catheter. A central venous catheter inserted percutaneously into the upper right subclavian vein with an intraluminal device is assigned code 05H63DZ (see Table 28.15). This code is found in the Medical Surgery section under Upper Veins and Insertion.

Table 28.15 Structure of Code 05H63DZ

Section	Body System	Root Operation	Body Part	Approach	Device	Qualifier
Medical and Surgical	Upper Veins	Insertion	Subclavian Vein, Right	Percutaneous	Intraluminal Device	No Qualifier
0	5	H	6	3	D	Z

Inspection procedures are those that visually and/or manually explore a body part. This may be achieved with or without the assistance of optical instrumentation. Manual exploration may be done either directly or through intervening body layers. Exploratory laparoscopy is an example of an inspection procedure. An exploratory laparoscopy performed percutaneously to inspect the ovary is assigned code 0UJ34ZZ (see Table 28.16). The coder can begin to locate this procedure in the alphabetic index under Inspection.

According to coding guideline *B3.11a.* Inspection Procedures, the inspection of body parts performed in order to achieve the objective of a procedure is not coded separately. One example of this practice is fiberoptic bronchoscopy performed for irrigation of the bronchus, in which only the irrigation procedure is coded.

If multiple tubular body parts are inspected, the most distal body part inspected is coded. If multiple nontubular body parts in a region are inspected, the body part that specifies the entire area inspected is coded, according to coding guideline *B3.11b.* For example, in the case of cystourethroscopy with inspection of the bladder and ureters, the procedure is coded to the ureter body part value.

Exploratory laparotomy with general inspection of abdominal contents is coded to the peritoneal cavity body part value.

When both an inspection procedure and another procedure are performed on the same body part during the same episode and the inspection procedure is performed using a different approach than the other procedure, the inspection procedure is coded separately, according to coding guideline *B3.11c.* For example, an endoscopic inspection of the duodenum is coded separately when open excision of the duodenum is performed during the same procedural episode.

Map procedures are performed for the purpose of locating the route of passage of electrical impulses and/or locating functional areas in a body part. This procedure is performed only on the cardiac conduction mechanism

inspection Procedure that visually and/or manually explores a body part, with or without the assistance of optical instrumentation.

map Procedure performed for the purpose of locating the route of passage of electrical impulses and/or locating functional areas in a body part.

Table 28.16 Structure of Code 0UJ34ZZ

Section	Body System	Root Operation	Body Part	Approach	Device	Qualifier
Medical and Surgical	Female	Inspection	Ovary	Percutaneous	No Device	No Qualifier
0	U	J	3	4	Z	Z

Table 28.17 Structure of Code 02K83ZZ

Section	Body System	Root Operation	Body Part	Approach	Device	Qualifier
Medical and Surgical	Heart and Great Vessels	Map	Conduction Mechanism	Percutaneous	No Device	No Qualifier
0	2	K	8	3	Z	Z

CODING TIP ▶

Map procedures are performed only on the cardiac conduction mechanism and the central nervous system.

occlusion Procedure that completely closes a natural or artificially created orifice or lumen of a tubular body part.

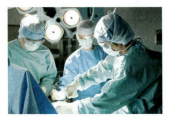

Medical and surgical procedures are classified by body system for the purposes of ICD-10-PCS coding.

reattachment Procedure that puts back in or on all or a portion of a separated body part to its normal location or another suitable location.

and the central nervous system. Percutaneous mapping of the conduction mechanism of the cardiac system is coded 02K83ZZ (see Table 28.17).

Occlusion procedures completely close an orifice or a lumen of a tubular body part. This may be either a natural or artificially created orifice. An example of an occlusion procedure is a tubal ligation. A percutaneous endoscopic tubal ligation of both fallopian tubes utilizing an intraluminal device is coded 0UL74DZ (see Table 28.18).

The code 0UL can be built by locating the term "Occlusion" under the Female Reproductive System of Medical and Surgical procedures. The remaining characters to fully describe this procedure are found within the 0UL table for this procedure.

According to coding guideline *B3.12* for occlusion versus restriction for vessel embolization procedures, if the objective of an embolization procedure is to completely close a vessel, the root operation Occlusion is coded. If the objective of an embolization procedure is to narrow the lumen of a vessel, the root operation Restriction is coded. For example, tumor embolization is coded to the root operation Occlusion, because the objective of the procedure is to cut off the blood supply to the vessel.

Embolization of a cerebral aneurysm is coded to the root operation Restriction, because the objective of the procedure is not to close off the vessel entirely but to narrow the lumen of the vessel at the site of the aneurysm where it is abnormally wide.

Reattachment procedures put back in or on all or a portion of a separated body part to its normal location or another suitable location. This may or may not involve reestablishing vascular circulation and nervous pathways. An example of a reattachment procedure is the reattachment of a severed limb. For reattachment of the right ring finger, the code is 0XMS0ZZ (see Table 28.19).

The first three characters of 0XMS0ZZ can be found by locating the term "Reattachment" in the alphabetic index. The remaining codes can be constructed from the 0XM table.

Table 28.18 Structure of Code 0UL74DZ

Section	Body System	Root Operation	Body Part	Approach	Device	Qualifier
Medical and Surgical	Female Reproductive System	Occlusion	Fallopian Tubes, Bilateral	Percutaneous Endoscopic	Intraluminal Device	No Qualifier
0	U	L	7	4	D	Z

Table 28.19 Structure of Code 0XMS0ZZ

Section	Body System	Root Operation	Body Part	Approach	Device	Qualifier
Medical and Surgical	Anatomic Regions, Upper Extremities	Reattachment	Ring Finger, Right	Open	No Device	No Qualifier
0	X	M	S	0	Z	Z

Release is a procedure that frees a body part from an abnormal physical constraint. Although none of the body part is removed with this procedure, sometimes it is necessary to take out some of the restraining tissue. Release of carpal tunnel is an example of a release procedure, assigned code 01N54ZZ (see Table 28.20) if performed via a percutaneous endoscopic approach.

This procedure is found under Peripheral Nervous System and Release of the Medical and Surgical section. The 4th character 5 identifies the median nerve as the body part operated on. The 5th character represents the open procedure performed. There is no device or qualifying factor in this procedure; therefore; Z is added to both the 6th and 7th positions to complete the code.

According to coding guideline B3.13 for release procedures, the body part value coded is the body part being freed, not the tissue being manipulated or cut to free the body part. Lysis of intestinal adhesions is coded to the specific intestine body part value. If the sole objective of the procedure is to free a body part without cutting it, the root operation is Release, according to coding guideline B3.14. If the sole objective of the procedure is to separate or transect a body part, the root operation is Division. An example of this is freeing a nerve root from surrounding scar tissue by severing it to relieve pain.

Removal is a procedure that takes a device out or off of a body part. If a new device is put in following removal, the procedure for putting in the new device is coded to the root operation performed. However, if the device is taken out and a similar device is put in without cutting or puncturing the skin or mucous membrane, the procedure is not considered a removal but, rather, should be coded as change. Removal of a drainage tube is an example of a removal procedure. This procedure can be coded by looking in the index for the removal of a device from the anatomic location specified in the medical record for this procedure. In this example, an external drainage tube is removed from the abdominal wall, which is assigned code 0WPFX0Z (see Table 28.21).

Table 28.20 Structure of Code 01N54ZZ

Section	Body System	Root Operation	Body Part	Approach	Device	Qualifier
Medical and Surgical	Peripheral Nervous System	Release	Median Nerve	Percutaneous Endoscopic	No Device	No Qualifier
0	1	N	5	4	Z	Z

Example: Destruction of sigmoid lesion and bypass of sigmoid colon are coded separately.

d. The intended root operation is attempted using one approach but is converted to a different approach.

Example: Laparoscopic cholecystectomy converted to an open cholecystectomy is coded as percutaneous endoscopic inspection and open resection.

According to coding guideline B3.3, if the intended procedure is discontinued, the procedure is coded to the root operation performed. If a procedure is discontinued before any other root operation is performed, the root operation inspection of the body part or anatomic region inspected is coded. An example is a planned aortic valve replacement procedure that is discontinued after the initial thoracotomy and before any incision is made in the heart muscle, when the patient becomes hemodynamically unstable. This procedure is coded as an open inspection of the mediastinum.

> **CODING TIP** ▸
>
> If the intended procedure is discontinued, code the procedure to the root operation performed. If a procedure is discontinued before any other root operation is performed, code the root operation Inspection of the body part or anatomic region inspected.

The specific body part on which the procedure was performed is identified in character 4. Values for this character vary by body system.

According to coding guideline B4.1a., if a procedure is performed on a portion of a body part that does not have a separate body part value, the body part value corresponding to the whole body part should be coded. For example, a procedure performed on the alveolar process of the mandible is coded to the mandible body part.

If the prefix "peri-" is combined with a body part to identify the site of the procedure, the procedure is coded to the body part named, according to coding guideline B4.1b. For example, a procedure site identified as perirenal is coded to the kidney body part.

If a specific branch of a body part does not have its own body part value in PCS, the body part is coded to the closest proximal branch that has a specific body part value, according to coding guideline B4.2, for branches of body parts. For example, a procedure performed on the mandibular branch of the trigeminal nerve is coded to the trigeminal nerve body part value.

According to coding guideline B4.3, body part values are available for a limited number of body parts. If the identical procedure is performed on contra-lateral body parts, and a bilateral body part value exists for that body part, a single procedure is coded using the bilateral body part value. If no bilateral body part value exists, each procedure is coded separately using the appropriate body part value. An example of this coding guidelines application can be seen in identical procedures performed on both fallopian tubes, which is coded once using the body part value Fallopian Tube, Bilateral. The identical procedure performed on both knee joints is coded twice using the body part values Knee Joint, Right, and Knee Joint, Left.

According to coding guideline B4.4, the coronary arteries are classified as a single body part that is further specified by the number of sites treated, not by the names or number of arteries. Separate body part values are used to specify the number of sites treated when the same procedure is performed on multiple sites in the coronary arteries. For example, angioplasty of two distinct sites in the left anterior descending coronary artery with placement of two stents is coded as Dilation of Coronary Arteries, Two Sites, with Intraluminal Device.

Angioplasty of two distinct sites in the left anterior descending coronary artery, one with a stent placed and one without, is coded separately as Dilation of Coronary Artery, One Site with Intraluminal Device, and Dilation of Coronary Artery, One Site with no device.

According to coding guideline B4.5, a procedure performed on tendons, ligaments, bursae, and fascia supporting a joint are coded to the body part in the respective body system that is the focus of the procedure. Procedures performed on joint structures themselves are coded to the body part in the Joint body systems. A repair of the anterior cruciate ligament of the knee is coded to the knee bursae and ligament body part in the Bursae and Ligaments body system. Knee arthroscopy with shaving of articular cartilage is coded to the knee joint body part in the Lower Joints body system.

According to coding guideline B4.6, if a procedure is performed on the skin, subcutaneous tissue, or fascia overlying a joint, the procedure is coded to the following body parts:

- Shoulder is coded to the upper arm.
- Elbow is coded to the lower arm.
- Wrist is coded to the lower arm.
- Hip is coded to the upper leg.
- Knee is coded to the lower leg.
- Ankle is coded to the foot.

If a body system does not contain a separate body part value for fingers, procedures performed on the fingers are coded to the body part value for the hand. If a body system does not contain a separate body part value for toes, procedures performed on the toes are coded to the body part value for the foot, according to coding guideline B4.7. An example of this can be seen in an excision of a finger muscle, which is coded to one of the hand muscle body part values in the Muscles body system.

Character 5 in the Medical and Surgical section is used to report the approach or technique to reach the site of the procedure. Three components are addressed by the approach values: access location, method, and type of instrumentation. The values for character 5 identify the approaches as open, percutaneous, percutaneous endoscopic, via natural or artificial opening, via natural or artificial opening endoscopic, via natural or artificial opening endoscopic with percutaneous endoscopic assistance, or external.

Table 28.30 Structure of Code 0UT90ZZ

Section	Body System	Root Operation	Body Part	Approach	Device	Qualifier
Medical and Surgical	Female Reproductive System	Resection	Uterus	Open	No Device	No Qualifier
0	U	T	9	0	Z	Z

An *open approach* cuts through the skin or mucous membrane and any other body layers necessary to expose the site of the procedure. The access location is the skin or mucous membrane, plus any other body layers. The method is cutting. No instrumentation is used. An example of a procedure performed with an open approach is an abdominal hysterectomy. The code for this procedure is 0UT90ZZ (see Table 28.30).

A *percutaneous approach* involves entry, by puncture or minor incision, of instrumentation through the skin or mucous membrane and any other body layers necessary to reach the site of the procedure. The access location is the skin or mucous membrane, plus any other body layers. The method is puncture or minor incision. Instrumentation is used without visualization. An example of a procedure performed with the percutaneous approach is a needle biopsy, which is reported with code 0FB13ZX (see Table 28.31).

According to coding guideline *B5.4*, percutaneous procedure via device, procedures performed percutaneously via a device placed for the procedure are coded to the approach Percutaneous. An example can be seen in the fragmentation of a kidney stone performed via percutaneous nephrostomy, which is coded to the approach Percutaneous.

A *percutaneous endoscopic approach* involves entry, by puncture or minor incision, of instrumentation through the skin or mucous membrane and any other body layers necessary to reach and visualize the site of the procedure. The access location is the skin or mucous membrane, plus any other body layers. The method is puncture or minor incision. Instrumentation is used with visualization. An example of a procedure performed with the percutaneous endoscopic approach is an arthroscopy. The complete code for a visual inspection of the lower knee joint by percutaneous endoscopy is 0SJD4ZZ (see Table 28.32).

Table 28.31 Structure of Code 0FB13ZX

Section	Body System	Root Operation	Body Part	Approach	Device	Qualifier
Medical and Surgical	Hepatobiliary System and Pancreas	Excision	Liver, Right Lobe	Percutaneous	No Device	Diagnostic
0	F	B	1	3	Z	X

Table 28.32 Structure of Code 0SJD4ZZ

Section	Body System	Root Operation	Body Part	Approach	Device	Qualifier
Medical and Surgical	Lower Joints	Inspection	Knee Joint, Left	Percutaneous Endoscopic	No Device	No Qualifier
0	S	J	D	4	Z	Z

The **approach via natural or artificial opening** is an approach with entry of instrumentation through a natural or artificial external opening to reach the site of the procedure. The access location is a natural or artificial external opening. The method is direct entry. Instrumentation is used without visualization. An example of a procedure performed via natural or artificial opening approach is the placement of a Foley catheter. The code for Foley catheter placement is 0T9B70Z (see Table 28.33).

Via natural or artificial opening endoscopic approach is the entry of instrumentation through a natural or artificial external opening to reach and visualize the site of the procedure. The access location is a natural or artificial external opening. The method is direct entry with puncture or minor incision for instrumentation only. Instrumentation is used with visualization. An example of a procedure performed via natural or artificial opening endoscopic approach is endoscopic retrograde cholangiopancreatography (ERCP). A dilation of the common bile duct via natural or artificial opening via endoscopy can be located under Hepatobiliary System and Pancreas within the Medical Surgical section. The complete code for this procedure is 0F798ZZ (see Table 28.34).

Open with percutaneous endoscopic assistance approach involves cutting through the skin or mucous membrane and any other body layers necessary to expose the site of the procedure and entry, by puncture or minor incision, of instrumentation through the skin or mucous membrane and any other body layers necessary to aid in the performance of the procedure. The access location is the skin or mucous membrane, plus any other body layers. The method is cutting. Instrumentation is used with visualization. An example of a procedure performed by the open with percutaneous endoscopic assistance approach is a laparoscopic-assisted vaginal hysterectomy. The code for this procedure is 0UT9FZZ (see Table 28.35).

approach via natural or artificial opening Approach with entry of instrumentation through a natural or artificial external opening to reach the site of the procedure.

Table 28.33 Structure of Code 0T9B70Z

Section	Body System	Root Operation	Body Part	Approach	Device	Qualifier
Medical and Surgical	Urinary System	Drainage	Bladder	Via Natural or Artificial Opening	Drainage Device	No Qualifier
0	T	9	B	7	0	Z

Table 28.34 Structure of Code 0F798ZZ

Section	Body System	Root Operation	Body Part	Approach	Device	Qualifier
Medical and Surgical	Hepatobiliary System and Pancreas	Dilation	Common Bile Duct	Via Natural or Artificial Opening Endoscopic	No Device	No Qualifier
0	F	7	9	8	Z	Z

Table 28.35 Structure of Code 0UT9FZZ

Section	Body System	Root Operation	Body Part	Approach	Device	Qualifier
Medical and Surgical	Female Reproductive System	Resection	Uterus	Via Natural or Artificial Opening with Percutaneous Endoscopic Assistance	No Device	No Qualifier
0	U	T	9	F	Z	Z

According to coding guideline *B5.2,* Open approach with percutaneous endoscopic assistance, procedures performed using the open approach with percutaneous endoscopic assistance are coded to the approach Open. An example of this can be seen in an open laparoscopic-assisted appendectomy, which is coded 0DTJ0ZZ (see Table 28.36).

External approach procedures are performed directly on the skin or mucous membrane and procedures performed indirectly by the application of external force through the skin or mucous membrane. The access location is the skin or mucous membrane. The method is direct or indirect application. No instrumentation is used. An example of a procedure performed with an external approach is extracorporeal shockwave lithotripsy of a right renal pelvis calculus, which is coded 0TF3XZZ (see Table 28.37).

According to coding guideline *B5.3a.* External approach, procedures performed within an orifice on structures that are visible without the aid of any instrumentation are coded to the approach External. An example of this can be seen in a resection of the tonsils. The complete code for this procedure is 0CTPXZZ (see Table 28.38).

Table 28.36 Structure of Code 0DTJ0ZZ

Section	Body System	Root Operation	Body Part	Approach	Device	Qualifier
Medical and Surgical	Gastrointestinal System	Resection	Appendix	Open	No Device	No Qualifier
0	D	T	J	0	Z	Z

Table 28.37 Structure of Code 0TF3XZZ

Section	Body System	Root Operation	Body Part	Approach	Device	Qualifier
Medical and Surgical	Urinary System	Fragmentation	Kidney Pelvis, Right	External	No Device	No Qualifier
0	T	F	3	X	Z	Z

Table 28.38 Structure of Code 0CTPXZZ

Section	Body System	Root Operation	Body Part	Approach	Device	Qualifier
Medical and Surgical	Mouth and Throat	Resection	Tonsils	External	No Device	No Qualifier
0	C	T	P	X	Z	Z

Procedures performed indirectly by the application of external force through the intervening body layers, such as closed reduction fractures, are coded to the approach External, according to coding guideline *B5.3b*.

Character 6 is used to report devices that remain following completion of the procedure. The four general types of devices that are specified through character 6 values are biological or synthetic material that takes the place of all or a portion of a body part; biological or synthetic material that assists or prevents a physiological function; therapeutic material that is not absorbed or eliminated by or incorporated into a body part; and mechanical or electronic appliances used to assist, monitor, take the place of, or prevent a physiological function. Table 28.39

Table 28.39 Device Values of Root Operations

Root Operations That *May* Have Device Values	Root Operations That *Must* Have Device Values
Alteration	Change
Bypass	Insertion
Creation	Removal
Dilation	Replacement
Drainage	Revision
Fusion	
Occlusion	
Reposition	
Restriction	

identifies root operations that have device values and those that do not have device values.

According to general coding guideline *B6.1a.*, a device is coded only if a device remains after the procedure is completed. If no device remains, the device value No Device is coded. Coding guideline *B6.1b.* states that materials such as sutures, ligatures, radiological markers, and temporary postoperative wound drains are considered integral to the performance of a procedure and are not coded as devices. According to coding guideline *B6.1c.*, procedures performed on a device only and not on a body part are specified in the root operations Change, Irrigation, Removal, and Revision and are coded to the procedure performed. An example of this can be seen in the irrigation of a percutaneous nephrostomy tube, which is coded to the root operation Irrigation of indwelling device in the Administration section.

According to coding guideline *B6.2*, Drainage device, a separate procedure to put in a drainage device is coded to the root operation Drainage with the device value Drainage Device.

Character 7 specifies values for qualifiers. These values are unique to individual procedures. A comprehensive overview of the character meanings and values for the Medical and Surgical section is provided in Table 28.40.

Table 28.40 Character Meanings and Values of the Medical and Surgical Section

Character	Meaning	Values		
1	Section	0 Medical and Surgical		
2	Body system	0 Central Nervous System	C Mouth and Throat	Q Lower Bones
		1 Peripheral Nervous System	D Gastrointestinal System	R Upper Joints
		2 Heart and Great Vessels	F Hepatobiliary System and Pancreas	S Lower Joints
		3 Upper Arteries	G Endocrine System	T Urinary System
		4 Lower Arteries	H Skin and Breast	U Female Reproductive System
		5 Upper Veins	J Subcutaneous Tissue and Fascia	V Male Reproductive System
		6 Lower Veins	K Muscles	W Anatomic Regions, General
		7 Lymphatic and Hemic Systems	L Tendons	X Anatomic Regions, Upper Extremities
		8 Eye	M Bursae and Ligaments	Y Anatomic Regions, Lower Extremities
		9 Ear, Nose, Sinus	N Head and Facial Bones	
		B Respiratory System	P Upper Bones	

3	Root operation	0 Alteration	C Extirpation	P Removal
		1 Bypass	D Extraction	Q Repair
		2 Change	F Fragmentation	R Replacement
		3 Control	G Fusion	S Reposition
		4 Creation	H Insertion	T Resection
		5 Destruction	J Inspection	V Restriction
		6 Detachment	K Map	W Revision
		7 Dilation	L Occlusion	U Supplement
		8 Division	M Reattachment	X Transfer
		9 Drainage	N Release	Y Transplantation
		B Excision		
4	Body part	Body part values vary by body system.		
5	Approach	0 Open		
		3 Percutaneous		
		4 Percutaneous Endoscopic		
		7 Via Natural or Artificial Opening		
		8 Via Natural or Artificial Opening Endoscopic		
		F Via Natural or Artificial Opening Endoscopic with Percutaneous Endoscopic Assistance		
		X External		
6	Device	Device values vary by root operation.		
7	Qualifier	Qualifier values vary by root operation.		

Think About It 28.1

also available in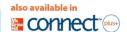

Detailed knowledge of anatomy and physiology is necessary for coding the Medical and Surgical section in ICD-10-PCS. Match the following anatomic structures to the corresponding body parts.

_____ 1. Trapezoid bone   **A.** Sternum

_____ 2. Vomer   **B.** Lumbar spinal cord

_____ 3. Xiphoid process   **C.** Carpal

_____ 4. Choroid plexus   **D.** Cerebral ventricle

_____ 5. Cauda equina   **E.** Nasal bone

Assign ICD-10-PCS codes for the following situations, applying any appropriate sequencing guidelines.

1. Hysteroscopy with intraluminal lithotripsy of left fallopian tube calcification   _____

2. Tracheoscopy with intraluminal dilation
   of tracheal stenosis   _____

3. Open fracture reduction, right tibia   _____

4. Placement of intraluminal plug into the
   right lacrimal duct via natural opening   _____

5. Suture of scalp laceration   _____

6. Mid-shaft amputation of the right
   humerus   _____

28.2 Obstetrics Section

During pregnancy, the course of fetal development may change or appear to be at risk for various reasons. These changes might warrant the use of electrode monitoring devices or other means to measure physiological responses in the fetus. Other methods of evaluation can be done for diagnostic reasons and further management of care—such as an amniocentesis, especially in an older pregnant woman who carries higher risk of something going wrong with the fetus during pregnancy. In the event of complications, interventions such as insertions, inspections, removal, repair, repositioning, or resection may be required. If the fetus is spontaneously aborted or there is a need to terminate the pregnancy due to complications or other preferences, this section of the ICD-10-PCS also provides codes for the products of conception that have been terminated, extracted, or delivered.

All codes in the Obstetrics section have a 1st character value of 1. The 2nd character value to identify the body system for the Obstetrics section is 0 for pregnancy. The designation of pregnancy for the body system is important, as the procedures in this section are performed on the products of conception, not on the pregnant female. To code procedures on the pregnant female, the coder must go to the Medical and Surgical section. Gestational age of the products of conception does not have any impact on the procedure code assignment, as this is considered to be part of the diagnosis; ICD-10-PCS does not include diagnosis information in the procedure codes.

> **CODING TIP ▸**
>
> Procedures in the Obstetrics section are performed on the products of conception, not on the pregnant female.

According to coding guideline *C1, Products of conception*, procedures performed on the products of conception are coded to the Obstetrics section. Procedures performed on the pregnant female other than the products of conception are coded to the appropriate root operation in the Medical and

Surgical section. An amniocentesis is coded to the products of conception body part in the Obstetrics section. Repair of obstetric urethral laceration is coded to the urethra body part in the Medical and Surgical section.

The root operations for the Obstetrics section are change, drainage, abortion, extraction, delivery, insertion, inspection, removal, repair, reposition, resection, and transplantation. Two of these root operations, abortion and delivery, are unique to the obstetrics section. The definitions for the terms "change," "drainage," "extraction," "insertion," "inspection," "removal," "repair," "reposition," "resection," and "transplantation" are identical to the definitions in the Medical and Surgical section.

According to coding guideline *C2, Procedures following delivery or abortion*, procedures performed following a delivery or an abortion for curettage of the endometrium or evacuation of retained products of conception are coded in the Obstetrics section, to the root operation Extraction and the body part Products of Conception, Retained. Diagnostic or therapeutic dilation and curettage performed during times other than the postpartum or post-abortion period are all coded from the Medical and Surgical section, to the root operation Extraction and the body part Endometrium.

Abortion is defined as a procedure to artificially terminate a pregnancy. There is a subdivision according to whether a laminaria or an abortifacient is used versus performing the procedure by mechanical means. An example of an abortion procedure is a vacuum aspiration transvaginal abortion, which is reported with code 10A07Z6 (see Table 28.41).

Delivery procedures are those that assist the passage of products of conception from the genital canal. For coding purposes, delivery procedures apply only to manually assisted vaginal deliveries. A manually assisted delivery is an example of a procedure coded as a delivery, 10E0XZZ (see Table 28.42).

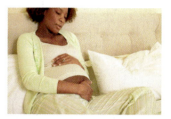

Deliveries are among the procedures coded in the Obstetrics section of ICD-10-PCS.

CODING TIP ▶

The root operation Delivery applies only to manually assisted vaginal deliveries for coding purposes.

Table 28.41 Structure of Code 10A07Z6

Section	Body System	Root Operation	Body Part	Approach	Device	Qualifier
Obstetrics	Pregnancy	Abortion	Products of Conception	Via Natural or Artificial Opening	No Device	Vacuum
1	0	A	0	7	Z	6

Table 28.42 Structure of Code 10E0XZZ

Section	Body System	Root Operation	Body Part	Approach	Device	Qualifier
Obstetrics	Pregnancy	Delivery	Products of Conception	External	No Device	No Qualifier
1	0	E	0	X	Z	Z

Body parts for the Obstetrics section are products of conception, retained products of conception, and ectopic products of conception. The approaches used in the Obstetrics section are open, open endoscopic, percutaneous, percutaneous endoscopic, via natural or artificial opening, via natural or artificial opening endoscopic, and external. Abortion procedures using laminaria or abortifacient are done using the approach Via Natural or Artificial Opening. The Obstetrics section defines three device values: monitoring electrode, other device, or no device. Qualifiers in the Obstetrics section identify the type of extraction, type of cesarean section, or type of fluid taken out during a drainage procedure. The qualifiers used in this section are classical, low cervical, extraperitoneal, low forceps, mid forceps, high forceps, vacuum, internal version, other, and fetal blood. An overview of the values and character meanings for the Obstetrics section is provided in Table 28.43.

Table 28.43 Character Meanings and Values for the Obstetrics Section

Character	Meaning	Values	
1	Section	1 Obstetrics	
2	Body system	0 Pregnancy	
3	Root operation	2 Change	J Inspection
		9 Drainage	P Removal
		A Abortion	Q Repair
		D Extraction	S Reposition
		E Delivery	T Resection
		H Insertion	Y Transplantation
4	Body part	0 Products of Conception	
		1 Products of Conception, Retained	
		2 Products of Conception, Ectopic	
5	Approach	0 Open	7 Via Natural or Artificial Opening
		2 Open Endoscopic	8 Via Natural or Artificial Opening Endoscopic
		3 Percutaneous	X External
		4 Percutaneous Endoscopic	
6	Device	3 Monitoring Electrode	
		Y Other Device	
		Z No Device	
7	Qualifier	0 Classical	5 High Forceps
		1 Low Cervical	6 Vacuum
		2 Extraperitoneal	7 Internal Version
		3 Low Forceps	8 Other
		4 Mid Forceps	9 Fetal Blood

Assign ICD-10-PCS codes for the following situations, applying any appropriate sequencing guidelines.

1. Drainage of fetal blood; open procedure _____

2. Extraction of an ectopic pregnancy via natural opening _____

3. Open endoscopic repair of the endocrine system of the products of conception; by other device _____

4. Insertion of a monitoring electrode; products of conception via natural opening _____

5. Abortion via natural or artificial opening using an abortifacient _____

Beyond the Code: Why is a pregnant female not the focus of procedures in the Obstetrics section?

28.3 Placement Section

During and after surgery, many devices may be needed to offer support and ensure safe healing of the body region or opening (orifice). Such devices include braces, splints, casts, dressings, pressure devices, and packing materials for wounds. These can be placed for a variety of reasons, including protection, immobilization, stretching, compression, or packing. In ICD-10-PCS, placement codes can be found under the main categories Anatomic Regions and Anatomic Orifices. Codes in the Placement section are used to report the placement of a device in or on a body region. For example, a dressing or bandage may need to be placed after abdominal surgery. This is coded 2W23X4Z (see Table 28.44).

All codes in the Placement section have a 1st character value of 2. There are two different value options in the Placement section. They are assigned to identify either the anatomic regions or the anatomic orifices.

The root operations of change and removal are defined the same as they are for the Medical and Surgical section. However, change and removal root operations have different character values assigned in the Placement section than they do in the Medical and Surgical section. Also, there are five root

Table 28.44 Structure of Code 2W23X4Z

Section	Body System	Root Operation	Body Region	Approach	Device	Qualifier
Placement	Anatomic Regions	Dressing	Abdominal Wall	External	Bandage	No Qualifier
2	W	2	3	X	4	Z

Table 28.45 Structure of Code 2W10X6Z

Section	Body System	Root Operation	Body Region	Approach	Device	Qualifier
Placement	Anatomic Regions	Compression	Head	External	Pressure Dressing	No Qualifier
2	W	1	0	X	6	Z

compression Application of pressure on a body region without incision or puncture.

operations in the Placement section that do not appear in the Medical and Surgical section: compression, dressing, immobilization, packing, and traction.

Compression is the application of pressure on a body region. These *procedures* do not involve making an incision or a puncture. An example of a compression procedure is the application of a pressure dressing. The complete code for the placement of a compression dressing to the head is 2W10X6Z (see Table 28.45).

Dressing is the procedure of putting material on a specified body region for the purpose of protecting that region. These procedures also do not involve any incision or puncture. Application of a sterile dressing to a wound is an example of a dressing procedure. A bandage dressing on the left lower leg is coded 2W2RX4Z (see Table 28.46).

Immobilization procedures are performed to limit or prevent motion of a specific body region. It is important to note the difference in splints and braces used for immobilization versus those used for rehabilitation purposes, as they are coded in different sections. An example of an immobilization procedure is the application of a finger splint. A left finger splint is coded 2W3KX1Z (see Table 28.47).

Packing is the procedure of putting a material into a body region or orifice. The procedure is performed without any incision or puncture.

Table 28.46 Structure of Code 2W2RX4Z

Section	Body System	Root Operation	Body Region	Approach	Device	Qualifier
Placement	Anatomic Regions	Dressing	Lower Leg, Left	External	Bandage	No Qualifier
2	W	2	R	X	4	Z

Table 28.47 Structure of Code 2W3KX1Z

Section	Body System	Root Operation	Body Region	Approach	Device	Qualifier
Placement	Anatomic Regions	Immobilization	Finger, Left	External	Splint	No Qualifier
2	W	3	K	X	1	Z

Table 28.48 Structure of Code 2W40X5Z\

Section	Body System	Root Operation	Body Region	Approach	Device	Qualifier
Placement	Anatomic Regions	Packing	Had	External	Packing Material	No Qualifier
2	W	4	0	X	5	Z

Placement of nasal packing is an example of a packing procedure and is coded 2W40X5Z (see Table 28.48).

Traction procedures are performed by application of a pulling force on a specific body region in a distal direction. The procedures coded in the Placement section use mechanical traction apparatuses. An example of a traction procedure is the use of a motorized split-traction table to perform lumbar traction and is coded 2W65X0Z (see Table 28.49).

Body region values reported in character 4 identify body regions for the anatomic region body system or natural orifices for the anatomic orifices body system. The only valid approach for the Placement section is external, since all procedures in the section are either performed directly on the skin or mucous membranes or performed indirectly through application of an external force through the skin or mucous membrane.

Device values reported in character 5 of the Placement section include traction apparatus, splint, cast, brace, bandage, packing material, pressure

> **CODING TIP ▶**
>
> The only valid approach for the Placement section is external, since all procedures in the section are either performed directly on the skin or mucous membranes or performed indirectly through application of an external force through the skin or mucous membrane.

dressing, intermitted pressure device, stereotactic apparatus, wire, other device, and no device. If traction is performed manually, there is no device specified. If a device requires extensive design, fabrication, or fitting, the procedure is not considered to be placement, but rather it should be reported in the Rehabilitation section. There are no qualifiers specified for the Placement section, so this value will always be reported as no qualifier. Table 28.50 provides an overview of the character meanings and values for the Placement section.

Table 28.49 Structure of Code 2W65X0Z

Section	Body System	Root Operation	Body Region	Approach	Device	Qualifier
Placement	Anatomic Regions	Traction	Back	External	Traction Apparatus	No Qualifier
2	W	6	5	X	0	Z

Table 28.50 Character Meanings and Values for the Placement Section

Character	Meaning	Values	
1	Section	2 Placement	
2	Body System	W Anatomic Regions Y Anatomic Orifices	
3	Root Operation	**Body System W**	**Body System Y**
		0 Change 1 Compression 2 Dressing 3 Immobilization 4 Packing 5 Removal 6 Traction	0 Change 4 Packing 5 Removal
4	Body Region	**Body System W**	**Body System Y**
		0 Head F Hand, Left 1 Face G Thumb, Right 2 Neck H Thumb, Left 3 Abdominal Wall J Finger, Right K Finger, Left 4 Chest Wall L Lower Extremity, Right 5 Back 6 Inguinal Region, Right M Lower Extremity, Left 7 Inguinal Region, Left N Upper Leg, Right 8 Upper Extremity, Right P Upper Leg, Left 9 Upper Extremity, Left Q Lower Leg, Right A Upper Arm, Right R Lower Leg, Left B Upper Arm, Left S Foot, Right C Lower Arm, Right T Foot, Left D Lower Arm, Left U Toe, Right E Hand, Right V Toe, Left	0 Mouth and Pharynx 1 Nasal 2- Ear 3 Anorectal 4 Female Genital Tract 5 Urethra
5	Approach	X External	

Character	Meaning	Values		
6	Device	Body System W		Body System Y
		0 Traction Apparatus	7 Intermittent Pressure Device	5 Packing Material
		1 Splint	8 Stereotactic Apparatus	
		2 Cast		
		3 Brace	9 Wire	
		4 Bandage	Y Other Device	
		5 Packing Material	Z - No Device	
		6 Pressure Dressing		
7	Qualifier	Z No Qualifier		

Think About It 28.3

also available in McGraw Hill connect plus+

Assign ICD-10-PCS codes for the following situations, applying any appropriate sequencing guidelines.

1. Mechanical traction of entire left leg _____

2. Removal of packing material from pharynx _____

3. Change of nasal packing material _____

4. Application of traction apparatus to left lower extremity _____

5. Placement of packing to female genital tract _____

Beyond the Code: Why are some devices that are applied reported as rehabilitation, rather than placement?

28.4 Administration Section

Throughout the course of treating a patient preoperatively, intra-operatively or postoperatively, the administration of medications or other biological products may be necessary to correct some abnormal physiological response. Surgery may not be involved, yet certain conditions warrant the use of various substances. Substances may be administered via an open approach, through a percutaneous route, externally, or through a natural or artificial opening in the body. Procedures in the Administration section include putting in or on a therapeutic, prophylactic, protective, diagnostic, nutritional, or physiological substance. All codes in the Administration section have a 1st character value of 3. There are three values available for character 2, which identify the procedures as being performed on the

Table 28.51 Structure of Code 3E0T3CZ

Section	Body System	Root Operation	Body System/Region	Approach	Substance	Qualifier
Administration	Physiological Systems and Anatomic Regions	Introduction	Peripheral Nerves and Plexus	Percutaneous	Regional Anesthetic	No Qualifier
3	E	0	T	3	C	Z

circulatory system, an indwelling device, or physiological systems and anatomic regions. Introduction, irrigation, and transfusion are the three root operations coded in the Administration section.

Introduction procedures involve putting in or on therapeutic, diagnostic, nutritional, physiological, or prophylactic substances. They do not include blood or blood products. An example of an introduction procedure is a nerve block injection; a nerve block injection of the peripheral nerves and plexus with a regional anesthetic agent is coded 3E0T3CZ (see Table 28.51).

Irrigation procedures are those in which a cleansing substance is put in or onto the body. The cleansing substance may be a cleansing substance or a dialysate. An example of an irrigation procedure is flushing of the eye. External eye irrigation is coded to 3E1CX8Z (see Table 28.52).

Transfusion procedures are those that put in blood or blood products. The substance administered is a blood product or a stem cell substance. An example is transfusion of red cells. Percutaneous transfusion of autologous red blood cells into a peripheral vein is coded 30233N0 (see Table 28.53).

Table 28.52 Structure of Code 3E1CX8Z

Section	Body System	Root Operation	Body System/Region	Approach	Substance	Qualifier
Administration	Physiological Systems and Anatomic Regions	Irrigation	Eye	External	Irrigating Substance	No Qualifier
3	E	1	C	X	8	Z

Table 28.53 Structure of Code 30233N0

Section	Body System	Root Operation	Body System/Region	Approach	Substance	Qualifier
Administration	Circulatory	Transfusion	Peripheral Vein	Percutaneous	Red Blood Cells	Autologous
3	0	2	3	3	N	0

Character 4 values for body system/region vary with the body system value. Administration procedures on the circulatory system may be performed on a peripheral vein, a central vein, a peripheral artery, a central artery, or the circulatory system of products of conception. The value of "none" is reported for irrigation procedures on indwelling devices.

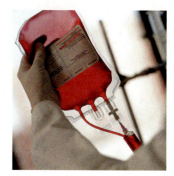

Transfusions of blood or blood products are coded in the Administration section.

> **CODING TIP ▶**
>
> The value of "none" is reported for character 4 when reporting irrigation procedures on indwelling devices.

Introduction or irrigation procedures are used to administer substances to physiological systems and anatomic regions. They are performed on body systems and regions that are identified with values to report:

- skin and mucous membranes
- subcutaneous tissue
- muscle
- peripheral vein
- central vein
- peripheral artery
- central artery
- coronary artery
- heart
- nose
- bone marrow
- ear, eye, mouth, and pharynx
- products of conception
- respiratory tract
- upper GI
- lower GI
- biliary and pancreatic tract
- genitourinary tract
- pleural cavity
- peritoneal cavity
- male reproductive
- female reproductive
- cranial cavity and brain
- spinal canal
- epidural space
- peripheral nerves and plexus
- joints
- bones
- lymphatics
- cranial nerves, an
- pericardial cavity

Approaches reported in character 5 include values for open, percutaneous, via natural or artificial opening, via natural or artificial opening endoscopic, and external.

Substance values for character 6 also vary with the body system value. Substances administered via transfusion in the circulatory system include

- embryonic stem cells
- bone marrow
- whole blood
- serum albumin
- frozen plasma
- fresh plasma
- plasma cryoprecipitate
- red blood cells
- frozen red cells
- white cells
- platelets
- globulin
- fibrinogen
- antihemophilic factors
- factor IX
- cord blood stem cells, and
- hematopoietic stem cells

Indwelling devices only have irrigating substances by means of the irrigation procedure. Introduction or irrigation procedures are used to administer substances to physiological systems and anatomic regions, which include those specified as

- antineoplastic
- thrombolytic
- anti-infective
- anti-inflammatory
- serum
- toxoid
- vaccine
- adhesion barrier
- nutritional substance
- electrolytic and water balance substance
- irrigating substance
- dialysate
- embryonic stem cells
- local anesthetic
- regional anesthetic
- inhalation anesthetic
- somatic stem cells

- intracirculatory anesthetic
- other therapeutic substance
- radioactive substance
- contrast agent
- other diagnostic substance
- sperm, pigment
- analgesics
- hypnotics
- sedatives
- platelet inhibitor
- fertilized ovum
- antiarrhythmic
- gas
- destructive agent
- pancreatic islet cells
- hormone
- immunotherapeutic, and
- vasopressor

Qualifier values for character 7 identify the specific substance being administered, or whether the substance is autologous versus non-autologous. An overview of the character meanings and values is provided in Table 28.54.

Table 28.54 Character Meanings and Values of the Administration Section

Character	Meaning	Values
1	Section	3 Administration
2	Body System	0 Circulatory 3 Indwelling Device E Physiological Systems and Anatomic Regions
3	Root Operation	0 Introduction 1 Irrigation 2 Transfusion
4	Body System/Region	Body system/region varies with body system value.
5	Approach	0 Open 3 Percutaneous 7 Via Natural or Artificial Opening 8 Via Natural or Artificial Opening Endoscopic X External
6	Substance	Substance varies with body system value.

Table 28.56 Structure of Code 4A1D7BZ

Section	Body System	Root Operation	Body System	Approach	Function/ Device	Qualifier
Measurement and Monitoring	Physiological Systems	Monitoring	Urinary	Via Natural or Artificial Opening	Pressure	No Qualifier
4	A	1	D	7	B	Z

The 4th character value identifies the body system measured or monitored. Physiological devices determine measurements for the central nervous system, peripheral nervous system, cardiac system, respiratory system, and musculoskeletal system. Measurement and monitoring of physiological systems are performed on a greater number of systems, which include the following:

- Central nervous
- Peripheral nervous
- Cardiac
- Arterial
- Venous
- Circulatory
- Lymphatic
- Visual
- Olfactory
- Respiratory
- Gastrointestinal
- Biliary
- Urinary
- Musculoskeletal
- Products of conception, cardiac
- Products of conception, nervous
- None

Character 5 values specify the approach. All measurements made by physiological devices use an external approach. Measurement and monitoring of physiological systems may be done by open, percutaneous, percutaneous endoscopic, via natural or artificial opening, via natural or artificial opening endoscopic, or external approach.

A function being measured and devices used for measurement and monitoring are represented by character 6. Sometimes a device is left in the patient following the measurement or monitoring. If this is the case, a code from the Medical and Surgical section should also be assigned to report insertion of the device.

Physiological devices used for measurements include pacemakers, defibrillators, and stimulators. Functions measured and monitored in physiological systems include the following:

- Acuity
- Capacity
- Conductivity
- Contractility
- Electrical activity
- Flow
- Metabolism
- Mobility
- Motility
- Output
- Pressure
- Rate
- Resistance
- Rhythm
- Secretion
- Sound
- Pulse
- Temperature
- Volume
- Total activity
- Sampling and pressure
- Action currents
- Sleep
- Saturation

The qualifier in character 7 provides values for further specificity of the body part. The value of Z should be reported for measurements using physiological devices. Qualifier values for measurement and monitoring of physiological systems include the following:

- Central
- Peripheral
- Portal
- Pulmonary
- Stress
- Right heart
- Left heart
- Bilateral

Checking Your Understanding

Select the letter that best answers the question or completes the sentence.

1. *[LO 28.2]* The root operation delivery applies to

   a. cesarean section.
   b. manually assisted vaginal delivery.
   c. abortion procedures.
   d. all of these procedures.

2. *[LO 28.1]* The 1st character value for the Medical and Surgical section is

   a. 0.
   c. 2.
   b. 1.
   d. 3.

3. *[LO 28.3]* Which root operation is the procedure of putting material on a specified body region for the purpose of protecting that region?

   a. traction
   b. packing
   c. immobilization
   d. dressing

4. *[LO 28.5]* You are coding a record for a patient who had a monitoring procedure done and the device is left in the patient. How should you report this?

   a. Use a qualifier.
   b. Use an additional code from the Medical and Surgical section to report insertion of the device.
   c. Only assign a code from the Medical and Surgical section to report insertion of the device. The monitoring procedure can be reported using a qualifier in that section.
   d. The monitoring procedure code includes insertion of devices that are left in, so nothing different needs to be done.

5. *[LO 28.1]* What is the root operation that involves cutting a portion of a body part out or off without replacement of the part?

   a. division
   b. removal
   c. excision
   d. resection

6. *[LO 28.4]* Which of the following is not a root operation for the Administration section?

   a. drainage
   b. introduction
   c. irrigation
   d. transfusion

7. *[LO 28.5]* What is the 1st character for codes in the Measurement and Monitoring section?

   a. 1
   c. 3
   b. 2
   d. 4

8. *[LO 28.3]* In which section is the root operation of immobilization located?

   a. Obstetrics
   c. Placement
   b. Medical and Surgical
   d. Measurement and Monitoring

9. *[LO 28.4]* Which section should be used to code a blood transfusion?

   a. Administration
   b. Measurement and Monitoring
   c. Medical and Surgical
   d. Placement

10. *[LO 28.2]* Which of the following procedures should be coded in the Obstetrics section?

    a. dilation and curettage following abortion
    b. dilation and curettage for dysfunctional uterine bleeding
    c. total abdominal hysterectomy
    d. All of these procedures should be coded in the Obstetrics section.

Online Activity

[LO 28.1] A high level of knowledge of anatomy and physiology is necessary for coding the Medical and Surgical section in ICD-10-PCS. It may require coders to use additional resources to support their existing knowledge. A wide variety of resources are available to promote understanding of anatomy and physiology and address various learning styles.

Search online to see what resources best fit your needs and discuss three of the resources that you found. Review the body part key in Appendix C of the code book as you perform your search to determine if those resources go into sufficient detail to support the needs of coders using ICD-10-PCS.

Real-World Application: Case Study

[LO 28.1] Code the procedure(s) for the following operative report:

> **Preoperative Diagnosis:** Melena.
> **Postoperative Diagnosis:** Colitis.
> **Procedure:** Colonoscopy with biopsy.
> **Anesthesia:** IV Versed.
> **Procedure:** The risks and benefits of the procedure were explained to the patient, and appropriate consent was obtained. The patient was taken to the endoscopy and was placed in left lateral Sims position. IV Versed was administered for monitored sedation. Digital rectal examination was performed with no masses and a boggy prostate noted. The colonoscope was inserted in the rectum and advanced, under direct vision, to the cecum. Several areas of ulceration, edema, and mucosal abnormalities were visualized. Multiple random biopsies were taken of the left and right colon to verify the diagnosis of colitis.
> Patient was transferred back to his room in stable condition.

Table 29.16 Structure of Code 6A930ZZ

Section	Physiological Systems	Root Operation	Body System	Duration	Qualifier	Qualifier
Extracorporeal Therapies	Physiological Systems	Shock Wave Therapy	Musculoskeletal	Single	No Qualifier	No Qualifier
6	A	9	3	0	Z	Z

duration of the Extracorporeal Therapy procedures are reported either as single or multiple with character 5. There are no qualifiers specified for character 6 in the Extracorporeal Therapies section, so this value will always be reported with a value of Z, which represents "no qualifier."

Qualifiers in character 7 are used to identify blood products that are separated in pheresis procedures as erythrocytes, leukocytes, platelets, plasma, cord blood stem cells, and hematopoietic stem cells. Additional qualifier values for character 7 in this section are used to identify sites on which ultrasound therapy was performed, including the head and neck vessels, heart, peripheral vessels, or other vessels. The remainder of the procedures that are performed in the Extracorporeal Therapies section do not have values assigned for qualifiers, so the value of Z should be assigned to represent "no qualifier." Character meanings and values for the Extracorporeal Therapies section are provided in Table 29.17.

CODING TIP ▶

There are no qualifiers specified for character 6 in the Extracorporeal Therapies section, so this value will always be reported with a value of Z, which represents "no qualifier."

Table 29.17 Character Meanings and Values for the Extracorporeal Therapies Section

Character	Meaning	Values	
1	Section	6 Extracorporeal Therapies	
2	Physiological Systems	A Physiological Systems	
3	Root Operation	0 Atmospheric Control	5 Pheresis
		1 Decompression	6 Phototherapy
		2 Electromagnetic Therapy	7 Ultrasound Therapy
		3 Hyperthermia	8 Ultraviolet Light Therapy
		4 Hypothermia	9 Shock Wave Therapy
4	Body System	0 Skin	3 Musculoskeletal
		1 Urinary	5 Circulatory
		2 Central Nervous	Z None
5	Duration	0 Single	
		1 Multiple	
6	Qualifier	Z No Qualifier	

(continued)

Character	Meaning	Values	
7	Qualifier	0 Erythrocytes	6 Peripheral Vessels
		1 Leukocytes	7 Other Vessels
		2 Platelets	T Stem Cells, Cord Blood
		3 Plasma	V Stem Cells, Hematopoietic
		4 Head and Neck Vessels	Z No Qualifier
		5 Heart	

Assign ICD-10-PCS codes for the following situations, applying any appropriate sequencing guidelines.

1. Circulatory phototherapy, single treatment _____

2. Single hypothermia treatment for temperature imbalance _____

3. Multiple UV light treatments _____

4. Multiple electromagnetic therapy treatments on the central nervous system _____

5. Multiple decompression treatments for elimination of undissolved gas from the circulatory system _____

Beyond the Code: What kind of documentation issues may be encountered related to coding hyperthermia in patients receiving cancer treatment? How might you prevent or address them to ensure accurate coding in the Extracorporeal Therapies section versus the Radiation Oncology section?

29.3 Osteopathic Procedures

Osteopathic medicine addresses concerns with disturbances in the musculoskeletal system. Conditions for which these procedures need to be performed may result from accidents, injuries, surgery, or other abnormal metabolic or diseased states. Mechanical manipulations and other therapeutic modalities can be combined with pharmacotherapy to achieve the best results for those patients in need of these services. It is hoped that the outcome of these interventions will eliminate or alleviate somatic dysfunction and any associated disorders.

All codes in the Osteopathic section have a 1st character value of 7. The 2nd character value of W represents anatomic regions for this section. Treatment is the only root operation for the Osteopathic section. Treatment is defined as manual elimination or alleviation of somatic dysfunction and related disorders. **Osteopathic treatment** for fascial release of the abdomen is an example. This procedure is coded to 7W00X1Z (see Table 29.18).

Body regions on which osteopathic treatment are performed are reported by values for character 4, which represent the head, cervical, thoracic, lumbar, sacrum, pelvis, lower extremities, upper extremities, rib cage, or abdomen. The approach, reported by character 5, is reported with the value of X for all procedures in this section, as all are performed externally.

osteopathic treatment
Manual elimination or alleviation of somatic dysfunction and related disorders in the musculoskeletal system.

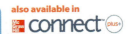
Assign ICD-10-PCS codes for the following situations, applying any appropriate sequencing guidelines.

1. Collection of cerebrospinal fluid _____

2. Therapeutic massage of the rectum; male reproductive _____

3. Near infrared spectroscopy of the circulatory system _____

4. Sperm collection; male reproductive _____

5. Yoga therapy _____

Beyond the Code: What kind of nontraditional treatments are you aware of that are performed in your area? What kind of documentation requirements should be considered for those specific treatments?

29.5 Chiropractic Procedures

chiropractic Manual manipulations that involve a directed thrust to move a joint past the physiological range of motion, without exceeding the anatomic limit.

According to ICD-10-PCS, **chiropractic** procedures involve manual manipulations defined as a directed thrust to move a joint past the physiological range of motion, without exceeding the anatomic limit. This may be necessary for patients who are trying to heal postoperatively or as an alternative to surgery. Many patients seeking chiropractic services have been in automobile accidents or occupational accidents that cause a great deal of pain and immobility, time away from work, and decreased quality of life.

All codes in the Chiropractic section have a 1st character value of 9. The value of W, which identifies anatomic regions, is the only option for character 2 in this section. There is also only one root operation value, B, which represents manipulation, for character 3 in the Chiropractic section.

Character 4 values identify the body region for the procedure, including head, cervical, thoracic, lumbar, sacrum, pelvis, lower extremities, upper extremities, rib cage, and abdomen. All procedures reported in the Chiropractic section are performed with an external approach, which is coded with the value of X for character 5. Methods are reported with character 6, which includes values to identify methods that include non-manual, indirect visceral, extra-articular, direct visceral, long lever specific contact, long and short lever specific contact, mechanically assisted, and other methods. No qualifiers have been specified for the Chiropractic section, so the value for character 7 is always Z to identify the qualifier as "none."

Table 29.22 provides character meanings and values for codes in the Chiropractic section.

CODING TIP ▶

There is only one value for characters 1, 2, 3, 5, and 7 in the Chiropractic section.

Table 29.22 Character Meanings and Values for the Chiropractic Section

Character	Meaning	Values	
1	Section	9 Chiropractic	
2	Anatomic Regions	W Anatomic Regions	
3	Root Operation	B Manipulation	
4	Body Region	0 Head	5 Pelvis
		1 Cervical	6 Lower Extremities
		2 Thoracic	7 Upper Extremities
		3 Lumbar	8 Rib Cage
		4 Sacrum	9 Abdomen
5	Approach	X External	
6	Method	B Non-manual	G Long Lever Specific Contact
		C Indirect Visceral	J Long and Short Lever Specific Contact
		D Extra-articular	K Mechanically Assisted
		F Direct Visceral	L Other Method
7	Qualifier	Z None	

Think About It 29.5

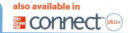
also available in

Assign ICD-10-PCS codes for the following situations, applying any appropriate sequencing guidelines.

1. Direct visceral manipulation of the sacrum _____

2. Mechanically assisted procedure for lumbar spine _____

3. Treatment of sacrum using a long and short lever specific contact _____

4. Lumbar manipulation using a long lever specific contact _____

5. Extra-articular treatment of the knee _____

Beyond the Code: ICD-10-PCS procedures were created for use in the inpatient setting. What kind of chiropractic procedures might you expect to code in an inpatient setting?

Chapter Summary

Learning Outcome	Key Concepts/Examples
29.1 Identify character values for coding extracorporeal assistance and performance procedures. **(pages 533–536)**	• All codes in the Extracorporeal Assistance and Performance section have a 1st character value of 5. • Assistance, performance, and restoration are the three values for character 3, root operation.
29.2 Define root operations for extracorporeal therapy procedures. **(pages 536–541)**	• All codes in the Extracorporeal Therapies section have a 1st character value of 6. • There are 10 values for the root operation, which include atmospheric control, decompression, electromagnetic therapy, hyperthermia, hypothermia, pheresis, phototherapy, ultrasound therapy, ultraviolet light therapy, and shock wave therapy. • There are no qualifiers specified for character 6 in the Extracorporeal Therapies section, so this value will always be reported with a value of Z, which represents "no qualifier."
29.3 Discuss procedures that are performed as osteopathic manipulation treatments. **(pages 541–543)**	• All codes in the Osteopathic section have a 1st character value of 7. • Treatment is the only root operation for the Osteopathic section. • All procedures in the Osteopathic section are performed externally.
29.4 Build codes for procedures in the Other Procedures section for nontraditional methods of treatment. **(pages 543–546)**	• All codes in the Other Procedures section have a 1st character value of 8. • Physiological systems and anatomic regions are performed using methods that include acupuncture, therapeutic massage, collection, computer-assisted procedure, robotic-assisted procedure, near infrared spectroscopy, and other methods.
29.5 Select the appropriate method of manipulation for chiropractic procedures. **(pages 546–547)**	• All codes in the Chiropractic section have a 1st character value of 9. • There is only one value for characters 1, 2, 3, 5, and 7 in the Chiropractic section.

Applying Your Skills

Identify the section and root operation for each of the following procedures; then assign ICD-10-PCS codes.

Procedure	Section	Root Operation	ICD-10-PCS Code
1. *[LO 29.1]* CPAP for 8 hours	_____	_____	_____
2. *[LO 29.2]* Multiple extracorporeal UV treatments of the skin	_____	_____	_____
3. *[LO 29.3]* Indirect osteopathic treatment of the rib cage	_____	_____	_____
4. *[LO 29.4]* Collection of breast milk	_____	_____	_____
5. *[LO 29.5]* Mechanically assisted chiropractic manipulation of the pelvis	_____	_____	_____
6. *[LO 29.1]* Performance of single urinary filtration	_____	_____	_____
7. *[LO 29.2]* Single extracorporeal hyperthermia treatment	_____	_____	_____
8. *[LO 29.3]* Low velocity–high amplitude osteopathic treatment of the head	_____	_____	_____
9. *[LO 29.4]* Yoga therapy	_____	_____	_____
10. *[LO 29.5]* Direct visceral chiropractic manipulation of the cervical spine	_____	_____	_____
11. *[LO 29.1]* Single extracorporeal restoration of cardiac rhythm	_____	_____	_____
12. *[LO 29.2]* Single extracorporeal platelet pheresis	_____	_____	_____
13. *[LO 29.3]* Osteopathic lumbar fascial release	_____	_____	_____
14. *[LO 29.4]* Therapeutic external prostate massage	_____	_____	_____
15. *[LO 29.5]* Indirect visceral chiropractic manipulation of the abdomen	_____	_____	_____
16. *[LO 29.1]* Intermittent performance of extracorporeal cardiac pacing	_____	_____	_____
17. *[LO 29.2]* Single extracorporeal ultrasound treatment of the heart	_____	_____	_____
18. *[LO 29.3]* Osteopathic lumbar pump of the thoracic region	_____	_____	_____
19. *[LO 29.4]* Removal of sutures from the forehead	_____	_____	_____
20. *[LO 29.5]* Long lever specific contact chiropractic manipulation of the left leg	_____	_____	_____

Checking Your Understanding

Select the letter that best answers the question or completes the sentence.

1. *[LO 29.2]* A procedure performed in a hyperbaric chamber to eliminate undissolved gas from body fluids using extracorporeal means is
   a. atmospheric control.
   b. decompression.
   c. pheresis.
   d. ultrasound therapy.

2. *[LO 29.4]* How many root operations are in the Other Procedures section?
   a. 0
   b. 1
   c. 2
   d. 6

3. *[LO 29.1]* Which root operation is assigned for a failed attempt at external cardioversion?
   a. assistance
   b. performance
   c. restoration
   d. attempt

4. *[LO 29.3]* What is the only root operation in the Osteopathic section?
   a. adjustment
   b. manipulation
   c. restoration
   d. treatment

5. *[LO 29.5]* Which characters in the Chiropractic section have only one value?
   a. 1
   b. 1 and 2
   c. 1, 2, 3, 5, and 7
   d. 1–7

6. *[LO 29.4]* What is the 1st character value for the Other Procedures section?
   a. 6
   b. 7
   c. 8
   d. 9

7. *[LO 29.1]* Which value for character 5 may be assigned for the performance of non-mechanical ventilation?
   a. single
   b. continuous
   c. intermittent
   d. less than 24 consecutive hours

8. *[LO 29.5]* What is the only root operation in the Chiropractic section?
   a. adjustment
   b. manipulation
   c. restoration
   d. treatment

9. *[LO 29.3]* What is the 1st character value for the Osteopathic section?
   a. 6
   b. 7
   c. 8
   d. 9

10. **[LO 29.2]** How many body systems are specified for the Extracorporeal Therapies section?

   a. 0
   b. 1
   c. 3
   d. 6

Online Activity

[LO 29.1, LO 29.2] This chapter presents some procedures that may not have been covered in detail in a regular medical terminology course. Identify three procedures that are unfamiliar to you and search for information about them online, using reputable medical websites. Summarize your findings about each procedure in a brief report.

Real-World Application: Case Study

[LO 29.5] Using ICD-10-PCS, code the procedure(s) for the following chiropractic progress note.

S : Patient with continued neck pain following automobile accident two days ago. States pain is decreasing, but still experiences tightness.

O: Examination of the cervical spine reveals moderate muscle tension of the cervical spine with C1 and C4 subluxation.

A: Cervical strain with C1 and C5 subluxation

P : Short lever adjustment of C1 and C5 was performed. Re-evaluation and additional adjustment tomorrow.

30

ICD-10-PCS SECTIONS B–H

Learning Outcomes *After completing this chapter, students should be able to*

30.1 Classify imaging procedures according to root type.

30.2 Apply rules for coding nuclear medicine procedures.

30.3 Describe radiation oncology modalities.

30.4 Define the components of physical rehabilitation and diagnostic audiology coding.

30.5 Discuss the rationale for coding mental health procedures.

30.6 Identify types of substance abuse treatment.

Key Terms

beam radiation therapy
biofeedback
brachytherapy
cochlear implant
counseling
crisis intervention
detoxification
diagnostic audiology
electroconvulsive therapy
fluoroscopy
hypnosis
individual psychotherapy
isotope
light therapy
medication management
modality
motor
narcosynthesis
pharmacotherapy
physical rehabilitation
psychological tests
radionuclide
radiopharmaceutical
stereotactic radiosurgery
substance abuse

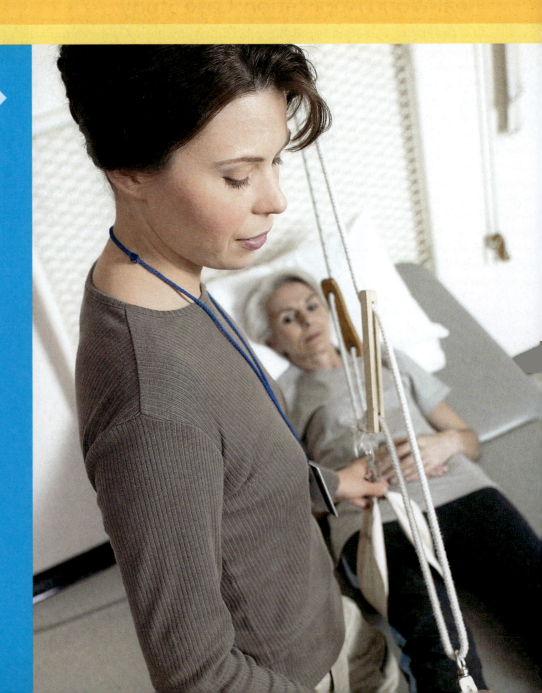

Introduction

The third set of sections of ICD-10-PCS, sections B–H, provides codes for procedures classified as imaging, nuclear medicine, radiation oncology, physical rehabilitation and diagnostic audiology, mental health, and substance abuse treatment. As in Sections 0–9, the section value of the ICD-10-PCS code is identified first by the coder, defining the general type of procedure performed and determining the values for the 2nd through 7th characters of the ICD-10-PCS code. The values for these characters can vary depending on the section into which the procedure is classified, because the factors of each type of procedure vary, but they typically identify such factors as body system and root operation. Like the rest of ICD-10-PCS, coding from sections B–H requires a step-by-step identification of the procedure and building of the corresponding ICD-10-PCS code.

30.1 Imaging Section

Codes in the Imaging section describe procedures used to view or generate images of parts of the body. All codes in the Imaging section have a 1st character value of B. 2nd character values represent body systems, which include the following:

1. Central nervous system
2. Heart
3. Upper arteries
4. Lower arteries
5. Veins
6. Lymphatic system
7. Eye
8. Ear, nose, mouth, and throat
9. Respiratory system
10. Gastrointestinal system
11. Hepatobiliary system and pancreas
12. Endocrine system
13. Skin, subcutaneous tissue, and breast
14. Connective tissue
15. Skull and facial bones
16. Non-axial upper bones
17. Non-axial lower bones
18. Axial skeleton, except skull and facial bones
19. Urinary system
20. Female reproductive system
21. Male reproductive system
22. Anatomic regions
23. Fetus and obstetrical

Character 3 in the Imaging section has values to represent the root type for the procedure. The values represent procedures performed by means

- Central nervous system
- Heart
- Veins
- Lymphatic and hematologic system
- Eye
- Ear, nose, mouth, and throat
- Respiratory system
- Gastrointestinal system
- Hepatobiliary system and pancreas
- Endocrine system
- Skin, subcutaneous tissue, and breast
- Musculoskeletal system
- Urinary system
- Male reproductive system
- Anatomic regions

Character 3 identifies the root type for nuclear medicine procedures. Values for this character specify the root types as planar nuclear medicine imaging, tomographic (tomo) nuclear medicine imaging, positron emission tomographic (PET) imaging, nonimaging nuclear medicine uptake, nonimaging nuclear medicine probe, nonimaging nuclear medicine assay, or systemic nuclear medicine therapy.

- *Nonimaging nuclear medicine assay* is the introduction of radioactive materials into the body for the study of body fluids and blood elements, by the detection of radioactive emissions.
- *Nonimaging nuclear medicine probe* is the introduction of radioactive materials into the body for the study of distribution and fate of certain substances by the detection of radioactive emissions; or, alternatively, measurement of absorption of radioactive emissions from an external source.
- *Nonimaging nuclear medicine uptake* introduces radioactive materials into the body for measurements of organ function, from the detection of radioactive emissions.
- *Planar nuclear medicine imaging* is the introduction of radioactive materials into the body for single plane display of images developed from the capture of radioactive emissions.
- *Positron emission tomographic (PET) imaging* introduces radioactive materials into the body for three-dimensional display of images developed from the simultaneous capture, 180 degrees apart, of radioactive emissions.
- *Systemic nuclear medicine therapy* is the introduction of unsealed radioactive materials into the body for treatment.
- *Tomographic (tomo) nuclear medicine imaging* introduces radioactive materials into the body for three-dimensional display of images developed from the capture of radioactive emissions

The values for body parts in character 4 are specified for each body system. The **radionuclide,** or source of radiation, is specified through values for character 5, which include the following:

radionuclide Source of radiation.

- Technetium 99m (Tc-99m)
- Cobalt 58 (Co-58)
- Samarium 153 (Sm-153)
- Krypton (Kr-81m)
- Carbon 11 (C-11)
- Cobalt 57 (Co-57)
- Indium 111 (In-111)
- Iodine 123 (I-123)
- Iodine 131 (I-131)
- Iodine 125 (I-125)
- Fluorine 18 (F-18)
- Gallium 67 (Ga67)
- Oxygen 15 (O-15)
- Phosphorus 32 (P-32)
- Strontium 89 (Sr-89)
- Rubidium 82 (Rb-82)
- Nitrogen 13 (N-13)
- Thallium 201 (Tl-201)
- Xenon 127 (Xe-127)
- Xenon 133 (Xe-133)
- Chromium 51 (Cr-51)
- Other radionuclide
- None

Characters 6 and 7 are both identified as qualifiers for the Nuclear Medicine section. No values are specified for these characters, so they should both be reported with the value of Z for "none." Table 30.2 provides character meanings and values for the Nuclear Medicine section.

CODING TIP ▶

If more than one **radiopharmaceutical** is used for nuclear medicine procedures, more than one code should be assigned.

radiopharmaceutical
Radioactive drug that is implanted.

Table 30.2 Character Meanings and Values for the Nuclear Medicine Section

Character	Meaning	Values	
1	Section	C Nuclear Medicine	
2	Body System	0 Central Nervous System	F Hepatobiliary System and Pancreas
		2 Heart	
		5 Veins	G Endocrine System
		7 Lymphatic and Hematologic System	H Skin, Subcutaneous Tissue, and Breast
		8 Eye	P Musculoskeletal System
		9 Ear, Nose, Mouth, and Throat	T Urinary System
			V Male Reproductive System
		B Respiratory System	W Anatomic Regions
		D Gastrointestinal System	

(continued)

isotope Atom having the same atomic number (same name) but a different mass number than similar atoms.

CODING TIP ▸

Whereas the modality is identified in character 3 for the root type in the Radiation Oncology section, character 5 values provide further specification of the modality.

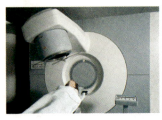

Radiation oncology procedures are classified by body system, type of radiation, treatment site, radiation substance used, and whether the treatment is intra-operative.

- Low dose rate (LDR)
- Intra-operative radiation therapy (IORT)
- Stereotactic other photon radiosurgery
- Plaque radiation
- Isotope administration
- Stereotactic particulate radiosurgery
- Stereotactic gamma beam radiosurgery
- Laser interstitial thermal therapy

The **isotope** that is introduced in the procedure is specified through character 6 values, which include the following:

- Cesium 137 (Cs-137)
- Iridium 192 (Ir-192)
- Iodine 125 (I-125)
- Palladium 103 (Pd-103)
- Californium 252 (Cf-252)
- Iodine 131 (I-131)
- Phosphorus 32 (P-32)
- Strontium 89 (Sr-89)
- Strontium 90 (Sr-90)
- Other isotope
- None

Character 7 is a qualifier that has two possible values. The value of 0 represents intra-operative, and the value of Z represents none. Values and character meanings for the Radiation Oncology section codes are provided in Table 30.3.

Table 30.3 Character Meanings and Values for the Radiation Oncology Section

Character	Meaning	Values	
1	Section	D Radiation Oncology	
2	Body System	0 Central and Peripheral Nervous System	G Endocrine System
		7 Lymphatic and Hematologic System	H Skin
		8 Eye	M Breast
		9 Ear, Nose, Mouth, and Throat	P Musculoskeletal System
		B Respiratory System	T Urinary System
		D Gastrointestinal System	U Female Reproductive System
		F Hepatobiliary System and Pancreas	V Male Reproductive System
			W Anatomic Regions
3	Root Type	0 Beam Radiation	
		1 Brachytherapy	
		2 Stereotactic Radiosurgery	
		Y Other Radiation	

(continued)

Character	Meaning	Values	
4	Treatment Site	Treatment sites are specified for each body system.	
5	Modality Qualifier	0 Photons <1 MeV 1 Photons 1–10 MeV 2 Photons >10 MeV 3 Electrons 4 Heavy Particles (Protons, Ions) 5 Neutrons 6 Neutron Capture 7 Contact Radiation 8 Hyperthermia 9 High Dose Rate (HDR) B Low Dose Rate (LDR)	C Intra-operative Radiation Therapy (IORT) D Stereotactic Other Photon Radiosurgery F Plaque Radiation G Isotope Administration H Stereotactic Particulate Radiosurgery J Stereotactic Gamma Beam Radiosurgery K Laser Interstitial Thermal Therapy
6	Isotope	7 Cesium 137 (Cs-137) 8 Iridium 192 (Ir-192) 9 Iodine 125 (I-125) B Palladium 103 (Pd-103) C Californium 252 (Cf-252) D Iodine 131 (I-131)	F Phosphorus 32 (P-32) G Strontium 89 (Sr-89) H Strontium 90 (Sr-90) Y Other Isotope Z None
7	Qualifier	0 Intraoperative Z None	

Think About It 30.3

also available in **McGraw Hill connect** plus+

Assign ICD-10-PCS codes for the following situations, applying any appropriate sequencing guidelines.

1. Brachytherapy; lymphatics of the abdomen with high dose radiation and cesium 137 (cs-137) _____

2. Stereotactic radiosurgery of the inguinal lymphatics using gamma beam _____

3. Electron beam radiation of the nose _____

4. Photon beam radiation of the adrenal glands using <1 MeV photons _____

5. Stereotactic particulate radiosurgery of the gallbladder _____

Beyond the Code: Find information about what services and procedures are provided at a radiation oncology facility in your area. Describe your findings.

30.4 Physical Rehabilitation and Diagnostic Audiology Section

Physical rehabilitation spans a wide range of services used to improve and restore function and mobility to the body. **Diagnostic audiology,** classified with physical rehabilitation in ICD-10-PCS, refers to the use of diagnostic tests to determine the extent and nature of hearing loss in order to manage or treat it.

All codes in the Physical Rehabilitation and Diagnostic Audiology section have a 1st character value of 2. The 2nd character value in this section represents the section qualifier. There are two section qualifiers: rehabilitation, which is identified by the value of 0, and diagnostic audiology, which is identified by the value of 1. The root type, body system and region, type qualifier, and equipment values in this section are dependent on the section qualifier.

> **CODING TIP ▸**
>
> Because two types of services are classified in one section, the root type, body system and region, type qualifier, and equipment values in this section are dependent on the section qualifier of rehabilitation versus diagnostic audiology.

Character 3 represents the root type, for which values are dependent on the section qualifier of rehabilitation versus diagnostic audiology. There are four basic classifications for the root type values, which are assessment, caregiver training, fitting, and treatment. Root types for rehabilitation include speech assessment, motor and/or nerve function assessment, activities of daily living assessment, speech treatment, motor treatment, activities of daily living treatment, hearing treatment, cochlear implant treatment, vestibular treatment, device fitting, and caregiver training.

- *Activities of daily living assessment* measures the functional level for activities of daily living.
- *Activities of daily living treatment* facilitates functional competence for activities of daily living through exercise and other activities.
- *Caregiver training* involves training in activities that support the patient's optimal level of function.
- *Cochlear implant* treatment is an application of techniques used to improve the communication abilities of individuals with cochlear implants.
- *Device fitting* involves fitting of a device designed to facilitate or support achievement of a higher level of function.
- *Hearing treatment* applies techniques to improve, augment, or compensate for hearing and related functional impairment.
- *Motor and/or nerve function assessment* measures motor, nerve, and related functions.
- *Motor treatment* increases or facilitates motor function through exercise or other activities.

- *Speech assessment* measures speech and related functions.
- *Speech treatment* is the application of techniques to improve, augment, or compensate for speech and related functional impairment.
- *Vestibular treatment* involves the application of techniques to improve, augment, or compensate for vestibular and related functional impairment.

Root types for diagnostic audiology include hearing assessment, hearing aid assessment, and vestibular assessment.

- *Hearing aid assessment* measures the appropriateness and/or effectiveness of a hearing device.
- *Hearing assessment* measures hearing and related functions.
- *Vestibular assessment* measures vestibular system and related functions.

Character 4 values represent the body systems and region for rehabilitation, which include the following:

- Neurological system—head and neck
- Neurological system—upper back/upper extremity
- Neurological system—lower back/lower extremity
- Neurological system—whole body
- Circulatory system—head and neck
- Circulatory system—upper back/upper extremity
- Circulatory system—lower back/lower extremity
- Circulatory system—whole body
- Respiratory system—head and neck
- Respiratory system—upper back/upper extremity
- Respiratory system—lower back/lower extremity
- Respiratory system—whole body
- Integumentary system—head and neck
- Integumentary system—upper back/upper extremity
- Integumentary system—lower back/lower extremity
- Integumentary system—whole body
- Musculoskeletal system—head and neck
- Musculoskeletal system—upper back/upper extremity
- Musculoskeletal system—lower back/lower extremity
- Musculoskeletal system—whole body
- Genitourinary system
- None

There are no body systems or regions specified for diagnostic audiology, so the character 4 value assigned is Z, to indicate "none."

CODING TIP ▸

There are no body systems or regions specified for diagnostic audiology, so the character 4 value assigned is Z, to indicate "none."

Character 5 identifies the type qualifier. The values of this character vary according to the root type, and include the following:

- *Acoustic reflex decay* measures reduction in size/strength of acoustic reflex over time. Site of lesion testing is included.
- *Acoustic reflex patterns* defines the site of a lesion, based on the presence/absence of acoustic reflexes with ipsilateral versus contralateral stimulation.
- *Acoustic reflex threshold* determines minimal intensity that acoustic reflex occurs with ipsilateral and/or contralateral stimulation.
- *Aerobic capacity and endurance* measures autonomic responses to positional changes; perceived exertion, dyspnea, or angina during activity; performance during exercise protocols; standard vital signs; and blood gas analysis or oxygen consumption.
- *Alternate binaural or monaural loudness balance* determines the auditory stimulus parameter that yields the same objective sensation. This includes sound intensities that yield the same loudness perception.
- *Anthropometric characteristics* measures edema, body fat composition, height, weight, length, and girth.
- *Aphasia (assessment)* measures expressive and receptive speech and language function, including reading and writing.
- *Aphasia (treatment)* applies techniques for the purpose of improving, augmenting, or compensating for receptive/expressive language impairments.
- *Articulation/phonology (assessment)* measures speech production.
- *Articulation/phonology (treatment)* applies techniques for the purpose of correcting, improving, or compensating for speech productive impairment.
- *Assistive listening device* assists in the use of an effective and appropriate assistive listening device/system.
- *Assistive listening system/device selection* measures the effectiveness and appropriateness of assistive listening systems/devices.
- *Assistive, adaptive, supportive, or protective devices* facilitate or support achievement of a higher level of function in wheelchair mobility; bed mobility; transfer or ambulation ability; bath and showering ability; dressing; grooming; personal hygiene; and play or leisure.
- *Auditory evoked potentials* measures electric responses produced by the cranial nerve VIII and brainstem following auditory stimulation.
- *Auditory processing (assessment)* is an evaluation of the ability to receive and process auditory information and comprehension of spoken language.
- *Auditory processing (treatment)* involves application of techniques to improve the receiving and processing of auditory information and comprehension of spoken language.
- *Augmentative/alternative communication system (assessment)* determines the appropriateness of aids, techniques, symbols, and/or strategies to augment or replace speech and enhance communication, including the use of telephones, writing equipment, emergency equipment, and TDD.

- *Augmentative/alternative communication system (treatment)* is treatment using augmentative communication devices and aids.
- *Aural rehabilitation* involves the application of techniques for the purpose of improving the communication abilities associated with hearing loss.
- *Aural rehabilitation status* measures the impact of a hearing loss, including evaluation of receptive and expressive communication skills.
- *Bathing/showering* involves obtaining and using supplies; soaping, rinsing, and drying body parts; maintaining bathing position; and transferring to and from bathing positions.
- *Bathing/showering techniques* address activities that facilitate obtaining and using supplies, soaping, rinsing and drying body parts, maintaining bathing position, and transferring to and from bathing positions.
- *Bed mobility (assessment)* addresses transitional movement within bed.
- *Bed mobility (treatment)* involves exercise or activities for the purpose of facilitating transitional movements within bed.
- *Bedside swallowing and oral function* involve assessment of bedside swallowing, which includes sucking, masticating, coughing, and swallowing, and oral function, which includes assessment of musculature for controlled movements, structures, and functions to determine coordination and phonation.
- *Bekesy audiometry* is performed using an instrument that provides a choice of discrete or continuously varying pure tones; choice of pulsed or continuous signal.
- *Binaural electroacoustic hearing aid check* determines mechanical and electroacoustic function of bilateral hearing aids using hearing aid test box.
- *Binaural hearing aid (assessment)* measures the candidacy, effectiveness, and appropriateness of hearing aids. Bilateral hearing aid fit is measured.
- *Binaural hearing aid (treatment)* assists in achieving maximum understanding and performance.
- *Bithermal, binaural caloric irrigation* measures the rhythmic eye movements stimulated by changing the temperature of the vestibular system.
- *Bithermal, monaural caloric irrigation* measures the rhythmic eye movements stimulated by changing the temperature of the vestibular system in one ear.
- *Brief tone stimuli* measure specific central auditory process.
- *Cerumen management* involves an examination of external auditory canal and tympanic membrane and the removal of cerumen from external ear canal.
- *Cochlear implant* measures candidacy for cochlear implant.
- *Cochlear implant rehabilitation* applies techniques to improve the communication abilities of individuals with cochlear implants, including programming the device and providing patients/families with information.
- *Communicative/cognitive integration skills (assessment)* measures ability to use higher cortical functions, including orientation, recognition,

- *Visual reinforcement audiometry* involves behavioral measures using non-speech and speech stimuli to obtain frequency/ear-specific information on auditory status, including a conditioned response of looking toward a visual reinforcer (e.g., lights, animated toy) every time auditory stimuli are heard.
- *Vocational activities and functional community or work reintegration skills (assessment)* measure environmental, home, and work (job/school/play) barriers that keep patients from functioning optimally in their environment. The measurements also assess vocational skills and interests, work environment (job/school/play), injury potential and injury prevention or reduction, ergonomic stressors, transportation skills, and ability to access and use community resources.
- *Vocational activities and functional community or work reintegration skills (treatment)* involve activities to facilitate vocational exploration, body mechanics training, job acquisition, and environmental or work (job/school/play) task adaptation. The activities address injury prevention and reduction, ergonomic stressor reduction, job coaching and simulation, work hardening and conditioning, driving training, transportation skills, and use of community resources.
- *Voice (assessment)* measures vocal structure, function, and production.
- *Voice (treatment)* uses techniques to improve the voice and vocal function.
- *Voice prosthetic (assessment)* determines the appropriateness of a voice prosthetic/adaptive device to enhance or facilitate communication.
- *Voice prosthetic (treatment)* involves the use of electrolarynx and other assistive, adaptive, supportive devices.
- *Wheelchair mobility (assessment)* measures fit and functional abilities within a wheelchair in a variety of environments.
- *Wheelchair mobility (treatment)* manages, maintains, and controls the operation of a wheelchair, scooter, or other device in and on a variety of surfaces and environments.
- *Wound management* involves non-selective and selective debridement (enzymes, autolysis, sharp debridement), dressings (wound coverings, hydrogel, vacuum-assisted closure), topical agents, and other methods.

Diagnostic audiology involves the use of a variety of devices to determine and treat hearing loss. Character 6 specifies equipment, with values that are dependent on the section qualifier of rehabilitation versus diagnostic audiology. Equipment character values for rehabilitation include the following:

- Audiometer
- Sound field/booth
- Tympanometer
- Electroacoustic immittance/acoustic reflex
- Hearing aid selection/fitting/test
- Electrophysiologic
- Vestibular/balance

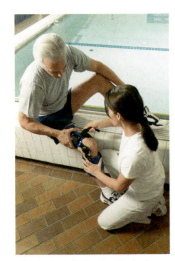

Physical rehabilitation includes a variety of services because there are a wide range of injuries and conditions that can be treated through rehabilitation.

- Cochlear implant
- Physical agents
- Mechanical
- Electrotherapeutic
- Orthosis
- Assistive, adaptive, supportive, or protective
- Aerobic endurance and conditioning
- Mechanical or electromechanical
- Somatosensory
- Audiovisual
- Assistive listening
- Augmentative/alternative communication
- Biosensory feedback
- Computer
- Speech analysis
- Voice analysis
- Aerodynamic function
- Prosthesis
- Speech prosthesis
- Swallowing
- Cerumen management
- Other equipment
- None

Equipment character values for diagnostic audiology include the following:

- Occupational hearing
- Audiometer
- Sound field/booth
- Tympanometer
- Electroacoustic immittance/acoustic reflex
- Hearing aid selection/fitting test
- Otoacoustic emission (OAE)
- Electrophysiologic
- Vestibular/balance
- Cochlear implant
- Audiovisual
- Assistive listening
- Computer
- Other equipment
- None

There are no qualifiers specified for the Physical Rehabilitation and Diagnostic Audiology section, so the value reported for this character is Z to indicate "none." Table 30.4 outlines character meanings and values for codes in the Physical Rehabilitation and Diagnostic Audiology section.

Table 30.4 Character Meanings and Values in the Physical Rehabilitation and Diagnostic Audiology Section

Character	Meaning	Values	
1	Section	F Physical Rehabilitation and Diagnostic Audiology	
2	Section Qualifier	0 Rehabilitation 1 Diagnostic Audiology	
3	Root Type	Section Qualifier 0	Section Qualifier 1
		0 Speech Assessment	3 Hearing Assessment
		1 Motor and/or Nerve Function Assessment	4 Hearing Aid Assessment
		2 Activities of Daily Living Assessment	5 Vestibular Assessment
		6 Speech Treatment	
		7 Motor Treatment	
		8 Activities of Daily Living Treatment	
		9 Hearing Treatment	
		B Cochlear Implant Treatment	
		C Vestibular Treatment	
		D Device Fitting	
		F Caregiver Training	
4	Body System and Region	Section Qualifier 0	Section Qualifier 1
		0 Neurological System—Head and Neck	Z None
		1 Neurological System—Upper Back/Upper extremity	
		2 Neurological System—Lower Back/Lower Extremity	
		3 Neurological System—Whole Body	
		4 Circulatory System—Head and Neck	
		5 Circulatory System—Upper Back/Upper Extremity	
		6 Circulatory System—Lower Back/Lower Extremity	
		7 Circulatory System—Whole Body	
		8 Respiratory System—Head and Neck	
		9 Respiratory System—Upper Back/Upper Extremity	

(continued)

Character	Meaning	Values	
		Section Qualifier 0	Section Qualifier 1
		B Respiratory System—Lower Back/Lower Extremity	
		C Respiratory System—Whole Body	
		D Integumentary System—Head and Neck	
		F Integumentary System—Upper Back/Upper Extremity	
		G Integumentary System—Lower Back/Lower Extremity	
		H Integumentary System—Whole Body	
		J Musculoskeletal System—Head and Neck	
		K Musculoskeletal System—Upper Back/Upper Extremity	
		L Musculoskeletal System—Lower Back/Lower Extremity	
		M Musculoskeletal System—Whole Body	
		N Genitourinary System	
		Z None	
5	Type Qualifier	Values for type qualifiers are located in the tables section of the ICD-10-PCS manual.	
6	Equipment	Section Qualifier 0	Section Qualifier 1
		1 Audiometer	0 Occupational Hearing
		2 Sound Field/Booth	1 Audiometer
		3 Tympanometer	2 Sound Field/Booth
		4 Electroacoustic Immittance/Acoustic Reflex	3 Tympanometer
		5 Hearing Aid Selection/Fitting/Test	4 Electroacoustic ImmitTance/Acoustic Reflex
		7 Electrophysiologic	5 Hearing Aid Selection/Fitting/Test
		8 Vestibular/Balance	6 Otoacoustic Emission (OAE)
		9 Cochlear Implant	7 Electrophysiologic
		B Physical Agents	8 Vestibular/Balance
		C Mechanical	9 Cochlear Implant
		D Electrotherapeutic	
		E Orthosis	
		F Assistive, Adaptive, Supportive, or Protective	

(continued)

Character	Meaning	Values	
		Section Qualifier 0	Section Qualifier 1
		G Aerobic Endurance and Conditioning	K Audiovisual
		H Mechanical or Electromechanical	L Assistive Listening
		J Somatosensory	P Computer
		K Audiovisual	Y Other Equipment
		L Assistive Listening	Z None
		M Augmentative/ Alternative Communication	
		N Biosensory Feedback	
		P Computer	
		Q Speech Analysis	
		S Voice Analysis	
		T Aerodynamic Function	
		U Prosthesis	
		V Speech Prosthesis	
		W Swallowing	
		X Cerumen Management	
		Y Other Equipment	
		Z None	
7	Qualifier	Z None	

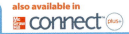

Think About It 30.4

also available in

Assign ICD-10-PCS codes for the following situations, applying any appropriate sequencing guidelines.

1. Speech assessment for aphasia utilizing computer equipment _____

2. Motor and nerve function assessment of muscle performance of the lower back with prosthesis _____

3. Voice assessment and analysis _____

4. Biosensory feedback motor speech treatment _____

5. Aerobic endurance and conditioning for the respiratory system; whole body therapeutic exercise _____

Beyond the Code: Why do you think no values are assigned to character 4 for the diagnostic audiology section qualifier of the Physical Rehabilitation and Diagnostic Audiology section?

30.5 Mental Health Section

Services for mental health include medication management, clinical treatments, and a wide variety of behavioral therapies. All codes in the Mental Health section have a first character value of G. While other sections use character 2 for the purpose of identifying the body system, the Mental Health section does not specify a body system, so the value reported is Z to reflect "none."

> **CODING TIP ▸**
>
> The Mental Health section does not specify a body system, so the value for character 2 is reported as Z to reflect "none."

Character 3 in the Mental Health section specifies the type of procedure with values to identify psychological tests, crisis intervention, medication management, individual psychotherapy, counseling, family psychotherapy, electroconvulsive therapy, biofeedback, hypnosis, narcosynthesis, group psychotherapy, or light therapy.

- *Biofeedback* involves the provision of information from monitoring and regulating physiological processes, along with cognitive-behavioral techniques to improve patient functioning or well-being. Some examples of biofeedback are EEG, EMG, blood pressure, and skin temperature.

- *Counseling* applies psychological methods to treating an individual with normal developmental issues and psychological problems to increase function, improve well-being, alleviate distress or maladjustment, or resolve crises.

- *Crisis intervention* is defined as treating a traumatized, acutely disturbed, or distressed individual for the purpose of short-term stabilization. This may involve counseling, psychotherapy, or coordinating care among other providers.

- *Electroconvulsive therapy* is a procedure that applies controlled electrical voltages for the purpose of treating a mental health disorder. The procedure includes appropriate sedation and other preparation of the individual.

- *Family psychotherapy* is a method of treatment including one or more family members of a patient with a mental health disorder by means of behavioral, cognitive, psychoanalytic, psychodynamic, or psychophysiological treatment in order to improve functioning or well-being.

- *Group psychotherapy* involves the treatment of two or more individuals with mental health disorders through behavioral, cognitive, psychoanalytic, psychodynamic, or psychophysiological methods for the purpose of improving functioning or well-being.

- *Hypnosis* is a procedure that induces a state of heightened suggestibility using auditory, visual, and tactile techniques in order to elicit an emotional or behavioral response.

biofeedback Technique of learning to control one's own body by monitoring brain waves, blood pressure, or other physiological measurement for the purpose of improving functioning or well-being.

counseling Applying psychological methods for the purpose of treating an individual with normal developmental issues and psychological problems to improve well-being and alleviate distress.

crisis intervention Treating a traumatized, acutely disturbed, or distressed individual for the purpose of short-term stabilization.

electroconvulsive therapy Procedure that applies controlled electrical voltages for the purpose of treating a mental health disorder.

hypnosis Procedure that induces a state of heightened suggestibility using auditory, visual, and tactile techniques in order to elicit an emotional or behavioral response.

individual psychotherapy
Treatment of an individual with a mental health disorder by behavioral, cognitive, psychoanalytic, psychodynamic, or psychophysiological means to improve functioning or well-being.

light therapy Application of specialized light treatments for the purpose of improving functioning or well-being.

medication management Monitoring and necessary adjustments of medications prescribed to treat a mental health disorder.

narcosynthesis Procedure in which intravenous barbiturates are administered for the purpose of releasing suppressed or repressed thoughts.

psychological tests Standardized psychological measurement instruments administered and interpreted to assess psychological function.

- *Individual psychotherapy* is the treatment of an individual with a mental health disorder by behavioral, cognitive, psychoanalytic, psychodynamic, or psychophysiological means to improve functioning or well-being.
- *Light therapy* involves the application of specialized light treatments for the purpose of improving functioning or well-being.
- *Medication management* is simply the monitoring and necessary adjustment of medications that are prescribed to treat a mental health disorder.
- *Narcosynthesis* is a procedure in which intravenous barbiturates are administered for the purpose of releasing suppressed or repressed thoughts.
- *Psychological* **tests** are standardized tests and measurement instruments administered and interpreted to assess psychological function.

Character 4 in the Mental Health section is called a type qualifier. The type qualifier provides further specificity about the root type. Physiological type qualifiers are developmental, personality and behavioral, intellectual and psychoeducational, neuropsychological, and neurobehavioral and cognitive status.

- *Developmental type* qualifier identifies an age-normed developmental status of cognitive, social, and adaptive behavior skills.
- *Personality and behavioral* refer to mood, emotion, behavior, social functioning, psychopathological conditions, personality traits, and characteristics.
- *Intellectual and psychoeducational* identify intellectual abilities, academic achievement, and learning capabilities, which include behaviors and emotional factors affecting learning.
- *Neuropsychological* is thinking, reasoning and judgment, acquired knowledge, attention, memory, visual spatial abilities, language functions, and planning.
- *Neurobehavioral and cognitive status* includes performance of a neurobehavioral status exam, interview(s), and observation to make a clinical assessment of thinking, reasoning and judgment, acquired knowledge, attention, memory, visual spatial abilities, language functions, and planning.

Individual psychotherapy type qualifiers are interactive, behavioral, cognitive, interpersonal, psychoanalysis, psychodynamic, supportive, cognitive-behavioral, and psychophysiological.

- *Interactive* uses primarily physical aids and other forms of non-oral interaction with a patient who is physically, psychologically or developmentally unable to use ordinary language for communication. This may include the use of toys in symbolic play.
- *Behavioral* is primarily for the purpose of behavioral modification. Methods include modeling and role-playing, positive reinforcement of target behaviors, response cost, and training of self-management skills.
- *Cognitive* is primarily for correction of cognitive distortions and errors.

- *Cognitive-behavioral* combines cognitive and behavioral treatment strategies in order to improve functioning. This includes an examination of maladaptive responses in order to determine how cognitions relate to behavior patterns in response to an event. The method uses learning principles and information-processing models.

- *Interpersonal therapy* helps an individual change interpersonal behaviors in order to reduce psychological dysfunction. Methods include exploratory techniques, encouragement of affective expression, clarification of patient statements, analysis of communication patterns, use of therapy relationship, and behavior change techniques.

- *Psychoanalysis* uses methods of obtaining a detailed accounting of past and present mental and emotional experiences in order to determine the source and eliminate or diminish the undesirable effects of unconscious conflicts. This is accomplished by making the individual aware of their existence, origin, and inappropriate expression in emotions and behavior.

- *Psychodynamic* is the exploration of past and present emotional experiences for the purpose of understanding motives and drives using insight-oriented techniques to reduce the undesirable effects of internal conflicts on emotions and behavior. This method uses techniques such as empathetic listening, clarifying self-defeating behavior patterns, and exploring adaptive alternatives.

- *Psychophysiological* monitors and alters physiological processes for the purpose of helping the individual associate physiological reactions combined with cognitive and behavioral strategies to gain improved control of these processes to help the individual cope more effectively.

- *Supportive* is the formation of a therapeutic relationship for the primary purpose of providing emotional support in order to prevent further deterioration in functioning during periods of particular stress. This method is often used in conjunction with other therapeutic approaches.

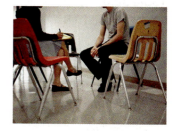

Therapies to monitor and improve mental health include various types of counseling, drug treatments, and treatments such as light therapy and hypnosis.

Counseling type qualifiers are educational, vocational, and other counseling. Vocational counseling is the exploration of vocational interests, aptitudes, and required adaptive behavior skills to develop and carry out a plan for achieving a successful vocational placement. Methods include enhancing work-related adjustment and pursuing viable options in training education or preparation. There is only one value specified for the family psychotherapy type qualifier, which is other family psychotherapy.

Electroconvulsive therapy type qualifiers are unilateral-single seizure, unilateral-multiple seizure, bilateral-single seizure, bilateral-multiple seizure, and other electroconvulsive therapy. There is only one value specified for biofeedback type qualifier, which is other biofeedback. There are no type qualifiers specified for the root operations of crisis intervention, medication management, hypnosis, narcosynthesis, group psychotherapy, and light therapy. The Mental Health section does not specify any qualifiers, so the value reported in characters 5–7 is always Z, to reflect "none." Character meanings and values for the Mental Health section are identified in Table 30.5 with details of the type qualifier provided in Table 30.6.

Root types, reported in character 3, include values for detoxification services, individual counseling, group counseling, individual psychotherapy, family counseling, medication management, and pharmacotherapy.

detoxification Process of counteracting or eliminating a toxic substance, as in treatment for drug addiction.

- *Detoxification* services involve cleansing the body of alcohol and/or drugs. This is not a treatment modality, but it helps the patient physically and psychologically stabilize until the body becomes free of drugs and the effects of alcohol.
- *Family counseling* applies psychological methods, including one or more family members, to treat an individual with addictive behavior. This method provides support and education for family members of addicted individuals. The rationale is that family member participation is a critical area of substance abuse treatment.
- *Group counseling* applies psychological methods to treat two or more individuals with addictive behaviors. It provides structured group counseling sessions and healing power through the connection with others.
- *Individual counseling* is the application of psychological methods for the purpose of treating an individual with addictive behavior. It involves several different techniques, which apply various strategies to address drug addiction.
- *Individual psychotherapy* treats an individual with an addictive behavior by behavioral, cognitive, psychoanalytic, psychodynamic, or psychophysiological means.
- *Medication management* involves monitoring and adjusting replacement medications used in addiction treatment.

pharmacotherapy Uses replacement medications for the treatment of addiction.

- *Pharmacotherapy* uses replacement medications for the treatment of addiction.

Character 4 values report type qualifiers. The type qualifiers are defined according to root types, and the values are not consistent across different groupings of root types.

Qualifier values for detoxification services, individual counseling, group counseling, and individual psychotherapy include the following:

- Cognitive
- Behavioral

- Cognitive-behavioral
- 12-step
- Interpersonal
- Vocational
- Psychoeducation
- Motivational enhancement
- Confrontational
- Continuing care
- Spiritual
- Pre/post-test infectious disease

The type qualifier for family counseling is other family counseling. Medication management and pharmacotherapy type qualifiers include the following:

- Nicotine replacement
- Methadone maintenance
- Levo-alpha-acetylmethadol (LAAM)
- Antabuse
- Naltrexone
- Naloxone
- Clonidine
- Bupropion
- Psychiatric medication
- Other replacement medication

The Substance Abuse Treatment section does not specify any qualifiers, so the value reported in characters 5–7 is always Z, to reflect "none." Table 30.7 provides character meanings and values for the Substance Abuse Treatment section.

Table 30.7 Character Meanings and Values for the Substance Abuse Section

Character	Meaning	Values
1	Section	H Substance Abuse
2	Body System	Z None
3	Root Type	2 Detoxification Services
		3 Individual Counseling
		4 Group Counseling
		5 Individual Psychotherapy
		6 Family Counseling
		8 Medication Management
		9 Pharmacotherapy

Character	Meaning	Values		
4	Type Qualifier	Root Types 2–5	Root Type 6	Root Types 8–9
		0 Cognitive 1 Behavioral 2 Cognitive-Behavioral 3 12-step 4 Interpersonal 5 Vocational 6 Psychoeducation 7 Motivational Enhancement 8 Confrontational 9 Continuing Care B Spiritual C Pre/Post-test Infectious Disease	3 Other Family Counseling	0 Nicotine Replacement 1 Methadone Maintenance 2 Levo-alpha-acetyl-methadol (LAAM) 3 Antabuse 4 Naltrexone 5 Naloxone 6 Clonidine 7 Bupropion 8 Psychiatric Medication 9 Other Replacement Medication
5	Qualifier	Z None		
6	Qualifier	Z None		
7	Qualifier	Z None		

Think About It 30.6

also available in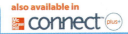

Assign ICD-10-PCS codes for the following situations, applying any appropriate sequencing guidelines.

1. Substance abuse treatment by psychiatric medication management _____

2. Motivational enhancement individual psychotherapy _____

3. Substance abuse pharmacotherapy treatment using Antabuse _____

4. Substance abuse detoxification services _____

5. Substance abuse group counseling using 12-step program _____

Beyond the Code: Why do you think that pharmacotherapy and medication management are classified separately? Justify your answer.

Chapter Summary

Learning Outcomes	Key Concepts / Examples
30.1 Classify imaging procedures according to root type. **(pages 553–555)**	• All codes in the Imaging section have a 1st character value of B. • Imaging procedures include plain radiography, fluoroscopy, computerized tomography (CT scan), magnetic resonance imaging (MRI), and ultrasound.
30.2 Apply rules for coding nuclear medicine procedures. **(pages 555–558)**	• All codes in the Nuclear Medicine section have a 1st character value of C. • If more than one radiopharmaceutical is used for nuclear medicine procedures, more than one code should be assigned.
30.3 Describe radiation oncology modalities. **(pages 559–561)**	• All codes in the Radiation Oncology section have a 1st character value of D. • Although the modality is identified in character 3 for the root type in the Radiation Oncology section, character 5 values provide further specification of the modality.
30.4 Define the components of physical rehabilitation and diagnostic audiology coding. **(pages 562–576)**	• All codes in the Physical Rehabilitation and Diagnostic Audiology section have a 1st character value of 2. • The root type, body system and region, type qualifier, and equipment values in the Physical Rehabilitation and Diagnostic Audiology section are dependent on the section qualifier of rehabilitation versus diagnostic audiology. • There are no body systems or regions specified for diagnostic audiology, so the character 4 value assigned is Z, to indicate "none."
30.5 Discuss the rationale for coding mental health procedures. **(pages 577–581)**	• All codes in the Mental Health section have a 1st character value of G. • The Mental Health section does not specify a body system, so the value for character 2 is reported as Z to reflect "none."
30.6 Identify types of substance abuse treatment. **(pages 581–584)**	• All codes in the Substance Abuse Treatment section have a 1st character value of H. • Like the Mental Health section, the substance section does not specify a body system, so the value for character 2 is reported as Z to reflect "none." • The type qualifiers reported in character 4 are defined according to root types, and the values are not consistent across different groupings of root types.

Applying Your Skills

Identify the section and root operation for each of the following procedures; then assign ICD-10-PCS codes.

Procedure	Section	Root Operation	ICD-10-PCS Code
1. *[LO 30.5]* Management of medication used for treatment of a mental health disorder	_____	_____	_____
2. *[LO 30.4]* Assessment for specified central auditory processing disorder	_____	_____	_____
3. *[LO 30.1]* Chest x-ray, PA and lateral	_____	_____	_____
4. *[LO 30.6]* Alcohol detoxification	_____	_____	_____
5. *[LO 30.2]* Bone scan of both lower legs with technetium 9m	_____	_____	_____
6. *[LO 30.3]* Gamma knife treatment for brain cancer	_____	_____	_____
7. *[LO 30.6]* Use of a 12-step program for group counseling in substance abuse treatment	_____	_____	_____
8. *[LO 30.4]* Assessment of the home for barriers related to activities of daily living	_____	_____	_____
9. *[LO 30.5]* Bilateral-single seizure electroconvulsive therapy for treatment of a mental health disorder	_____	_____	_____
10. *[LO 30.4]* Caregiver training for assistive listening communication skills	_____	_____	_____
11. *[LO 30.1]* Pregnancy sonogram in the first trimester, single gestation	_____	_____	_____
12. *[LO 30.5]* Hypnosis for weight loss	_____	_____	_____
13. *[LO 30.2]* Whole body PET scan	_____	_____	_____
14. *[LO 30.4]* Oscillating tracking to assess for vestibular disorder	_____	_____	_____
15. *[LO 30.6]* Monitoring a patient using Habitrol	_____	_____	_____
16. *[LO 30.3]* HDR brachytherapy treatment with iridium 192 for cervical cancer	_____	_____	_____
17. *[LO 30.1]* CT of head with and without Isovue 370 contrast	_____	_____	_____
18. *[LO 30.1]* MRI of the left breast with and without contrast	_____	_____	_____
19. *[LO 30.4]* Fitting of binaural hearing aidd	_____	_____	_____
20. *[LO 30.6]* Family counseling for substance abuse	_____	_____	_____

Checking Your Understanding

Select the letter that best answers the question or completes the sentence.

1. *[LO 30.3]* Which type of radiation oncology may be delivered in the form of a seed implant?

    a. beam radiation therapy
    b. brachytherapy
    c. stereotactic radiosurgery
    d. none of these

2. *[LO 30.1]* Which procedure is a digital display of multiplanar images reformatted by a computer, which is developed by capturing multiple exposures of external ionizing radiation?

    a. computerized tomography
    b. fluoroscopy
    c. magnetic resonance imaging
    d. ultrasonography

3. *[LO 30.5]* Which procedure involves the application of specialized light treatments for the purpose of improving functioning or well-being?

    a. biofeedback
    b. electroconvulsive therapy
    c. light therapy
    d. narcosynthesis

4. *[LO 30.2]* Introduction of radioactive materials into the body to study the distribution and fate of certain substances by the detection of radioactive emissions or, alternatively, the measurement of the absorption of radioactive emissions from an external source is

    a. nonimaging nuclear medicine assay.
    b. nonimaging nuclear medicine probe.
    c. nonimaging nuclear medicine uptake.
    d. planar nuclear medicine imaging.

5. *[LO 30.4]* Which of the following is the application of techniques for the purpose of improving, altering, or augmenting impaired orofacial myofunctional patterns and related speech production errors?

    a. aphasia treatment
    b. articulation/phonology treatment
    c. communicative/cognitive integration skills treatment
    d. orofacial myofunctional treatment

6. *[LO 30.1]* Which of the following is a type of contrast used for imaging procedures, reported by character 5?

    a. ionizing
    b. enhanced
    c. low osmolar
    d. optical coherence

7. *[LO 30.6]* Which of the following treats an individual with an addictive behavior by behavioral, cognitive, psychoanalytic, psychodynamic, or psychophysiological means?

    a. individual psychotherapy
    b. individual counseling
    c. detoxification services
    d. pharmacotherapy

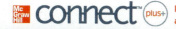

8. *[LO 30.3]* Which of the following is a type of stereotactic radiosurgery?

    a. wire
    b. ribbon
    c. gamma knife
    d. low-dose beam

9. *[LO 30.4]* Which of the following measures large and small muscle groups for controlled goal-directed movements?

    a. motor function assessment
    b. muscle performance assessment
    c. anthropometric characteristics
    d. coordination/dexterity assessment

10. *[LO 30.2]* If three different radiopharmaceuticals are used for a nuclear medicine procedure, how many codes should be assigned?

    a. 1
    b. 2
    c. 3
    d. 4

Online Activity

[LO 30.1, LO 30.2, LO 30.3] Using the Internet, do exploratory research about three procedures: stereotactic radiosurgery, tomographic (tomo) nuclear medicine imaging, and ultrasonography. Summarize your findings in a brief report. In your report, define each procedure and use the coding guidelines for ICD-10-PCS to identify information relevant to coding. You may also refer to ICD-10-PCS Appendix D: Type and Type Qualifier Definitions for Sections B-H.

Real-World Application: Case Study

[LO 30.1] Using ICD-10-PCS, code the procedure(s) for the following diagnostic imaging report.

Diagnostic Imaging Report

Exam: CT chest without contrast.

Indications: Consolidation versus mass in the left lower lobe revealed on chest x-ray.

Technique: Unenhanced spiral images were obtained through the chest.

Findings: Several, patchy air-space opacities identified in the left lower lobe, which appear to be most compatible with infiltrates. The remainder of the lung parenchyma is clear. Cardiac effusion and mediastinal lymphadenopathy noted.

Impression: Several, patchy air-space opacities in the left lower lobe, suggestive of pneumonia. Cardiac effusion and mediastinal lymphadenopathy also noted.

GLOSSARY

A

ABO isoimmunization Development of antibody against a blood antigen.

abrasion Rubbing or scraping of the surface layer of cells or tissue from an area of the skin or mucous membrane.

abuse Misuse or wrong use; excessive use of a substance; harm against another person.

accessory Gland, muscle, nerve, or other part that is associated in position or function to a more important structure.

accidental Unexpected or unforeseen; especially an occurrence of an injurious character.

active phase of labor Stage of labor in which the cervix begins to dilate and contractions are more intense and frequent.

Advance Beneficiary Notice (ABN) Written notice that is provided to patients before services are completed when Medicare may not pay for all or any of the services provided. Completed ABNs show a patient's acceptance of responsibility for payment.

aftercare Encounters following initial treatment when a patient needs to have additional care related to recovery or long-term effects of a disease.

agenesis Failure to develop any organ or any part during embryonic development.

alopecia Hair loss, which may be partial or complete and may be from natural or medicinal causes.

alphabetic index Alphabetic list of possible diagnosis codes, which should always be used first when locating an ICD-9-CM or ICD-10-CM diagnosis code.

alteration Operation that modifies the natural anatomic structure of a body part without affecting the function of the body part. Its principle purpose is to improve the appearance of the body part.

Alzheimer's dementia Dementia occurring with Alzheimer's disease; classified as early onset or late onset, depending on the person's age at onset. Early onset is before 65, and late onset is after 65.

Alzheimer's disease Progressive degenerative disease of the brain. First signs of the disease are memory loss and changes in personality. It progresses to profound dementia in 5 to 10 years.

ambiguous genitalia Appearing neither male nor female.

ambulatory payment classifications (APCs) Classifications of all hospital outpatient services. All CPT and HCPCS codes for procedures or services in an outpatient setting have associated APCs. Each APC has an assigned payment rate.

American Dental Association (ADA) Largest national dental society, founded in 1859. Leading source for oral health–related information, public health–related information, ethics, scientific advancement, and professional advocacy. The ADA developed the Current Dental Terminology (CDT).

American Health Information Management Association (AHIMA) National organization for health information management professionals; one of the cooperating parties for the ICD-9-CM.

American Hospital Association (AHA) National organization representing hospitals, healthcare networks, and their patients and communities; one of the cooperating parties for the ICD-9-CM.

American Medical Association (AMA) Society founded in 1847 and dedicated to promoting the art and science of medicine and improvements to public health. It educates the healthcare community; addresses ethical, financial, and political pressures within healthcare; advocates for physicians and their patients; and maintains the CPT code set.

American Public Health Association (APHA) Organization of public health professionals in existence since 1872.

amyelia Congenital absence of the spinal cord.

anaphylactic shock Extreme and sometimes fatal allergic reaction with circulatory failure.

and Term used in the coding manual to mean "and/or" when it appears in a title or narrative statement.

anencephaly Birth defect of the central nervous system in which all or most of the brain and spinal cord are missing.

aneurysm Weak area of an artery, which can suddenly rupture, causing extreme blood loss, damage to surrounding anatomic structures, and possibly death. It can be repaired through endovascular repair.

angina pectoris Severe acute chest pain caused by an inadequate supply of oxygen to part of the heart.

anomaly Structural abnormality, especially as a result of congenital defects.

aphakia Absence of the lens of the eye; may be from trauma or extraction of a cataract.

congenital Acquired in utero or at birth and progressing throughout the patient's life.

constitutional Symptom, such as fever, weight loss, or chills, that affects the general well-being of a patient.

consultation report Record included in a patient's chart if an attending physician requests a specialist to see a patient in order to provide an opinion or provide coverage for an aspect of care related to the consulting physician's area of specialization. The format is similar to a history and physical.

contact Patient encounter with a healthcare professional.

continuing education units (CEUs) Training required for coders who have successfully passed certification exams to keep skills current.

control Procedure to stop, or attempt to stop, postprocedural bleeding.

contusion Injury to tissue, usually without laceration; bruise; includes injuries of this type to the brain.

conventions Terms and symbols used to provide instructions for the use of diagnostic codes; located in the front of most ICD-9-CM, ICD-10-CM, and ICD-10-PCS manuals.

coronary artery bypass graft (CABG) A new vessel (vein or artery) grafted onto the heart to bridge the blockage of an artery.

corpus callosum Bridge of commissural fibers connecting the two cerebral hemispheres.

corrosion Burnlike injury due to chemicals.

counseling Application of psychological methods for the purpose of treating an individual with normal developmental issues and psychological problems to increase function, improve well-being, alleviate distress or maladjustment, or resolve a crisis.

cranial nerves Twelve paired nerves that start at the lower surface of the brain and pass through openings of the skull to the other parts of the body.

crisis intervention Treatment of a traumatized, acutely disturbed, or distressed individual for the purpose of short-term stabilization; may involve counseling, psychotherapy, or coordinating care among other providers.

Crohn's disease Inflammatory bowel disease with narrowing and thickening of the terminal small intestine.

Current Procedure Terminology (CPT) Code set created by the AMA to accurately describe services and provide a convenient method of communicating this information among providers, payers, administrators, and regulators.

cystocele Hernia of the bladder into the vagina; also known as vesical hernia.

D

Data Elements for Emergency Department Systems (DEEDS) Data set used to promote increased uniformity among data elements documented by emergency department physicians. It reports trauma registry data.

decompression Procedure involving elimination of undissolved gas from body fluids using extracorporeal means. It is performed in a hyperbaric chamber and is usually done to treat decompression sickness.

deep transverse arrest Occiput of the fetus turns and stops in the trasverse diameter of the pelvis during delivery.

defibrination syndrome of newborn Diffuse intravascular coagulation of a newborn.

delirium Disturbance of consciousness with a change in cognition.

demographic Statistical information on a patient, including gender, race, age, and location.

demyelinating Destroying or removing the myelin sheath of a nerve.

Department of Health and Human Services (HHS) US government agency for protecting the health of all Americans and providing essential human services; works with the AHA and cooperating parties for ICD-9-CM to maintain official guidelines and official advice on utilizing ICD-9-CM.

dependence Psychological craving for a substance.

dermatitis Bumps, rash, itchy, redness, swelling, oozing, or scarring of the skin brought on by an allergic reaction.

detachment Procedure in which all or a portion of an extremity is cut off. A qualifier should be used to specify the level at which detachment occurred, if available.

detoxification Process of counteracting or eliminating a toxic substance, as in treatment for drug addiction.

development disorder Disorder related to development, including speech and language disorders, disorder of scholastic skills, and pervasive developmental disorders.

device Equipment meant for a specific purpose; the 6th character of an ICD-10-PCS code in Sections 0–2. Section 4 has a 6th character, which is function/device.

diabetes mellitus disease process that impairs a body's ability to metabolize carbohydrates, fat, and proteins because of an insufficient secretion of insulin; includes type 1 and type 2 diabetes mellitus.

diagnosis Conclusion reached by a healthcare professional based on observation, history, and review of laboratory data. A coder should think of this as "why it was done."

diagnostic criteria Logical standards for coding specific disease entities.

diaphragmatic hernia Hernia in which the contents of the abdomen protrude into the chest through a weak spot in the diaphragm.

differential diagnoses Two or more contrasting or comparative diagnoses.

discharge summary Summary of a hospitalization, starting with the chief complaint or reason for admission and providing information about diagnostic testing, surgical procedures, and other treatments provided during the hospitalization; includes discharge disposition of the patient and follow-up care; also known as a final summary.

dislocation Displacement of any part of the body from its normal location, usually of a bone.

dissection Act of dividing into parts by one or more incisions.

disseminated intravascular coagulation Acute or chronic thrombotic and hemorrhagic disorder; uncontrolled systemic coagulation, resulting in thrombosis.

disseminated malignant neoplasm Malignant neoplasm that is scattered and distributed over a considerable area.

dorsopathy Disease of the back.

drainage Taking or letting fluids and/or gases out of the body.

Drug Registration and Listing System (DRLS) Database, created by the FDA, that lists the NDC and associated information, such as active ingredients, strength, dosage, and codes of manufactured drugs.

ductus arteriosus Fetal blood vessel that connects the left pulmonary artery directly to the descending aorta.

dyshidrosis Skin disease characterized by small blisters, especially on the hands and feet.

dysmenorrhea Painful and difficult menstruation.

dyspepsia Stomach condition marked by abdominal pain and bloating, also known as indigestion.

dysplasia Abnormality of development, often used when documenting in situ neoplasms.

dystocia Slow or difficult labor or delivery.

E

ecchymoses Escape of blood into tissues from a ruptured blood vessel; characterized by a livid black-and-blue or purple spot or area.

eccrine Sweat glands found all over the body.

eclampsia Convulsions in a pregnant woman associated with hypertension, proteinuria, or edema.

ectopic pregnancy Gestation outside the uterus; may be in a fallopian tube or the peritoneal cavity.

eczema Chronic skin disorder with scaly rashes and itching, which may be brought on by an allergic reaction.

effusion Collection of fluid that has escaped from blood vessels by rupture or exudation into a cavity or tissues.

electroconvulsive therapy Procedure that applies controlled electrical voltages for the purpose of treating a mental health disorder; includes appropriate sedation and other preparation of the individual.

electromagnetic therapy Use of electromagnetic rays to provide extracorporeal treatment.

electronic data interchange (EDI) Transmission of electronic medical insurance claims from providers to payers.

electronic health record (EHR) Medical record that is in a computerized system.

embolism Obstruction of a blood vessel by an embolus (clot).

embryonic cyst Abnormal, fluid-containing sac that develops from embryonic tissue.

emphysema Condition in which there is an increased accumulation of air in the organs and tissues, especially in the lungs, resulting in the loss of lung elasticity and decreased gas exchange.

encephalitis Inflammation of the brain.

encephalopathy Disease or disorder of the brain.

encounter Patient visit for medical treatment or procedure in an outpatient setting; may be diagnostic or screening.

endocarditis Inflammation of the lining of the heart.

endocrine System of glands that secrete or excrete hormones. Major glands of the system are the hypothalamus, pituitary, pineal, thyroid, parathyroids, thymus, adrenals, pancreas, ovaries, and testes.

endometriosis Presence of endometrial tissue in the abdomen outside the uterus, often resulting in severe pain and infertility.

enteritis Inflammation of the small intestine due to irritants, poisons, or viral or bacterial infection.

enterocele Hernia containing part of the intestine.

enthesopathy Disorder of the muscular or tendinous attachments to a bone.

epilepsy Disease marked by abnormal electrical discharges in the brain; can cause loss of consciousness, abnormal motor phenomena, or sensory disturbances. A single episode is called a seizure. Documentation of a seizure does not mean a diagnosis of epilepsy.

epispadias Condition in which the urethral opening is on the dorsum of the penis, manifested as a groove or cleft without a covering.

eponym Medical term based on or derived from a person's name. Many identify the person associated with the process or the disease.

erythematous Redness of the skin produced by congestion of the capillaries.

exchange transfusion Withdrawal of a small amount of blood and replacement with donor blood, repeated until a large portion of the blood has been replaced; primarily used for infants with erythroblastosis fetalis.

excision Procedure using a sharp instrument for cutting a portion of a body part out or off without replacement of the part.

excludes ICD-9-CM instruction that indicates a code should not be assigned because a different code may be more appropriate.

excludes1 ICD-10-CM instructional term indicating that the excluded code should not be assigned in conjunction with the code under which it is listed, as the two conditions do not occur together.

excludes2 ICD-10-CM instructional term indicating that the condition being excluded is not considered part of the condition for the code under which it is listed, but rather another code should also be assigned.

expandability One of the six major attributes that were goals of the development of the ICD-10-PCS. It ensures sufficient room for adding new values for characters as new procedures and technology are developed, allowing expansion to occur without disruption to the structures of the system.

exposure Contact with infectious disease or health risk.

external cause Cause of injury not stemming from the patient's status or condition. External cause codes are secondary codes that provide data for injury research and evaluation of strategies for injury prevention.

extirpation Procedure that takes or cuts solid matter out of a body part. Matter may be from a variety of origins and may or may not be embedded in the body part or the lumen of a tubular body part.

extracorporeal Outside the body.

extraction Procedure that uses force to pull or strip out or off all or a portion of a body part.

extrapyramidal Involving nerve tracts outside pyramidal tracts.

F

facesheet Document generally filed first or at the top of many types of healthcare encounters. Most inpatient facesheets include patient identification number, demographic information, insurance information, attending physician, admitting physician, and other pertinent data as determined by the facility. Physician office facesheets usually contain demographic information, employer information, insurance information, emergency contact information, and other data.

failure to thrive Term used to indicate an individual's weight or rate of weight gain is significantly lower than that of individuals of similar age and sex.

Fascicle V Surgical Procedures Document created by WHO for classification of medical and surgical procedures; the root of ICD-9-CM, Volume 3.

Federal Register Official publication for rules, proposed rules, and notices of federal agencies and organizations. Proposed ICD-9-CM changes are usually published in April, and final rule is published in August.

femoral hernia Hernia in which a portion of the intestine pushes through the fascia enclosing the femoral vessels and into the groin.

fetopelvic disproportion Condition in which the pelvis is unusually small or the fetus is unusually large.

fibrosis Condition marked by increased interstitial fibrous tissue, reactive process or in repair of something, rather than as part of normal tissue building.

final summary Summary of a hospitalization, starting with the chief complaint or reason for admission and providing information about diagnostic testing, surgical procedures, and other treatments provided during the hospitalization, including discharge disposition of the patient and follow-up care; also known as discharge summary.

first-listed diagnosis Main reason for the patient's visit; used in the outpatient setting rather than the term "principal diagnosis."

fissure Deep furrow or cleft between body parts or in the substance of an organ.

fluoroscopy Single-plane or bi-plane real-time display of an image that is developed from the capture of external ionizing radiation on a fluorescent screen; may be stored in a digital or analog format.

follow-up Visit after treatment is complete.

Food and Drug Administration (FDA) US government agency responsible for ensuring the safety and effectiveness of all drugs and medical supplies. It is also responsible for the safety of veterinary drugs, the nation's food supply, cosmetics, and products that emit radiation.

fragmentation Procedure to break solid matter in a body part into pieces; may be accomplished by physical force and may be done through direct application to the solid matter or indirectly through intervening body parts.

frostbite Destruction of skin and muscle tissue caused by prolonged exposure to freezing temperatures; commonly seen in hands and feet.

functional activity Effect associated with a neoplasm, such as decreased hormone production.

functioning properties Disabilities or functional impact of disease entities.

furuncle Infected hair follicle that spreads into the tissues around the follicle. It has a hard central core and forms pus; also known as a boil.

G

gastroenteritis Acute inflammation of the lining of the stomach and intestines. It is characterized by nausea, abdominal pain, diarrhea, and weakness and can be caused by food poisoning, the consumption of irritating food or drink, or psychological factors.

gastroesophageal reflux disease (GERD) Disease in which there is recurrent backwards flow of stomach acids into the esophagus, causing burning pain and discomfort and sometimes ulcers, neoplastic changes, and stricture.

Glasgow coma scale Scale used to document the conscious state of a patient; an integral part of trauma registry reporting.

glaucoma Group of eye diseases that cause increased intraocular pressure. This pressure changes the optic disk and causes a defect in the field of vision.

goiter Enlargement of the thyroid gland.

gout Metabolic disease marked by various combinations of hyperuricemia, recurrent accute inflammatory arthritis, deposits of urates in and around the joints, and uric acid urolithiasis. It can lead to deformity and disability and is associated with renal dysfunction and increased urea in the blood.

guidelines Instructions that are necessary to accurately report codes. They are usually found in the front of the ICD-9-CM, ICD-10-CM, and ICD-10-PCS manuals.

gynecomastia Enlargement of the breast in a male.

H

Healthcare Common Procedure Coding System (HCPCS) System used for reporting procedures, supplies, and nonphysician services that are not included in the CPT. It was established and is maintained by the CMS.

Health Care Financing Administration (HCFA) Previously the part of the US Department of Health and Human Services responsible for administering Medicare and Medicaid; now known as the Centers for Medicare and Medicaid Services (CMS).

Health Insurance Portability and Accountability Act of 1996 (HIPAA) US law providing uniform privacy, security, and electronic transaction standards regarding patients' medical records and other health-related information and allowing the continuation of health insurance after termination of employment for a prescribed period.

helminthiases Diseases or infections caused by parasitic worms, such as hookworm or roundworm.

hemangioma Extremely common benign tumor usually occurring in childhood or infancy. It is made up of blood vessels and typically occurs as a purple or red, slightly elevated area of the skin.

hemiparalysis Weakness or partial paralysis affecting one side of the body.

hemolytic Pertaining to the disruption of the integrity of the erythrocyte membrane, causing the release of hemoglobin.

hemolytic anemia Condition that is the result of red blood cells being destroyed or a reduction in their capacity.

hernia Bulge, or protrusion, through a weak spot of tissue due to increased pressure on the anatomic structure from pregnancy, obesity, heavy lifting, or aging.

hidradenitis Infection or inflammation of a sweat gland, usually of an apocrine type.

histologic type Cell type of a neoplasm.

history Patient's record of having a previous medical condition that is no longer active and for which the patient is no longer receiving treatment. The patient's family history and environmental history are included.

history and physical (H&P) Document that normally includes the chief complaint or reason for admission, past medical history, social history, surgical history, family history, review of symptoms, physical examination, assessment of the patient's problems, and plans for treatment.

Hodgkin's lymphoma Malignant lymphoma characterized by painless, progressive enlargement of the lymph nodes, spleen, and lymphoid tissue.

home health resource groups (HHRGs) Eighty case-mix groups available for patient classification based on clinical presentation, functional factors, and service utilization.

Huntington's disease Progressive neurodegenerative disorder, usually beginning in middle age and characterized by choreiform movements, emotional disturbances, and mental deterioration, leading to dementia.

hyaline membrane disease Respiratory disorder occurring in premature newborns. There is a deficiency in the surfactant coating the inner surface of the lungs, which cannot expand and contract properly; also called respiratory distress syndrome.

hydatidiform mole Mass in the uterus consisting of edematous degenerated chorionic villi. It typically develops after fertilization of an enucleate egg and may contain fetal tissue.

hydrocele Fluid-filled cavity or duct, especially in the scrotum.

hydrocephalus Enlarged head, especially forehead, due to excess cerebrospinal fluid in the cerebral ventricles.

hydronephrosis Condition of accumulation of excess urine in the kidneys due to obstruction in urine outflow. It is accompanied by atrophy of the kidney structure and cyst formation.

hyperalimentation Ingestion of excessive quantities of nutrients

hypercapnia Excess of carbon dioxide in the blood.

hypertension Elevated tension or pressure on arteries, veins, and capillaries. It can have life-threatening consequences, presenting increased risk factors for progressive and potentially life-threatening diseases such as stroke and heart disease.

hypertensive Suffering from persistent high arterial blood pressure; indicates a causal relationship to hypertension.

hyperthermia   Procedure to raise the body temperature using extracorporeal means.

hypnosis   Procedure that induces a state of heightened suggestibility using auditory, visual, and tactile techniques in order to elicit an emotional or behavioral response.

hypospadias   Urethral opening more proximal than normal on the ventral surface of the penis.

hypothermia   Procedure to lower the body temperature using extracorporeal means.

I

ICD-9-CM Coordination and Maintenance Committee   Established in 1985 by the Department of Health and Human Services to perform annual review and maintenance of the ICD-9-CM. Cooperating parties are the AHA, AHIMA, CMS, and National Center for Health Statistics.

ileitis   Inflammation of the ileum.

ill-defined condition   Condition that does not have a diagnosis code elsewhere classified.

immunodeficiency   State in which the immune response is unable to protect the body; caused by a decrease in or absence of leukocytes.

impingement syndrome   Disorder of the tendons of the rotator cuff muscles, which become irritated and inflamed as they pass through the subacromial space, resulting in pain, weakness, and loss of movement.

impetigo   Acute contagious staphylococcal or streptococcal skin disease, producing thick, yellow crusts.

in situ   Confined to the site of origin; non-invasive.

includes   Term accompanied by conditions that are examples of what may be included in a specific category.

individual psychotherapy   Treatment of an individual with a mental health disorder by behavioral, cognitive, psychoanalytic, psychodynamic, or psychophysiological means to improve functioning or well-being.

infarction   Sudden blockage of an artery.

inguinal hernia   Hernia in the inner groin.

inpatient prospective payment system (IPPS)   PPS for acute care hospital admissions, categorized into Medicare severity diagnosis-related groups (MS-DRGs).

inspection   Procedure to visually and/or manually explore a body part; may be achieved with or without optical instrumentation.

intentional   Done deliberately.

International Classification of Diseases   Coding system that contains both alphabetic and tabular lists of codes associated with medical diagnoses. The United States will utilize ICD-9-CM until September 30, 2013. On October 1, 2013, the United States will begin using ICD-10-CM.

International Classification of Diseases for Oncology (ICD-O)   Resource used for cancer registry reporting.

International Classification of Procedures in Medicine (ICPM)   Result of a modification of Fascicle V Surgical Procedures, published in 1978 by the WHO and adopted for use in 1979.

intracerebral   Situated or occurring within the brain.

intractable   Difficult to stop or control.

intrinsic circulating anticoagulants   Anticoagulants naturally produced by the body.

introduction   Procedure involving putting in or on therapeutic, diagnostic, nutritional, physiological, or prophylactic substances, not including blood or blood products.

intussusception   Slipping of one part of the intestines into another, usually producing an obstruction.

iron deficiency anemia   Anemia caused by low or absent iron stores and serum iron concentration. When used as a secondary diagnosis code to blood loss, care should be taken to mark as acute or chronic correctly.

irrigation   Procedure in which a cleansing substance is put in or onto the body; may be a cleansing substance or a dialysate.

ischemic   Caused by a lack of blood supply to a tissue.

isotope   Atom having the same atomic number (same name) but a different mass number from similar atoms.

J

jaundice   Yellowish pigmentation caused by the deposition of bile pigments following interference with the normal production and discharge of bile or excessive breakdown of red blood cells.

jejunitis   Inflammation of the jejunum.

K

Kaposi's sarcoma   Malignant neoplastic vascular proliferation characterized by bluish-red cutaneous nodules on the lower limbs.

keloid   Raised, irregular, lumpy, shiny scar due to excess collagen fiber production during healing of a wound.

keratosis   Excessive growth of the horny layers of the skin—for example, a wart or callus.

kyphosis   Exaggerated outward curvature of the thoracic region.

L

laryngitis   Inflammation of the larynx.

late effect   Additional treatment or impact on conditions later in life from a medical condition or injury. "Sequelae" is the term used by medical coders for late effects.

latent phase of labor First stage of labor, consisting of irregular contractions that become regular. The cervix begins to dilate; averages eight hours.

leukemia Progressive, malignant disease of blood-forming organs; can be acute or chronic.

light therapy Application of specialized light treatments for the purpose of improving functioning or well-being.

linearization Lists that are established for statistical reporting of mortality, morbidity, and other aspects in the upcoming ICD-11.

London Bills of Mortality System that tracked death from plague and other fatal illnesses. It was created in 1562, with official reporting beginning in 1603. This system was the root of medical coding.

lower urinary tract symptoms (LUTS) Group of common symptoms related to the lower urinary tract, such as poor urinary stream. It is found in category N40 of the ICD-10, along with instructional notes.

lymphangioma Benign tumor; congenital malformation of the lymphatic system.

lymphangitis Inflammation of one or more lymphatic vessels.

M

main term Key term that is used in the alphabetic index of the ICD-9 or ICD-10 to find the appropriate diagnosis code.

malabsorption Inadequate absorption of nutrient materials from the alimentary canal.

malignant Cancerous.

malnutrition Any disorder of nutrition; may be caused by unbalanced or insufficient diet or defective assimilation or utilization of nutrients.

malpresentation Abnormal presentation of the fetus at birth.

malunion Condition in which fragments of a fractured bone heal in a faulty position.

manifestation properties Signs, symptoms, and clinical findings.

map Procedure performed for the purpose of locating the route of passage of electrical impulses and/or locating functional areas in a body part. It is performed only on the cardiac conduction mechanism and the central nervous system.

measurement Process of determining physiological or physical function level at a point in time. A single reading constitutes a measure.

meconium Dark green, mucilaginous material in the intestine of a full-term fetus.

Medicaid Provides medical coverage for low-income individuals; created through Title XIX of the Social Security Act.

medical necessity Need for each procedure code to be justified by at least one diagnosis code.

Medicare Provides health coverage for the elderly and disabled; created through Title XVIII of the Social Security Act.

Medicare severity diagnosis-related groups (MS-DRGs) Categorization of IPPS that is associated with a standardized basic payment amount. Payment amount is based on average resources used to treat Medicare patients for diagnoses and procedures and has two parts: labor-related and non-labor share.

Medication Administration Record List of medications that has been ordered for the patient. It includes both routine and PRN medications and documents the time, dose, and route of medications administered.

medication management Monitoring and necessary adjustments of medications that were prescribed to treat a mental health disorder.

meningitis Bacterial or viral inflammation of the meninges.

meningocele Protrusion of the meninges from the spinal cord or brain through a defect in the vertebral column or cranium. It forms a cyst with cerebrospinal fluid.

mental retardation Intellectual ability equal to or less than an IQ of 70. It is accompanied by significant deficits in abilities. Diagnosis codes are assigned according to the level of retardation based on IQ scores.

metabolic Pertaining to a physical and chemical process whereby a body is maintained and the transformation that produces energy for the body.

metastasis Transfer of disease from one site to another not directly connected to the original site.

migraine Recurrent, severe headache, often accompanied by nausea and vomiting. It seems to occur more often with individuals who have a family history.

misadventure Unintended negative effect or mishap during surgical or medical care.

miscarriage Spontaneous abortion.

missed abortion Early fetal death prior to 20 weeks' gestation; the dead fetus is retained.

modality Form of use or application of a treatment.

molar pregnancy Conversion of fertilized ovum into a mole.

monitoring Determination of physiological or physical function level through repeated measurements over a period of time.

mood disorders Affective disorder classified by symptoms and severity.

morbidity Frequency at which complications occur after an operation or other medical treatment.

morphology Study of the form and structure of a particular organism, organ, or part.

motor   Of or referring to neural structures that transmit the signals that cause muscles to contract and glands to secrete.

multi-axial code   One of the six major attributes that were goals of the development of ICD-10-PCS. It is a code structure whose characters are independent yet maintain consistency within defined sections.

multiple myeloma   Multiple tumors made up of cells normally found in the blood marrow.

multiple sclerosis   Demyelinating disease characterized by hardened tissue in the brain or spinal cord. It causes partial or complete paralysis and jerky muscle tremors.

mycoses   Diseases caused by a fungus.

myelopathy   Disease or disorder of the spinal cord or bone marrow.

myocarditis   Inflammation of the heart muscle.

myocardial infarction (MI)   Sudden interruption of blood supply to part of the heart muscle due to an obstructed or constricted coronary artery; also known as a stroke.

myoneural junction   Junction of nerve fiber and muscle fiber plasma membrane; also known as neuromuscular junction.

N

narcosynthesis   Procedure in which intravenous barbiturates are administered for the purpose of releasing suppressed or repressed thoughts.

National Center for Health Statistics (NCHS)   Agency that compiles statistical information to guide actions and policies to improve the health of Americans. It established guidelines to develop ICD-10-PCS. It is one of the cooperating agencies for ICD-9-CM and, along with CMS, performs annual revisions of the ICD-9-CM.

National Drug Codes (NDC)   Unique, three-segment numbers that serve as universal product identifiers for human drugs.

National Electronic Disease Surveillance System (NEDSS)   Collection of data for disease trends and/or outbreaks; used by public health personnel to protect the nation's health.

National Hospital Ambulatory Medical Care Survey (NHAMCS)   Report of data that reflect utilization and provision of ambulatory care services in hospital emergency and outpatient services.

neglect   Disregard or failure to provide care to a person when one is able to or is responsible for the care.

neonatal   Period lasting from birth to one month of age.

neoplasm   Abnormal new tissue growth; may be benign or malignant.

nephrolithiasis   Condition marked by the presence of a kidney stone (renal calculi).

nephropathy   Disease or abnormal state of the kidney.

neuroendocrine tumors   Neoplasms that originate from the cells of the endocrine and nervous systems.

neuropathy   Functional disturbance or pathological change in the peripheral nervous system.

nevus   Congenital lesion of the skin; birthmark.

nocturnal enuresis   Nighttime urinary incontinence.

non-collision transport accident   Vehicular accident not involving collision. One example is a motorcyclist falling or being thrown from a motorcycle.

nonessential modifier   Term that may coexist with the main term but does not change the code assignment for the condition. It is indicated by parentheses in both the tabular list and alphabetic index.

nonunion   Total failure of a fracture to unite.

nosocomial   Acquired while in the hospital.

Not Elsewhere Classifiable (NEC)   Code assigned when there is more specific documentation but no code exists to the appropriate level of specificity.

Not Otherwise Specified (NOS)   Code assigned when more specific codes exist but documentation lacks specificity.

nursing notes   Documentation by nursing staff, including nursing assessments and treatments, vital signs, and other pertinent information.

nutritional   Related to the taking in and metabolizing of nutrients by a body to continue maintaining life and allowing for growth.

nutritional anemia   Anemia caused by inadequate intake of the nutrients needed for production of red blood cells and hemoglobin.

O

obesity   Excessive accumulation of fat that increases body weight beyond the limits of the skeletal and physical requirement.

objective   Type of documentation based on observation by a healthcare professional.

observation   Patient that is being observed for a condition that is suspected.

obstructive uropathy   Disease of the urinary tract in which the flow of urine is blocked, causing it to back up and injure a kidney.

occlusion   Procedure to completely close an orifice or a lumen of a tubular body part; may be either a natural or artificially created orifice.

open fracture   Fracture in which the skin is open and the fracture is exposed to external elements.

operative report   Report used for surgical procedure during the encounter. It includes information on pre- and postoperative diagnosis, the surgeon who performed the procedure, the type of anesthesia, the name of the procedure, the specimens sent to pathology, a narrative description of the procedure, the condition of patient following the procedure, and patient disposition following the procedure.

organic brain syndrome Mental dysfunction resulting from physical changes in brain structure; can be acute or chronic.

ossification Conversion of fibrous tissue or cartilage into bone or bony substance.

osteoarthritis Chronic inflammatory disease of the joints, with pain and loss of function. It typically has an onset during middle or old age.

osteomyelitis Inflammation of bone tissue caused by infection, which may remain localized or spread through bone to involve marrow, cortex, cancellous tissue, and periosteum.

osteopathic treatment Manual elimination or alleviation of somatic dysfunction and related disorders in the musculoskeletal system.

Outcome and Assessment Information Set (OASIS) Instrument used to document assessment of a patient's condition in the home health setting. It is used to determine the case-mix adjustment to the standard rate of pay.

P

palsy Paralysis.

parameters Thirteen main classification categories for the upcoming ICD-11.

paraplegia Loss of feeling and movement in both legs and trunk of the body.

parasite Organism that lives on or within another organism, the host, and gains benefits while the host suffers.

parentheses Punctuation, found in both the tabular list and alphabetic index, that surrounds nonessential modifiers.

Parkinson's disease Chronic, progressive disease linked to decreased dopamine. It is characterized by tremors of resting muscles, rigidity, slowness, impaired balance, and shuffling gait.

paroxysmal Spasm or convulsion.

pathological fracture Fracture of a bone already weakened by existing disease.

pedestrian Person involved in an accident who was not at the time of the accident riding in or on a motor vehicle, a railway car, a streetcar, an animal-drawn or other vehicle, a pedal cycle, or an animal.

pediculosis Infestation with lice.

pemphigus Group of autoimmune diseases marked by successive, recurring blisters on skin and mucous membranes, often in association with sensations of itching and burning.

performance Procedure that uses extracorporeal means to completely take over a physiological function.

pericarditis Inflammation of the pericardium, the covering of the heart.

perinatal Period beginning before birth and lasting 28 days after birth.

pervasive Characterized by impairment of development in multiple areas.

pes planus Flat foot with no plantar arch.

petechia Perfectly round, purplish red spot caused by intradermal or submucous hemorrhage.

pharmacotherapy Use of replacement medications for the treatment of addiction.

pharyngitis Inflammation of the pharynx.

pheresis Procedure involving extracorporeal separation of blood products; may be done as a treatment for a disease or removal of a blood product from a donor.

phototherapy Extracorporeal treatment procedure using light rays.

physical rehabilitation Restoration to physical health through training and therapy.

physician orders Prescribed medications, therapies, consultation requests, and other treatments documented by a physician.

pilonidal Of or involving the growth of hairs embedded under the skin.

placeholder "X" inserted into a diagnosis code to indicate unused digits; used when a code requires fewer than six digits but needs a 7th digit to convey specific information; also seen in some diagnosis codes to allow for future expansions of categories and subcategories.

placenta previa Abnormal implantation of the placenta near the uterine cervix; usually precedes the fetus at birth, causing severe maternal hemorrhage.

place of occurrence Location of a patient when an accident occurred.

plan Information about medications to be ordered, surgical procedures to be performed, or other treatment information.

plexus Network of lymphatic vessels, nerves, or veins.

pneumoconiosis Any chronic lung disease, such as asbestosis and silicosis, caused by long-term inhalation of particulate matter, such as coal dust; may be from organic or non-organic agents.

pneumonia Inflammation of the lungs, with congestion, usually caused by a bacterial or viral infection.

pneumonitis Inflammation of the lungs.

poisoning Occurs due to misuse or adverse effects of prescribed medication, accidental exposure to chemical toxins, food poisoning, or other methods; may be accidental or intentional. The substance that causes the poisoning destroys or impairs normal functioning.

portal hypertension Hypertension in the hepatic portal system, which carries blood to the liver from the stomach, intestine, pancreas, and spleen; caused by a venous obstruction or occlusion.

posthemorrhagic anemia Anemia occurring after hemorrhage; can be acute or chronic. A coder should take great care when coding to correctly code as chronic or acute as indicated by the patient record.

primary Original site and type of tumor.

primigravida Referring to a woman's first pregnancy.

principal diagnosis Main reason a patient has been admitted to a hospital for care.

prion Abnormal form of a normal cellular protein, causing a group of progressive neurodegenerative diseases.

procedure Treatment or medical service that was performed on a patient during a visit to the facility.

progress notes Notes written by physicians and other providers to document pertinent information during a hospital or long-term care stay, often in the SOAP format.

prolapse Falling or slipping of a body part from its normal position.

prolonged pregnancy Pregnancy that exceeds 42 weeks.

prospective payment system (PPS) System in which payment is made based on a predetermined, fixed amount. It is used for Medicare reimbursement and many other specific areas.

prurigo Any of various skin conditions of unknown cause with itching papules.

pruritus Any type of itch; may be caused by an infection, an allergy, skin irritation, a disease, or another reason.

psychological tests Standardized psychological tests and measurement instruments administered and interpreted to assess psychological function.

puerperium Period between childbirth and the return of the uterus to its normal size.

purpura Bleeding disorder characterized by initial areas turning purplish because of bleeding into the skin or mucus membrane.

pyelonephritis Inflammation of the kidney and renal pelvis, especially due to bacterial infection.

pyoderma Pus-producing infection of the skin, such as impetigo.

pyonephrosis Collection of pus in the kidney, usually caused by an obstruction.

Q

quadriplegia Loss of movement and feeling in the trunk and all four extremities.

qualifier Seventh character of an ICD-10-PCS code. Values are unique to individual procedures or treatments.

query Question asked of a physician regarding documentation for coding purposes.

R

radiculopathy Any pathological condition of the nerve roots.

radionuclide Source of radiation.

radiopharmaceutical Radioactive drug that is implanted in the body.

reattachment Procedure to put back in or on all or a portion of a separated body part to its normal location or other suitable location. It may or may not involve the reestablishment of vascular circulation and nervous pathways.

rectocele Hernia of the rectum through the intervening fascia into the vagina.

remission Period of abatement from symptoms of a disease.

replacement Procedure to put biological or synthetic material in or on to physically take the place of all or a portion of a body part.

reposition Procedure to move all or a portion of a body part to its normal location or other suitable location.

restoration Procedure that uses extracorporeal means to return, or attempt to return, physiological functions to the original state of function. The only restoration procedure is external cardioversion and defibrillation.

restriction Procedure involving partial closure of an orifice or a lumen of a tubular body part; may be a natural or artificially created orifice.

retroperitoneum Space between the peritoneum and the posterior abdominal wall.

Rh incompatibility Condition that develops when a pregnant woman has Rh-negative blood and the fetus has Rh-positive blood.

rhesus isoimmunization Development of antibodies against Rh antigens.

rheumatic Of the joints, muscles, and bones.

rheumatoid arthritis Inflammatory polyarthropy that affects the lungs, heart, and other organs and tissues; a disease of connective tissue, with arthritis as a major manifestation.

rhinitis Viral inflammation of the mucous membrane of the nose.

root operation Third character in Sections 0–9 of the ICD-10-PCS code. It identifies the basic type of service or procedure performed.

rosacea Red, inflamed cheeks, nose, and forehead; persistent erythematous rash.

routine and administrative examinations General checkups or pre-employment physicals.

Rule of Nines Method used to calculate the extent of a burn injury by assigning values of 9% to various surface areas of the body.

S

schizophrenia Psychotic disorder in which the individual loses contact with the environment and has a noticeable deterioration of function in everyday life. The disintegration of feeling, thought, and behavior, possibly with delusions and hallucinations.

sclerosis Thickening or hardening of a tissue due to overgrowth of fibrous tissue or increase in interstitial tissue.

screening Test performed in the absence of signs or symptoms of a disease.

secondary Tumor that has metastasized, or spread, from the original location to another site.

secondary diagnosis Diagnosis that impacts patient care because it requires clinical evaluation, therapeutic treatment, diagnostic procedures, an extended length of stay, or increased care and/or monitoring.

section Grouping of several categories of codes.

see Instructional term to tell coder to refer to another item.

see also Instructional term to tell coders to refer to another item.

sepsis Systemic inflammatory response syndrome (SIRS) secondary to an infection.

septic shock Circulatory failure associated with severe sepsis.

septicemia Systemic disease due to the presence of bacteria in the bloodstream.

sequela Additional treatment or impact on conditions later in life from a medical condition or an injury.

severe sepsis Sepsis associated with acute organ dysfunction.

severity of subtypes properties Extent, magnitude, or severity of a condition.

shock wave therapy Extracorporeal treatment by shock waves. It is thought to be helpful because it leads to revascularization in the tendons, which creates a blood supply to help with healing and the reduction of pain.

sickle cell anemia Chronic anemia characterized by the destruction of red blood cells and episodic blocking of blood vessels; usually seen in individuals of African or Mediterranean descent.

sigmoiditis Inflammation of the sigmoid colon.

sign Something objectively observable, possibly an indication of a disease process.

sinusitis Inflammation of the lining of a sinus.

SOAP note Acronym that stands for subjective, objective, assessment, and plan; one form of progress note.

Social Security Act Bill that created programs to aid numerous groups of Americans. It was signed into law in 1935. Several additions have been made, including those creating Medicare and Medicaid.

somatoform disorders Disorders in which an individual has physical complaints that have no organic or physiological explanation.

specific condition properties Properties of a condition that may require monitoring according to public health indicators.

spermatocele Benign cyst or tumor in the scrotum.

spina bifida Failure of one or more vertebral arches to close during fetal development, usually with hernial protrusion of the meninges and sometimes the spinal cord.

spirochetal Caused by a spiral bacterium.

spondylolisthesis Forward displacement of one of the lower lumbar, usually the fifth lumbar over the sacrum or the fourth lumbar over the fifth, causing nerve root compression and pain and/or weakness in the legs.

spondylolysis Any of several degenerative diseases causing disintegration or dissolution of a vertebra.

spontaneous abortion Abortion occurring naturally.

sprain Sudden twist or wrench of a joint, causing a stretch or tear in a ligament.

standardized terminology One of the six main attributes that were goals of the development of the ICD-10-PCS. It established terms for use in the ICD-10-PCS. Each has a unique meaning used to provide the code descriptions.

status (1) Code used to report that a patient either is a carrier of a disease or has the sequelae or residual of a past disease or condition. (2) State, particularly of a morbid condition.

steatorrhea Overactivity of any sebaceous gland; excess of fat in the stool.

stereotactic radiosurgery Procedure that involves delivery of a high-dose beam of radiation used for tumors of the head and neck.

stillbirth Birth of a dead fetus.

stress incontinence Involuntary leakage of urine from the bladder when involuntary pressure is exerted on the bladder by sneezing, coughing, laughing, or straining.

structural integrity One of the six main attributes that were goals of development of the ICD-10-PCS. It provides for expansion to occur without disrupting the structure of the system.

subarachnoid Space between the arachnoid and the pia mater in the tissue surrounding and protecting the brain and spinal cord.

subcategory Additional characters beyond the first three digits of a diagnosis code.

subdural Located under the dura mater.

subjective Statement, generally in a patient's own words, about why the patient is seeking care or how the patient feels.

subluxation Partial dislocation in which some contact between the joint surfaces remains.

submersion Remaining or being held under the surface of a liquid.

substance abuse Excessive and usually illegal use of a drug.

subterm Term listed below main terms in the alphabetic index; give greater specificity.

superficial injury Less severe injury that does not penetrate to bones or organs; abrasion or contusion.

symptom Manifestation of disease process subjectively reported by a patient. It may lead a physician to diagnose one or more disease processes.

systematic inflammatory response syndrome (SIRS) Systemic response to infection, burns, trauma, or other severe insults. The symptoms include fever, tachycardia, tachypnea, and leukocytosis.

systemic lupus erythematosus (SLE) Inflammatory, multisystemic, autoimmune disease of the connective tissue with no known cause, occurring chiefly in women. It is characterized by fever, skin lesions, joint pain or arthritis, and anemia and often affects the kidneys, spleen, and other organs.

T

table Section of ICD-10-PCS that must be consulted along with the index, which contains the remainder of the information needed to finish building a procedure code.

Table of Neoplasms Table that lists the types and location of neoplasms. It directs a coder to the appropriate diagnosis code.

tabular list List of disease classifications by etiology or site, supplementary classification, and appendices. It should be used after locating a possible diagnosis from ICD-9-CM, Volume 2, or ICD-10-CM.

temporal properties Characteristics of the patient's condition. Examples are onset characteristics and the duration or course of a disease or health condition.

terms Words or phrases that have been assigned standard meanings to reflect underlying concepts that are used in the ICD context. Examples are "includes" and "excludes."

terrorism Unlawful use of force or violence against persons or property to intimidate or coerce a government, the civilian population, or any segment thereof, in furtherance of political or social objectives.

tetralogy of Fallot Pulmonary stenosis, interventricular septal defect, dextro position of the aorta, and right ventricular hypertrophy occurring together.

Code on Dental Procedures and Nomenclature Current Dental Terminology (CDT); a standardized way of reporting dental procedures performed in the treatment of dental disease; developed by the ADA.

thrombosis Formation of a clot attached to a diseased blood vessel or heart lining.

thyroid Endocrine gland located in the neck.

thyrotoxic crisis or storm Acute, life-threatening hypermetabolic state caused by excessive release of thyroid hormones.

Title XIX Portion of the Social Security Act that created Medicaid in 1966.

Title XVIII Portion of the Social Security Act that created Medicare, introduced in 1965 and implemented in 1966.

tonsillitis Inflammation of the tonsils.

topography Site of a neoplasm.

tracheitis Inflammation of the trachea.

transfer Procedure to move all or a portion of a body part to another location to take over the function of all or a portion of a body part. The body part is not taken out in the process and remains connected to vascular and nervous supplies.

transfusion Procedure that puts in blood or blood products.

transient ischemic attack Brief episode of cerebral ischemia, often predictive of a serious stroke.

transient tachypnea of newborn Isolated wave of excessive rapidity of breathing in a newborn.

translocation Transfer of a part of a chromosome to a different location within the same chromosome, or the exchange of parts between two chromosomes.

transplantation Procedure to put in or on all or a portion of a living body part taken from another individual or an animal to physically take the place and/or function of all or a portion of a similar body part.

transport accident Accident involving a device designed primarily for, or used at the time primarily for, conveying persons or goods from one place to another; involves a vehicle, which is moving, running, or in use for transport purposes at the time the accident occurs.

transposition Transfer of a DNA segment to a new site on the same or another chromosome.

trauma registry List of statistical and demographic information from patients that were seen for trauma. Reporting of Glasgow coma scale diagnosis codes is an integral part of this registry.

treatment properties Identify pertinent interventions that are related to a diagnosis entity—for example, insulin treatment for a diabetic patient.

trisomy Presence of an extra chromosome, as in Down syndrome.

tubulo-interstitial nephritis Inflammation of the spaces between kidneys.

type 1 diabetes mellitus Diabetes characterized by the abrupt onset of symptoms. Most individuals are diagnosed with this type of diabetes around age 12, but it can begin at any age. It requires the use of insulin to properly process glucose.

type 2 diabetes mellitus Diabetes with a usual occurrence around age 50–60. Many cases can be controlled by diet, but insulin may also be needed to provide sufficient glucose metabolism. Usually, it is secondary to poor diet and obesity.

U

ulcerative colitis Serious inflammatory disease of the colon and rectum marked by ulcers of the intestinal lining and continual attacks of abdominal pain, diarrhea, and rectal bleeding; the cause is unknown.

ultrasound therapy Extracorporeal treatment using very high frequency sound waves. The procedure has shown efficacy in diabetic patients with peripheral neuropathies.

ultraviolet light therapy Extracorporeal treatment using electromagnetic rays at higher frequency than the violet end of the spectrum. It is effective for those with skin disorders, such as psoriasis.

umbilical hernia Abdominal hernia of newborns in which a section of the intestines bulges up through an opening between the abdominal muscles beneath or near the umbilicus.

uncertain behavior Neoplasm that cannot be determined to be either malignant or benign.

underdosing Taking a dose of medication that is less than what is prescribed.

Uniform Ambulatory Care Data Set (UACDS) Used to collect data that are relevant to the ambulatory care or outpatient setting.

Uniform Hospital Discharge Data Set (UHDDS) Standard data set for collection of data for Medicare and Medicaid.

unique definition One of the six main attributes that were goals of development of ICD-10-PCS. It was fulfilled by the process of custom-building codes to define each unique procedure. It provides consistency that does not allow for the recycling of codes to later be assigned to report a procedure that is defined differently in any way.

urosepsis Syndrome characterized by fever, chills, and hypertension resulting from microorganism invasion that starts in the urinary tract and moves to the bloodstream. It is nonspecific for coding and should prompt a provider query.

use Distinct version of ICD-11. The three versions are primary care, clinical, and research.

use additional code Instruction to assign a secondary code, following the disease code, for any manifestations that exist for the case being coded.

uterine inertia Weak or poorly coordinated uterine contractions during labor.

V

valgus deformity Permanent abnormal outward twist or bend of bone.

value Information conveyed by a particular character in an ICD-10-PCS code, which is defined as it relates to specific sections.

varus deformity Permanent abnormal inward twist or bend of bone.

vein Blood vessel carrying deoxygenated blood back to the heart.

ventral hernia Hernia in the midline of the abdomen, often resulting from a surgical incision or scar.

virus Minute infectious agent characterized by a lack of metabolism and the ability to replicate only while in host organisms.

vitiligo Nonpigmented, white patches on otherwise normal skin, thought to have an autoimmune mechanism.

W

wet lung syndrome Benign condition of a near-term infant who has respiratory distress syndrome after delivery; usually lasts three to five days.

with Term used in the alphabetic index immediately following a main term; terms listed may not be in alphabetic order.

World Health Assembly (WHA) Decision-making body of the World Health Organization. The ICD-11 final draft is due to be submitted to WHA by 2014.

World Health Organization (WHO) Directing and coordinating authority for health within the United Nations system.

Z

zoonotic Transferable from animals to humans under normal circumstances.

PHOTO CREDITS

Chapter 1

Opener: © Ingram Publishing RF; **3:** © Ingram Publishing RF; **5:** © Veer RF; **6:** © Ingram Publishing RF.

Chapter 2

Opener: © Blend Images RF; **14, 18:** © Ingram Publishing RF.

Chapter 3

Opener: © Getty RF; **27:** © Blend Images RF; **30:** © Getty RF.

Chapter 4

Opener: © Veer RF; **38, 46:** © Getty RF.

Chapter 5

Opener: © Getty RF; **54:** © The McGraw-Hill Companies, Inc. Rick Brady, photographer; **56:** © Ingram Publishing RF; **58:** © Getty RF; **62:** © Digital Vision/Getty RF; **64:** © Getty RF.

Chapter 6

Opener: © Getty RF; **75:** © Blend Images RF; **77:** © Veer RF; **78:** © Getty RF; **82, 85:** © Blend Images RF.

Chapter 7

Opener: © Blend Images RF; **93:** © Ingram Publishing RF; **95:** © Blend Images RF; **99:** © Veer RF; **101:** © Custom Medical Stock/Alamy RF.

Chapter 8

Opener: CDC; **113:** CDC; **8.1:** © Kathy Park Talaro; **8.2:** CDC; **8.3:** © Dr. Marazzi/SPL/Photo Researchers, Inc.; **8.4:** National Genome New Institute/NIH; **8.5:** © Eric Grave/Photo Researchers, Inc.

Chapter 9

Opener: CDC/Dr. Steve Kraus; **129:** Photograph by Judie Arnold; **131:** © SPL/Getty RF; **133:** © Blend Images RF.

Chapter 10

Opener: © Getty RF; **141:** © Getty RF; **145:** © Blend Images RF.

Chapter 11

Opener: © The McGraw-hill Companies, Inc.; **11.1:** © Meckes/Ottawa/Photo Researchers, Inc.; **11.3:** © The McGraw-Hill Companies, Inc.

Chapter 12

Opener: © The McGraw-Hill Companies, Inc. Gary He, photographer; **168, 169, 171:** © Getty RF; **173:** © Ingram Publishing RF.

Chapter 13

Opener: © Getty RF; **13 5:** © The McGraw-Hill Companies, Inc. Joe DeGrandis, photographer.

Chapter 14

Opener: © Alamy RF.

Chapter 15

Opener: © Getty RF.

Chapter 16

Opener: © Getty RF; **16.15:** © SIU Biomedical/Photo Researchers, Inc.

Chapter 17

Opener: © Medical/Getty RF; **17.1b:** © CNRI/SPL/Photo Researchers, Inc.

Chapter 18

Opener: © Alamy RF; **274:** © Blend Images RF; **279:** © Punchstock/Banana Stock RF.

Chapter 19

Opener: © Blend Images RF; **296:** © Barry Slaven, MD, PhD/Phototake; **297:** © Susan Leavines/Photo Researchers, Inc.

Chapter 20

Opener: © Getty RF; **20.1:** © NMSB/Custom Medical Stock Photo; **20.4:** © Scott Camazine/Alamy; **20.5:** © CNRI/Photo Researchers, Inc.

Chapter 21

Opener: © Stockbyte/Punchstock RF; **21.2:** © Dr. Marazzi/SPL/Photo Researchers, Inc.; **21.3:** © Mediscan/Visuals Unlimited; **21.8:** © Kenneth Greer/Visuals Unlimited; **21.9:** © Medical-on-line/Alamy.

Chapter 22

Opener: © The McGraw-Hill Companies, Inc. Photo by JW Ramsey; **22 2:** © Ralph Hutchings/Visuals Unlimited; **22.4:** © Dr. Michael Klein/Peter Arnold, Inc./Photolibrary.

Chapter 23

Opener: © Getty RF; **23.5a:** © Sheila Terry/Photo Researchers, Inc; **23.5b:** © SPL/Photo Researchers, Inc.; **23.5c:** © John Radcliffe Hospital/Photo Researchers, Inc.

Chapter 24

Opener: © Getty RF; **406:** © Getty RF; **414, 421:** © Ingram Publishing RF.

Chapter 25

Opener: © Getty RF; **443:** © Blend Images RF; **447:** © Getty RF; **452:** © Banana Stock/PictureQuest RF.

Chapter 26

Opener: © Getty RF; **460:** © Getty RF.

Chapter 27

Opener: © Getty/Image Source RF; **478:** © Getty RF;

Chapter 28

Opener: © Science Photo Library RF; **496:** © Digital Vision/Getty RF; **511:** © Brand X/Jupiter RF; **519:** © Getty RF.

Chapter 29

Opener: © Creatas/Punchstock RF; **537:** © Getty/Image Source RF; **544:** © Ingram Publishing/Superstock RF.

Chapter 30

Opener: © Ingram Publishing RF; **560:** © Getty/Image Source RF; **572:** © Ingram Publishing RF; **579:** © Getty RF.

Page numbers in **bold** indicate definitions of key terms.
Page numbers followed by *t* and *f* denote tables and figures, respectively.

Transport vehicles, definitions of, 407t–409t
Transposition, **321**
Trauma, 394–398; *see also* injuries
    birth, 297
    early complications of, 397
Trauma registry, **80**
Treatment properties, 6t, **7**
Trichorrhexis nodosa, 339
Tricuspid stenosis, 317
Trigeminal nerve disorders, 183
Trimesters, pregnancy, 267–268, 267t
Triploidy, 325
Tripping (falls), 412–414, 415t–416t
Trisomy, **325**
Truman, Harry, 24
TTN (transient tachypnea of newborn), **298**
Tubal ligation, 496, 496t
Tuberculosis (TB), 110
Tubulo-interstitial nephritis, **251,** 356
Tumor lysis syndrome, 147
Tumor markers, 85; *see also* neoplasms
Turner syndrome, 325
Tympanic membrane disorders, 195
Tympanometry, 571
Type I diabetes mellitus, **141**
Type II diabetes mellitus, **141**
Type qualifiers, 473
    mental health, 578–579, 580t–581t
    rehabilitation and audiology, 564–572
    substance abuse, 582–583
    table of, 479

U

UACDS (Uniform Ambulatory Care Data Set), **32**
UB-04 (CMS–1450) Claim Form, 24–25, 26f
UHDDS (Uniform Hospital Discharge Data Sets), **27,** 28, 64, 268
Ulcer(s)
    atherosclerotic, 211
    decubitus, 342f
    esophageal, 236
    female pelvic organs, 260
    in newborns, 302
    pressure, 46, 341, 342
Ulcerative colitis, **238,** 352
Ultrasonography, 554
Ultrasound therapy, **539,** 539t
Ultraviolet light therapy, **539,** 539t
Ultraviolet radiation, injuries due to, 337, 420
Umbilical cord complications, 277–278
Umbilical hernia, **238**
Uncertain behavior, **133**
Uncertain diagnosis, 55, 65, 66, 75
Underdosing, **390,** 390–393, 426–427
Underlying condition, 54
Underweight, 82
Uniform Ambulatory Care Data Set (UACDS), **32**

Uniform Hospital Discharge Data Sets (UHDDS), **27,** 28, 64, 268
Unique definitions, **469,** 470
Unknown or undetermined intent, 406
Unrelated diagnoses
    with aftercare, 99
    in pregnancy, 99
Upper respiratory system disorders, 221–222
    infections, 219
Ureteral disorders, 254, 322
Urethra, 257f
    disorders of, 255, 261, 322
    obstetric laceration, 511
Urethrocele, 260
Uric acid, 147
Urinary pressure, transurethral monitoring of, 523, 524t
Urinary system, 249, 249f; *see also* genitourinary system
    disorders of, 78, 252–255, 261, 322
Urinary tract infection (UTI), 111, 120, 255
Urine testing, abnormal findings, 84
Urolithiasis, 254
Urosepsis, 111, **112**
Urticaria, 335, 336–337
Urticaria neonatorum, 304
US Department of Health and Human Services (US DHHS), **4,** 5, 449, 456
Use (substance), **168**
Use additional code, 16f, **17,** 54, 55f
Uses (ICD-11), **6**
US National Committee on Vital and Health Statistics (NCVHS), 450, 456
US Public Health Services, 450, 456
Uterine inertia, **278**
Uterine malformations, 321
UTI (urinary tract infection), 111, 120, 255

V

V codes, 404, 409–413; *see also* external cause codes
V codes (ICD-9-CM), 92, 102
Vaccinations, 98
Vaginal adhesions, postoperative, 261
Vaginal malformations, 321
Vaginitis, 260
Valgus deformity, **354**
Value, **470**
Van accidents, 411
VAP (ventilator-associated pneumonia), 398
Varicose veins, 212, 273, 281
Varus deformity, **354**
Vascular disorders, 210–212; *see also* specific disorder
    congenital, 317–318
    connective tissue, 356
    male genitals, 256
Vasculitis, 341, 352

Vasospastic syndrome, 397
Veins, **203**
    disorders of, 211–212
        congenital, 317–318
        major systemic, 211f
Vena cava, malformations of, 318
Venous insufficiency, 212
Ventilator-associated pneumonia (VAP), 398
Ventilatory support, 571
Ventral hernia, **238**
Ventricular septal defect, 317, 318f
Verbal communication skills, 57–58
Vertebral disorders, 358–359
Vertiginous syndromes, 195, 397
Vesicoureteral reflux, 251
Vestibular assessment, 563, 565, 566, 571
Vestibular function disorders, 195
Veterans Administration, 450, 456
Villonodular synovitis, 352
Violence-related injuries, 395–396, 418, 423–424
Viral diseases, 114–117, 120; *see also* specific disease
    infectious agents, 120
    in newborns, 299
Virus, **114**
Vision sensitivity deficiencies, 192
Visual cortex disorders, 191
Visual disturbances, 192–193
Visual field defects, 192
Visual pathways, 191f
    disorders of, 191
Vitamin deficiencies, 145, 154, 168
Vitiligo, **341**
Vitreous body, 189f
    disorders of, 190–191
Vocal cord paralysis, 221
Vocational activities, 572
Vocational counseling, 579
Voice assessment, 572
Voice disorders
    assessment of, 563–572
    symptoms and signs, 80
Volcanic eruptions, 421–422
Volume 3 codes (ICD-9-CM), 455–466
    assignment of, 459–461
    background of, 450–451, 456–457
    format and structure, 451–452, 458–459, 458t
    HIPAA designation, 441, 442t, 461
    versus ICD-10-PCS, 478
    need to replace, 461–462
    settings using, 457
Vomiting
    in newborns, 304
    in pregnancy, 273
Vulva, 259, 260f

W

W codes, 404, 413–420; *see also* external cause codes
War, 425–427
Water pressure, effects of, 395, 416, 417

Water transport accidents, 412
Weapons-related injuries, 414–418
    assault, 423–424
    intentional self-harm, 423
    legal interventions, military, and terrorism, 426
    undetermined intent, 425
Wegener's granulomatosis, 356
Weight
    birth, 296t
    during pregnancy, 273
Weightlessness, 397, 422
West Nile virus infection, 114–115
Wet lung syndrome, **298**
Wheelchair mobility, 572
Whipple's disease, 243
White blood cell disorders, 159
Wilson-Mikity syndrome, 298
With, **16**
World Health Assembly (WHA), **4**
World Health Organization (WHO), **3,** 441, 456
Wounds; *see* injuries
Wrist injuries, 381
Written communication skills, 57–58

X

X codes, 420–423; *see also* external cause codes
Xeroderma pigmentosum, 324
Xerosis cutis, 342

Y

Y codes, 403, 423–433; *see also* external cause codes
Yellow nail syndrome, 339
"Young," in pregnancy, 272

Z

Z codes, 91–107; *see also* specific condition
    overview, 92–94
    aftercare, 99–100, 374–375
    communicable diseases, 97–98
    encounters in other circumstances, 101
    examinations, 94–96 (see also examinations)
    genetic disease, 97
    history, 101–102 (see also history)
    versus procedure codes, 93, 98
    psychosocial circumstances, 101
    reproduction, 99
    search terms for, 93–94
    socioeconomic circumstances, 101
    specific procedures, 99–100
Zoonotic diseases, **109,** 110